Contemporary Issues in Colorectal Cancer

A Nursing Perspective

Jones and Bartlett Series in Oncology

Contemporary Issues in Colorectal Cancer

A Nursing Perspective

Edited by

Deborah T. Berg, RN, BSN
Oncology Consultant
Derry, New Hampshire

JONES AND BARTLETT PUBLISHERS
Sudbury, Massachusetts
BOSTON   TORONTO   LONDON   SINGAPORE

World Headquarters
Jones and Bartlett Publishers
40 Tall Pine Drive
Sudbury, MA 01776
978-443-5000
info@jbpub.com
www.jbpub.com

Jones and Bartlett Publishers Canada
2406 Nikanna Road
Mississauga, ON L5C 2W6
CANADA

Jones and Bartlett Publishers International
Barb House, Barb Mews
London W6 7PA
UK

Production Credits
Acquisitions Editor: Penny M. Glynn
Associate Editor: Christine Tridente
Production Editor: AnnMarie Lemoine
Editorial Assistant: Thomas Prindle
Manufacturing Buyer: Amy Duddridge

Typesetting: Modern Graphics, Inc.
Text Design: Modern Graphics, Inc.
Cover Design: Anne Spencer/Philip Regan
Printing and Binding: Malloy Lithographing

Library of Congress Cataloging-in-Publication Data

Contemporary issues in colorectal cancer : a nursing perspective
/ edited by Deborah T. Berg.
     p. ; cm.
Includes bibliographical references and index.
    ISBN 0-7637-1475-5
    1. Colon (Anatomy)—Cancer—Nursing. 2.
Rectum—Cancer—Nursing.
    [DNLM: 1. Colorectal Neoplasms—nursing. WI 529 C761 2001]
I. Berg, Deborah T.
    RC280.C6 C683 2001
    616.99'4347—dc21

2001029459

The selection and dosage of drugs presented in this book are in accord with standards accepted at the time of publication. The authors, editors, and publisher have made every effort to provide accurate information. However, research, clinical practice, and government regulations often change the accepted standard in this field. Before administering any drug, the reader is advised to check the manufacturer's product information sheet for the most up-to-date recommendations on dosage, precautions, and contraindications. This is especially important in the case of drugs that are new or seldom used.

Printed in the United States of America
05 04 03 02 01   10 9 8 7 6 5 4 3 2 1

Thank you with all my heart.
To my husband, Ed
My daughters, Megan and Lauren
Your love, support, and patience are extraordinary.

CONTENTS

PREFACE

Colorectal cancer is one of the most common cancers in the United States. Though there is a declining incidence and an improving survival, this disease remains a significant health problem. Advances in the understanding of the development of colorectal cancer have greatly impacted screening, diagnostic, and new therapeutic approaches. The issues of colorectal cancer management have undergone significant changes in the last few years. Yet, there are no textbooks dedicated to addressing nursing care and management of patients at high risk for or with colorectal cancer. Nurses need up-to-date information to provide accurate patient education and competent nursing care to patients. The vision of *Contemporary Issues in Colorectal Cancer: A Nursing Perspective* is to fill this need not only by addressing the science, but also by providing practical information about patient care.

To help nurses interpret confusing and, at times, contradictory information, the reader will find chapters devoted to risk factors, screening, and prevention. The content also focuses on the treatment modalities of surgery, chemotherapy, and radiotherapy, with a review of current and emerging treatment options from a nursing perspective. The treatment recommendations are based on the National Comprehensive Cancer Network guidelines, not on individual practice settings. Novel treatments in clinical trials for patients with colorectal cancer are also investi-

gated. Quality of life, advanced symptom management, and survivorship are explored and offer insight into the colorectal cancer experience. Each chapter is thorough in its scope of history and current issues and suggests areas of future research in a concise yet thorough manner. A resource section, with information both specific to colorectal cancer and cancer in general, completes the topic areas. Though primarily for nurses, especially nurses working with cancer patients, other health professionals will find *Contemporary Issues* pertinent to their practice.

Contemporary Issues in Colorectal Cancer: A Nursing Perspective provides the basic information that oncology nurses and other health professionals need to have a comprehensive understanding of colon and rectal cancer. Within these pages, the reader will gain knowledge that can be shared with colleagues, patients, family, and friends. Accurate information is the cornerstone of quality care. Colorectal cancer is preventable, detectable, and treatable when we are all correctly informed about risk factors, prevention methods, screening recommendations, and appropriate treatment interventions. It is my goal to educate nurses in all aspects of the care of patients with colorectal cancer. Therefore, I would like to hear from the readers of this book to find out whether that goal is being met.

ACKNOWLEDGMENTS

When a book is completed, the author(s) or, in this case, the editor gets the credit for putting the whole thing together. With this book, I feel it is appropriate to acknowledge some of the support that made this tremendous project possible.

Thank you to my contributing authors. Your knowledge and willingness to share your expertise provided the most up-to-date information possible so the reader can provide accurate patient education and competent nursing care to patients and their families. This book would not be possible without each of you. To my father-in-law, Russell Peter Berg, for sharing his story and experience with colon cancer. You give the reader insight into what it takes to survive this disease. To my parents, Larry and Betty Anderson, for always encouraging me that you can do *it* if you try. And last, but certainly not least, to the editorial staff at Jones and Bartlett Publishers, especially Christine Tridente, AnnMarie Lemoine, and Peg Latham of Colophon. It was your time, patience, attention to detail, and persistence that made this a book of which to be proud.

CONTRIBUTORS

Deborah T. Berg, RN, BSN
Oncology Consultant
Derry, NH

Russell Peter Berg
Limington, ME

Kathy Christiansen, RN, BSN, OCN
Nurse Coordinator
Cancer Prevention and Hereditary Cancer
    Program
Methodist Cancer Center
Omaha, NE

Mary Ellen Crane, RN, BSN, CETN
*Patient Care Manager for the Wound Ostomy
    Continence Teams*
Visiting Nurses of Greater Philadelphia
Philadelphia, PA

Denise A. DeLollo RN, OCN
Community Outreach Nurse
Cancer Care Center
St. Peter's Hospital
Albany, NY

Tracy K. Gosselin, RN, MSN, AOCN
Nursing Program Manager
Department of Radiation Oncology
Duke University Medical Center
Durham, NC

Joyce P. Griffin-Sobel, RN, PhD, AOCN, CS
Oncology Advanced Practice Nurse
Cancer Institute of New Jersey
New Brunswick, NJ

Catherine M. Hogan, MN, RN, CS, AOCN
Clinical Assistant Professor of Medicine
Nurse Practitioner/Coordinator Hematologic
    Malignancies Program
The University of North Carolina at Chapel Hill
Chapel Hill, NC

Cynthia R. King, PhD, NP, MSN, RN, FAAN
Special Care Consultants
Rochester, NY

Yvonne Lassere, RN, OCN, CCRP
Research Nurse Supervisor
The University of Texas M.D. Anderson Cancer
    Center
Houston, TX

Neal J. Meropol, MD
Director
Gastrointestinal Cancer Program
Fox Chase Cancer Center
Philadelphia, PA

Marilyn Mulay, RN, MS, OCN
Administrative Director
Cancer Therapy Development Program
University of California at Los Angeles
Los Angeles, CA

Delores A. Saddler, RN, MSN, CGRN
Clinical Care Coordinator
Gastrointestinal Multidisciplinary Care Center
The University of Texas M.D. Anderson Cancer
    Center
Houston, TX

Margot R. Sweed, RN, CRNP, CNSN
Nurse Practitioner
Collaborative practice with Neal J. Meropol,
  MD
Gastrointestinal Cancer Program
Fox Chase Cancer Center
Philadelphia, PA

Anne R. Waldman, MSN, RN, C, AOCN
Oncology Clinical Nurse Specialist
Albert Einstein Cancer Center
Philadelphia, PA
Adjunct Faculty
LaSalle University
Philadelphia, PA

CHAPTER 1 | # Epidemiology and Risk of Cancer of the Colon or Rectum

Deborah T. Berg, RN, BSN

Introduction

Audrey Hepburn, Elizabeth Montgomery, Barbara Barrie, Thomas "Tip" O'Neil, and Jay Monahan. What do these people have in common? Famous? Yes, but there's something more. What if Darryl Strawberry, Eric Davis, Ruth Bader-Ginsburg, Ronald Reagan, and Charles Schultz are added to the list? Is the picture clearer? These individuals, plus hundreds of thousands of mothers, fathers, sisters, brothers, sons, and daughters, have been diagnosed with colorectal cancer (CRC). In fact, at the time of this writing, another 130,000 people will be added to this list when they are told they, too, have cancer of the colon or rectum.

CRC is moving from the shadows into the spotlight in terms of awareness. This is not a very "sexy" disease and not one you are apt to hear discussed at any social gathering, in part because of the taboos we were taught during our potty-training years. We do not talk about the stuff we eliminate from our body or the parts of the body that do this work. There are many reasons for this recent heightened attention, however, not the least of which are advocacy groups such as the Colon Cancer Alliance, the Wellness Community, and Katie Couric's crusade against the disease that prematurely claimed her husband's (Jay Monahan) life. They each want to spread awareness that screening and early detection work, treatments are better, and eating right and exercising regularly can dramatically decrease the risk of developing the disease.

The slogan for the first colorectal cancer awareness month was "Preventable. Treatable. Beatable." These words are true. With persistence and some consistent changes in our lifestyle, we can prevent this malignancy. CRC is the ideal cancer to screen because, if detected early, before it metastasizes, it can be cured. Survival rates correlate with the amount of disease at diagnosis. If it is found during its earliest stage, 90% of people diagnosed will still be alive in 5 years, yet only 37% of people are diagnosed when it is the most treatable.[1] Few men and women aged 50 or older are screened because they are not keen on, or are skittish about, the screening methods[2] (You plan on putting that tube where?!?). According to an article in *Time* magazine, it was that very fear that led to the death of Charles Schultz.[3] He resisted going for screening, even though he had a strong family history of colon cancer; his mother, two uncles, and an aunt had died of the disease. The article stated that by the time he finally agreed to be tested, the cancer had already metastasized; only about 8% to 9% of people live 5 years if they are diagnosed at this late stage.[3,4] As Katie Couric said in an interview, people are frightened by the tests used to screen for CRC, but it is more frightening to be told you have CRC; going for the test is inconvenient, but it is still less inconvenient than a premature death! CRC screening has a dual role: It can detect the cancer early, and it can prevent cancer from developing by the subsequent removal of one of the known causes—the adenomatous polyp. (See Chapters 2 and 4 for more information about screening and pathophysiology.)

Epidemiology

About 5.5% of Americans will develop CRC at some point during their lives. This means that for the average American the lifetime probability is 1 out of every 18 people.[1] As noted, it is estimated that 130,200 people will be diagnosed with this malignancy this year, while 56,300 will lose their battle with this disease (Figure 1.1). To put this in perspective, Shea Stadium in Flushing, New York, holds about 56,000 fans. If every person diagnosed with CRC wanted to go to a baseball game at Shea Stadium, there would need to be two games to accommodate all of them. In terms of death, everyone in the stadium for one of the games would lose their life to this disease.

The incidence of CRC began to decrease in the mid-1980s, and in the 6 years between 1990 and 1996, it decreased at a rate of 2.1% per year. This trend was observed in both men and women of all racial and ethnic groups, except for American Indian women, for whom data are insufficient.[1] Declining incidence is attributed to increased public and professional awareness about the disease, assimilation of the recommended dietary habits into our daily lives, and early detection. The publicity surrounding former president Ronald Reagan's diagnosis of CRC in 1982 was probably the beginning of this heightened awareness. After undergoing a sigmoidoscopy for rectal bleeding, during which polyps were noted in his sigmoid colon, he underwent a colonoscopy, where upon a localized malignant lesion was found in his proximal colon, the opposite side of the bowel from where the polyps were found.

Incidence	
Colon	93,800
Rectum	36,400
	130,200
Mortality	
Colon	47,700
Rectum	8,600
	56,300

Figure 1.1   Incidence and mortality of colon and rectal cancer: 2000.

Source: From Greenlee RT, Murray T, Bolden S, Wingo PA. Cancer statistics 2000. CA Cancer J Clin. 2000; 50(1):7–33.

This situation highlighted colon cancer and demonstrated the importance of visualizing the whole colon. The incidence of CRC dropped for the first time in 1986.

Looking at the population at large, more Americans die of lung cancer, but CRC is the second leading cause of cancer-related deaths. Looking at gender separately, CRC is third in mortality after lung and prostate cancer in men and lung and breast cancer in women. Death from CRC also declined on an average of 1.7% between 1990 and 1996.[1] The percentage of people alive at 5 years is also improving, though it is greatly influenced by the stage at the time of diagnosis. More than 90% of patients that are diagnosed with a lesion that is still within the colon live 5 years, while this number drops to about a 66% 5-year survival rate if the disease has spread to adjacent lymph nodes.[1,4] Despite improvements in incidence and mortality, CRC is a significant health problem, utilizing a significant proportion of our healthcare dollars.

What Should I Know about Cancer of the Colon and Rectum?

Etiology

The exact cause of cancers of the colon and rectum is unknown. Instead of attributing the incidence of CRC to one etiology, several related factors are being investigated. Risk factors are defined as something that has been proved scientifically to be associated with a higher-than-normal frequency of a certain disease. The main risk factors for CRC are age and family history.[4] In addition, the relative risk of developing CRC is associated with preexisting adenomatous polyps or adenomas, genetic predisposition, preexisting diseases of the bowel, and environmental factors such as nutrition, alcohol, sedentary lifestyle, and cigarette smoking. There are two main genetic syndromes

associated with CRC risk: familial adenomatous polyposis (FAP) and hereditary nonpolyposis colorectal cancer (HNPCC). All remaining cases are attributed to sporadic CRC, which may be caused by lifestyle or environmental exposures. People cannot change their genes, but they can influence their lifestyle to decrease the odds of their developing cancer (Figure 1.2). Each of these factors is discussed in the following sections.

Adenomatous Polyps or Adenomas

It is believed that cancers of the colon and rectum begin with the formation of a polyp. These preexisting clumps of cells are quite common, especially as we grow older, when we are more likely to produce polyps; that is, about 30% of people in their 50s produce polyps, but this increases to about 50% in people in their 70s.[5] Adenomas are classified by their structure as either pedunculated (stalked or tubular), sessile (flat or villous), or a combination of the two (tubulovillous). Most polyps do not became cancerous, but under the influence of a series of genetic events, the polyps can change. The theory is that the polyp enlarges, becomes more dysplastic, develops into carcinoma in situ, eventually invades into and/or through the colon wall, and spreads to distant sites. Only about 5% of all polyps become cancerous, with sessile polyps associated with a higher frequency of malignant transformation.[6] In addition to type of polyp, size is also a predictor of malignant transformation; polyps of less than 1 cm have about a 1% chance of being malignant, in contrast to polyps of greater than 2 cm, which have up to a 40% likelihood of malignant transformation.[4] In fact, if a polyp is going to become malignant, it can take 5 to 10 years. Therefore, there are plenty of opportunities to find and remove polyps before they become malignant, thus dramatically decreasing the risk of developing CRC.

Second most common cancer after lung cancer

- Colorectal cancer is cancer of the colon or rectum
- 130,200 people will be stricken this year
- 56,000 people will die this year because of it
- 90% of people with colorectal cancer are more than 50 years old
- Increased incidence above age 40
- Highest incidence between the ages of 65 and 74

Colorectal cancer affects us all

- Young people believe that it is a disease of the elderly
- Women believe that only men get it
- African Americans believe only whites get it
- Everyone believes that there is nothing you can do about it

Risk factors include:

- Age
- Diet high in animal fats and processed meat; low in fruits and vegetables
- Personal history of colorectal cancer, polyps, ulcerative colitis, or Crohn's disease
- Family history of colorectal cancer, polyps, or other cancers, e.g., breast, ovarian, uterine
- Sedentary lifestyle

Take action!

- Exercise regularly
- Keep weight at recommended levels
- Eat less red meat
- Eat more fruits and vegetables (5–6 servings each day)
- Take a multivitamin with folic acid and calcium
- Don't smoke
- Limit alcohol
- Consider 1 aspirin a day, if approved by your doctor

See your doctor as soon as possible for:

- Rectal bleeding
- Blood in your stool
- Abdominal cramping or pain
- Change in bowel habits lasting more than a few days
- Narrowing of the stool (ribbon-like)
- Weakness or fatigue
- Urge to have a bowel movement, even after just having one

Get checked!

- All men and women aged 50 or older should be screened
- Don't wait for your doctor to recommend screening; tell him/her *you* want it!
- Starting at age 40, rectal examination every year
- Starting at age 40, stool blood test every year
- Starting at age 50, flexible sigmoidoscopy every 3–5 years, *or*
- Starting at age 50, colonoscopy every 5–10 years
- Earlier and more frequent screening tests if family history of cancer at a young age

Figure 1.2   Fast facts that could save your life.

Beyond early detection of polyps while they are still benign, researchers are investigating ways to prevent polyps from forming, for example, with aspirin, nonsteroidal antiinflammatory agents, and cyclooxygenase (COX) inhibitors. It is hypothesized that these agents stop the production of an enzyme called COX-2 that the cancer cells need to grow. By blocking the enzyme, the cells on the lining of the colon may not form into a mass or polyp in the first place.[4] (See Chapter 3, Prevention Strategies and the Diet Connection.)

Intestinal Conditions

There is an increased risk of CRC in people with other comorbid conditions of the bowel. Inflammatory bowel disease, ulcerative colitis, and Crohn's disease are the conditions with a higher-than-normal incidence of CRC. There is a 30-fold increased risk of CRC in people with inflammatory bowel disease. The risk associated with colitis increases with the duration of active disease and the extent of dysplasia.[4,6] For example, 3% of people with ulcerative colitis are reported to develop CRC in the first decade after diagnosis; this exponentially increases with each decade to greater than 30% after three decades with the disease.[4] The risk of CRC is also higher than normal in patients with Crohn's disease, but to a lesser degree as compared with colitis.[4] The correlation between polyps and CRC was discussed previously with the risk predisposition associated with size and number of polyps. Moreover, survivors of CRC are at increased risk of developing other cancers as well as other malignant lesions in the bowel.[4]

Age

Colorectal cancer is thought to be a disease of the elderly, with a median age at the time of diagnosis of 70 for men and 73 for women.[7] Overall, the mean age at the time of diagnosis

is 60 to 65.[4] The risk increases after the age of 40 and continues to do so until the eighth or ninth decade of life, doubling each decade after the age of 50.[8] Though CRC is more common in people above the age of 50, young people are also affected.[6] About 3% of CRCs are diagnosed in people less than 40 years of age.[9] A recent report from surgeons at the University of Texas–Southwestern Medical Center (UT-SW) in Dallas documented a rising incidence of CRC among people aged 40 to 49.[10] In a retrospective study, the investigators looked at 1,128 patients diagnosed with CRC between 1978 and 1998. They looked at age at time of diagnosis for two time frames: 1978 to 1982 and 1983 to 1998. In the first time frame (1978–1982), 8.1% of the patients diagnosed with CRC were between 40 and 49 years of age. In the later time frame (1983–1998), the percentage had increased to 14.4% in people in their 40s. The results have two major implications. First, the investigators recommend that other institutions repeat their study in their own hospitals to verify the findings. Second, if the data are verified, the standard recommendation to initiate screening at the age of 50 may be out of date. It may be more appropriate to initiate screening at the age of 40.[10] As suggested, the probability of developing CRC varies during our lifetimes[1]:

Genders	Ages < 39 yr	Ages 40–59 yr	Ages > 60 yr
Males	1 in 1,579	1 in 124	1 in 29
Females	1 in 1,947	1 in 149	1 in 33

Interestingly, the National Cancer Data Base found an inverse relationship between age and stage of disease at diagnosis. Patients under the age of 50 presented with the more advanced stage III and IV diseases, while the elderly, those over the age of 80, presented with early-stage disease. This did not translate into a survival advantage, though, as younger patients had a 14% to 24% improvement in survival compared with the elderly adult. Even more surprising, the middle-aged elderly patient (70–79 years of age) had a 4% to 9% improvement in survival compared with the eldest of the elderly patients (age > 80).[11] Comorbid conditions, postoperative complications, and a possible disparity regarding postoperative systemic therapy and radiotherapy (older patients may not be offered adjuvant therapy) are likely explanations.[12,13] Several investigations report that careful selection of patients for surgery and systemic chemotherapy, based on functional (performance) status, not on age, is key to the elderly patient receiving the same therapeutic benefit as younger patients.[12–15]

Gender

CRC is a commonly diagnosed cancer in both men and women and is not an epidemiologic factor. Rectal and anal cancers are more common in men, while colon cancer is more common in women.[6,16]

Ethnicity/Race

CRC occurs in all ethnic and racial groups. There is a wide divergence seen between racial groups. In the United States, Alaskan Natives have the highest rates in men, followed by, in descending order, the Japanese, African American, non-Hispanic white, Chinese, Hawaiian, Hispanic, Filipino, Korean, and Vietnamese populations. The order is similar for women: Alaskan Natives, African American, Japanese, non-Hispanic white, Chinese, Hawaiian, Vietnamese, Hispanic, Korean, and Filipino populations, again in descending order. In American Indians in New Mexico, the rates are quite low

in both men and women.[17] In the African American population, the incidence of CRC has increased by 30% since the early 1970s, surpassing that seen in whites, and the mortality rate has increased in both men and women (47% and 16%, respectively) over the same time frame.[12] The pattern for mortality is similar to those for incidence, except that African Americans, Alaskan Natives, and Hispanic men and women, along with Hawaiian and Japanese men, have high mortality rates.[17] For example, the 5-year survival rate is 10% points lower for African Americans than for whites[1] (Figures 1.3 and 1.4).

The National Cancer Data Base reports that all ethnic groups present with similar stages of disease, except African Americans, who present more frequently with advanced-stage disease[11] (Figure 1.5). As with other cancers, the reasons they present with a later stage of disease are unclear. Poverty and poor access to medical care are often cited, but this does not answer why only *one* minority population would present with a later stage of disease. Other possible factors, such as genetic makeup or another as yet undiscovered factor, may be involved, and will provide long-needed answers.

Socioeconomic Status and Geography

A person's socioeconomic status does not appear to play a direct role in risk predisposition. Industrialized areas of the world—namely, the United States, Canada, Australia, New Zealand, the Scandinavian countries, Northern and Western Europe, and Israel—have more cases of CRC than underdeveloped or poorly industrialized areas in Asia, South America (except Argentina and Uruguay), and Africa (i.e., Gambia). When moving from an area of low risk to one of high risk, the person takes on the risk of the adopted country *if* they embrace the lifestyle and diet of the new area. Interestingly, this

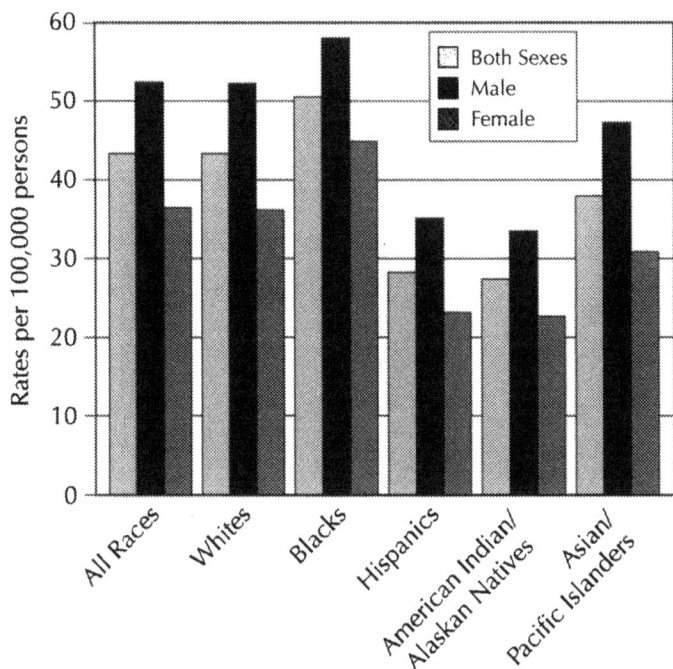

Figure 1.3   Colorectal cancer incidence by gender and ethnicity: 1990–1997

Source: Data from Colorectal cancer incidence and death rates by gender and race/ethnicity, 1990–1997. Available at: http://seer.cancer.gov/Publications/ReportCard/ArticleDataPoints/AllFigures.pdf

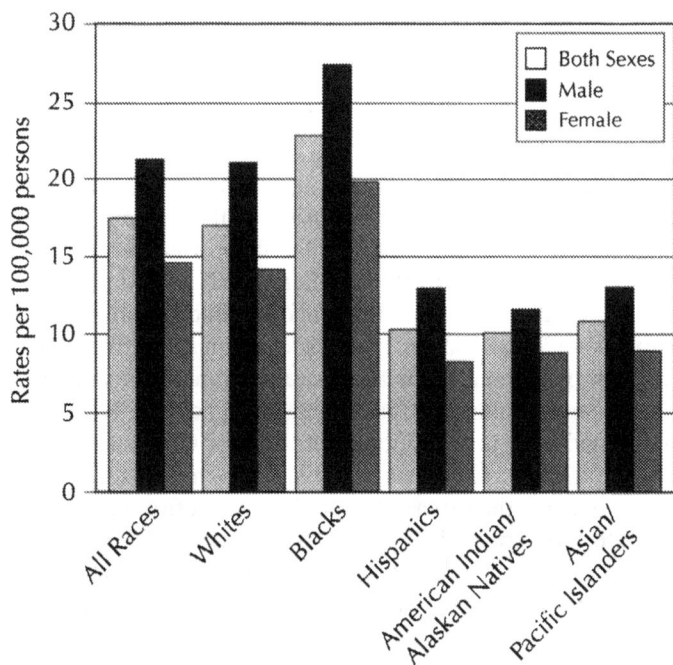

Figure 1.4   Colorectal cancer mortality by gender and ethnicity: 1990–1997

Source: Data from Colorectal cancer incidence and death rates by gender and race/ethnicity, 1990–1997. Available at: http://seer.cancer.gov/Publications/ReportCard/ArticleDataPoints/AllFigures.pdf

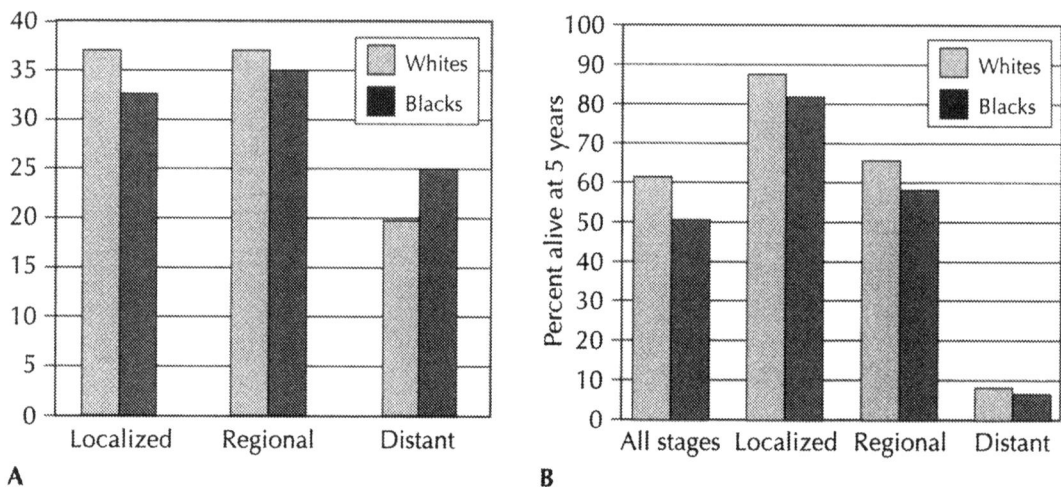

Figure 1.5   A: Distribution of colorectal cancer stage at diagnosis by race (1989–1995). **B:** Colorectal cancer survival by stage and race (1989–1995).

Source: From Greenlee RT, Murray T, Bolden S, Wingo PA. Cancer statistics 2000. CA Cancer J Clin. 2000; 50(1):7–33.

change in risk occurs rapidly, within the life-span of the migrant.[7] This points to the importance of environmental factors—such as the Western diet, known for being rich in animal fats, cholesterol, red meat, and refined sugar, but poor in fruits and vegetables—as key facets involved in the carcinogenesis of this cancer rather than socioeconomic status.[7]

In the United States, the highest incidence of CRC is noted in the states or areas with previous intense industrialization, for example, New Jersey, New York, and Massachusetts (Figure 1.6). However, there has not been a link between incidence and occupational exposure.[7]

Roetzheim and colleagues[18] recently reported that health insurance influenced patient outcomes. Patients who were uninsured had a mortality rate 64% higher than patients who were insured. Medicaid patients fared better than the uninsured, but their mortality rate was still 36% higher than patients with private insurance. Patients with health maintenance organizations (HMOs) had mortality rates 22% higher than patients with more traditional fee-for-service plans.[18] The availability of health insur-

ance may be influenced by a person's socioeconomic status.

Genetics

CRC develops because a collection of cells change as a result of some genetic mishap, either present since birth (germline defects) or due to a change in normal genes caused by age or toxic exposure to the numerous things traveling through the colon each day (somatic mutations). Therefore, CRC is believed to be caused by a mixture of genetic and environmental factors.[7] Two observations contribute to the conclusion that there is a genetic connection to CRC risk: increased frequency of CRC in people with a family history of CRC and families with clusters of family members affected by the disease.[4] A person with a first-degree relative with CRC has a two- to threefold increased risk of developing a large bowel cancer.[8] As outlined in the following table, the risk of developing CRC increases with the number of affected family members and in the presence of a genetic familial syndrome.[1,19]

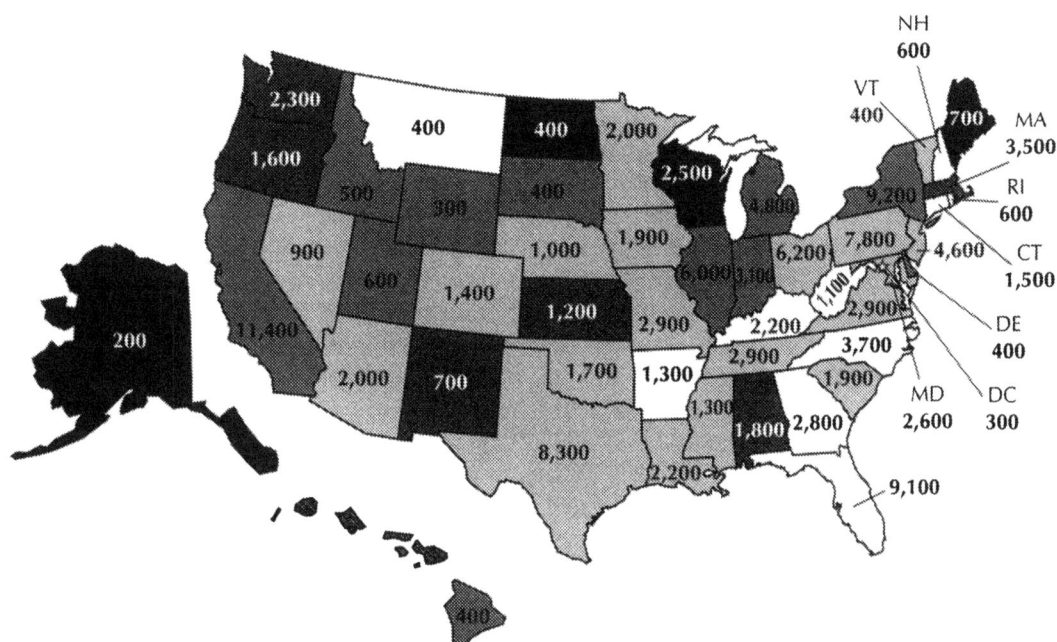

Figure 1.6 Incidence of colorectal cancer by state. Total in the United States: 130,200.

Source: Data from Greenlee RT, Murray T, Bolden S, Wingo PA. Cancer statistics 2000. CA Cancer J Clin. 2000; 50(1):7–33.

Overall risk	5.5%
Negative family history of colorectal cancer	2%

Positive family history

• One first-degree relative with CRC	6%
• One first-degree relative plus two second-degree relatives with CRC	8%
• One first-degree relative diagnosed < age 45	10%
• Two first-degree relatives with CRC	17%

Genetic syndromes

• HNPCC (genetic carrier)	70%
• FAP (genetic carrier)	100%

Note: A first-degree relative is a parent, sibling, or child; a second-degree relative is an aunt, uncle, or cousin. CRC, colorectal cancer; HNPCC, hereditary nonpolyposis colon cancer; FAP, familial adenomatous polyposis.

About 95% of CRCs are felt to be sporadic, that is, developing without an apparent genetic mutation. Interestingly, about 15% to 25% of these sporadic cases report a positive family history of CRC.[8,9,20] The remaining cases are felt to have a genetic factor, common exposure among family members, environmental consequences, or some combination of these. Genetic mutations have been identified in some cancer-prone families and account for 5% to 6% of all CRC. It is expected that there are also other as yet undiscovered major genetic mutations and background genetic factors that contribute to the development of CRC. As noted, there are two main hereditary polyposis syndromes: FAP and HNPCC. Other rare genetic syndromes include Gardner's, Turcot's, Peutz-Jeghers', and juvenile polyposis. The latter two are not cancer or precancerous conditions, but they put patients at a higher than normal risk of developing CRC.[21] The characteristics of these differ, but they share the polyp to adenoma to cancer sequence. (See Table 1.1 for characteristics of FAP and HNPCC.)

FAP is characterized by thousands of polyps, usually pediculated; therefore, there is an increased likelihood that one, or some, of them will become cancerous.[9] The polyps are not usually present at birth but do develop early (median age, 25 years) and are spread throughout the colon (pancolonic).[8] Individuals usually develop symptoms by the age of 33 years, are diagnosed with FAP by the age of 36, and develop CRC by the age of 42.[4] FAP accounts for 1% of CRC incidence, representing about 7,000 people.[8,22] The gene predisposing people to FAP is the adenomatous polyposis coli (APC) gene, found in about 80% of families with this syndrome.[23] This gene is reportedly a tumor-suppressor gene. Genetic testing should be considered in families with known FAP. The success of genetic testing improves if the affected relative has a positive test for APC.[23] Thus, if the affected relative is positive and a family member is negative, the family member will have the same risks as the average American.[23] Screening should begin at puberty.

Sigmoidoscopy, a valuable screening tool because the polyps are distributed throughout the entire bowel, is repeated frequently (every 1–2 years).[23] It is recommended that patients found to have FAP undergo a total colectomy with construction of an ileal pouch–anal anastomosis.[23] From the perspective of prevention, a demonstrated benefit has been documented in terms of decrease in size and number of polyps in patients treated with nonsteroidal antiinflammatory agents or celecoxib.[4,22]

HNPCC is another syndrome associated with a high risk of CRC. HNPCC is more common than FAP, occurring in 1% to 5% of CRC cases, or about 1 in every 500 people. Clinically, HNPCC looks like sporadic CRC.[22] The progression through the carcinogenesis sequence is accelerated in HNPCC compared with sporadic cancers.[23] Therefore, screening colonoscopies are done every 1 to 3 years. The recommended treatment is segmental colectomy with continued close monitoring, as 30% to 50% will develop a second colon cancer.[23]

The genetic changes that predispose for HNPCC are in the mismatch repair (MMR) genes (i.e., hMSH1, hMLH1, hPMS1, and

Table 1.1   Characteristics of Genetic Syndromes

Characteristic	HNPCC	Flat Adenoma	FAP	Gardner's Syndrome
Age at onset	Early	Late (7th decade)	Early (average, 42 yr)	Same as FAP
No. of adenomas/ polyps	<10	<100	100s–1,000s	Same as FAP
Tumor location	Right colon	Right colon	Random	Same as FAP
Genetic mutation	Mismatch repair genes (hMSH1, hMLH1, hPMS1, hPMS2)		Adenomatous polyposis coli gene	Adenomatous polyposis coli gene
Inheritance	Dominant		Dominant	Dominant
Extracolonic cancers	Endometrial and others	Periampullary	Periampullary; mandibular osteomas	Same as FAP with more evident and varied extracolonic cancers

Source: Data from Coia LR, Ellenhorn JDI, Ayoub JF. Cancer Management: A Multidisciplinary Approach, 4th ed. Available at: www.cancernetwork.com Accessed January 23, 2001; and Engelking C. Profiling colorectal cancer: Nature and scope of the disease. Dev Supportive Cancer Care. 1997; 1(2):1–40.

*h*PMS2). Normal MMR genes detect and correct any genetic errors during DNA replication. When the gene has been inactivated (mutated), these errors are not corrected. As a result, the genetic alterations lead to genetic instability, reflected in errors carried forward during DNA replication.[4] The gene carriers, unfortunately, are not conclusively known; thus, penetrance can only be estimated. Furthermore, only a few of the MMR genes have been identified, so some families may still have HNPCC but with an as yet unknown gene mutation.[23] For these reasons, the clinical diagnosis utilizes the Amsterdam Criteria, also known as the 1, 2, 3 Rule:

- 1 or more family members with CRC diagnosed before age 50
- 2 or more generations affected by CRC
- 3 or more relatives with a confirmed diagnosis of CRC, one of which must be a first-degree relative of the other two members

The Amsterdam Criteria are controversial, as they do not provide a means of diagnosis for some subpopulations, for example, people with small families or extracolonic tumors.[22] A less stringent criterion has been proposed (the Bethesda Guidelines) that would take into consideration HNPCC extracolonic tumors and microsatellite instability testing.[22] HNPCC is divided into two variants: Lynch I and Lynch II. Families with Lynch I have familial colorectal cancer only, while those with Lynch II have nonpolyposis CRC along with other forms of cancer, such as breast, uterine, ovarian, pancreatic, or gastric cancer.[6,9] Patients develop CRC at a young age, often in the right colon.[9]

Another genetic mutation, APC11307K, an alteration of the APC gene, has been described in some Jewish populations.[24] This mutation is found in about 6% of people from Eastern Europe of Ashkenazi Jewish descent, and confers a twofold increase in CRC risk.[24–27] Genetic testing for this mutation is extremely sensitive

and specific; therefore, a positive result is truly positive.[24–27] More research into this mutation and the afflicted population is needed to define mean age at onset, as well as the natural history of the disease in carriers.

Genetic testing for these syndromes is a possibility, as they are associated with different genetic mutations. As noted in Table 1.1, HNPCC is associated with a mutation in the MMR genes, and FAP is attributed to damage in the APC gene. Such genetic testing could provide a person with individualized risk avoidance, surveillance, and therapeutic options.

CASE STUDY

Question: You are reading the medical history of a patient with newly diagnosed metastatic colon cancer. In the chart you see the following diagram:

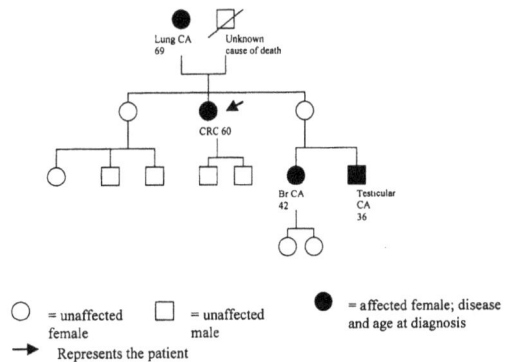

- Does this diagram represent a family with an hereditary CRC syndrome?
- What more do you need to know about the family history?
- What information can you provide the sons of the patient regarding their risk of developing CRC?

Lifestyle

People cannot change their genes, but they can change their lifestyle to improve their odds of not developing a cancer of the large bowel. Lifestyle factors such as diet, alcohol intake, and cigarette smoking have been demonstrated to have an impact on CRC risk.

"Food" for Thought

- How would you describe your diet?
- Would your food consumption put you at low or high risk for CRC?
- What about the diet of your family and friends?
- What about the diet of your patients?
- How would you describe your intake of alcohol?
- Are you a smoker?
- Do you exercise regularly?

DIET

Diets low in fruits, vegetables, and folate and high in fat and red meat reportedly facilitate the development of CRC. It is theorized that exogenous fats and cholesterol promote colonic tumors by inducing endogenous bile salts, neutral steroids, and fatty acids, which eventually break down the bacteria within the bowel. The bacterial degradation and the excretion of the bile salts, steroids, and fatty acids promote colonic mucosal cellular turnover and thus initiate or potentiate carcinogenesis.[16] In several studies, participants who consumed a diet high in fat or red meat had a 2 to 2.5 times higher risk of developing CRC than those who ate the least amounts of these products.[28] The risk appears to be associated with total fat intake rather than the specific type of fat consumed.[28] The average American gets about 37% of his or her calories from fat, whereas the recommendation is that this amount be no more than 30%. Fats in meats, whole milk, margarines, salad oils, mayonnaise products, and so on are the major sources of fat.[28]

Traditionally it was believed that diets high in fiber were protective, because the increased bulk from the fiber "swept out" toxins before they could damage the colonic lining. This theory has not held up against current research. Prospective studies have not shown the benefit of dietary fiber.[29,30] Because diets high in fiber contain other nutrients and are often low in fat, the specific item that provides the protection may not have been identified.[28]

In several reports, vegetables have been reported to be protective. Fruits, on the other hand, have been noted to have an inverse relationship, but the findings are inconsistent. In general, vegetables, fruits, and grains contain carotenoids, vitamins A and C, and other nutrients that confer the protective effect. These nutrients are highest in dark yellow–orange vegetables and fruits (e.g., carrots, sweet potatoes, cantaloupe) and green leafy vegetables (e.g., broccoli, collard greens, and spinach).[28]

Other nutrients, such as calcium salts, calcium-rich foods, and folic acid, have been shown to have a protective effect.[29] They decrease the cellular proliferation of the colonic lining and the carcinogenesis-promoting effects of bile and steroids.[16] Good sources of calcium include dairy products, okra, root vegetables, and dark green leafy vegetables.[28]

ALCOHOL CONSUMPTION AND CIGARETTE SMOKING

Though beer consumption has been linked to the development of rectal cancer, a relationship between alcohol consumption and development of CRC is inconsistent. A metaanalysis of 27 studies reported, at worst, a minimal association between alcohol consumption and incidence of CRC, without any direct association.[31]

Several studies have suggested a strong association between cigarette smoking and the development of gastrointestinal cancers, including CRC.[32,33] A recent report links cigarette smoking and microsatellite instability (MSI) in colon tumors. According to the results of a population-based study reported in the *Journal of the National Cancer Institute*, cigarette smoking may cause MSI.[34,35] This is an area that needs to be explored, as results may impact methods for prevention.

OBESITY AND PHYSICAL ACTIVITY

Obesity is another concomitant condition that has been associated with CRC. Though the direct effect is unclear, this is an area of active research.[4,36] Calle and colleagues reported that a high body mass index (obesity) was an independent risk factor for developing CRC, especially in men.[36] The link between physical activity and CRC risk is consistent.[7] Regular activity reduces the risk of CRC.[37,38]

ASPIRIN, NONSTEROIDAL ANTIINFLAMMATORY AGENTS, COX INHIBITORS, AND HORMONE-REPLACEMENT THERAPY

Aspirin, nonsteroidal antiinflammatory agents, and COX inhibitors, especially COX-2 inhibitor consumption, has been associated with a decreased risk of CRC.[7] The effect of these agents on prostaglandins and COX is an area of active research. Hormone-replacement therapy may also reduce the risk of CRC in women, though the exact mechanism is not yet understood.[39]

What Can Be Recommended?

The key to get the most benefit from "taking action" (see Figure 1.2) is to be consistent and persistent. It takes decades for CRC to develop; therefore, we need to make lifestyle changes a long-term habit to receive the full benefit. These actions also deliver other health benefits, such as a decreased risk of heart disease. Nutritionally, the American Cancer Society recommends that we eat a balanced diet consisting of 5 to 6 servings of fruits and yellow or green vegetables. An example of one serving is a medium-sized piece of fresh fruit or half a cup of solid vegetables, or a full cup of leafy vegeta-

bles. Most Americans fall very short of this goal, with most consuming 3.5 servings of fruits and vegetables each day. Reportedly, only about 23% of Americans achieve the desired goal.[29] Folic acid decreases the risk of developing CRC by 75%, according to the Nurses Health study, so including a multivitamin with folic acid could be beneficial.[5] For women, hormone-replacement therapy should be considered after a discussion with their physicians. Regular physical activity should be incorporated into your daily life.[4]

"Food" for Thought

- Does your food consumption put you at low or high risk for CRC?
- Do you plan on adapting your diet in any way?
- What about the diet of your family and friends?
- What recommendations about diet will you make to your patients?
- What about alcohol intake and smoking?
- Do you plan on taking any vitamin supplements?
- What about exercise? Will you make any changes to your routine?

The Role of the Nurse

Staying abreast of the data on risk predisposition and prevention is a challenge (Figure 1.7). The field of genetics is ever-changing, as is the understanding of carcinogenesis. As nurses are taking patients' medical histories, they must promptly identify patients and families at high risk of developing CRC by keeping in mind the hallmarks of inherited syndromes. General oncology nurses are not often well versed in the details of the inherited syndromes, but they should be educated about the available resources and how to access them. Individuals and/or families with an apparent genetic predisposition should be referred to a genetic coun-

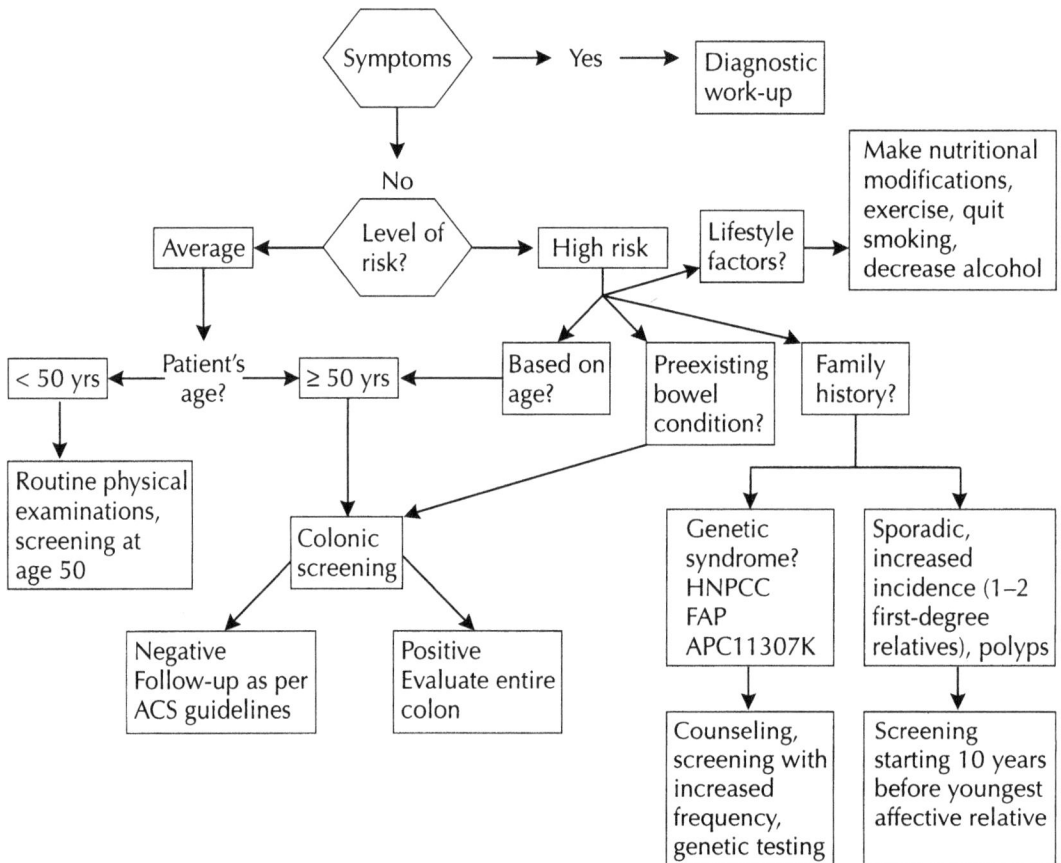

Figure 1.7 Risk assessment pathway.

Source: Data from Saddler DA, Ellis C. Colorectal cancer. Semin Oncol Nurs. 1999; 15(1):58–69.

selor and/or high-risk specialty clinic for further risk evaluation. Nurses with advanced degrees in genetics and oncology genetic counseling are already integrated in several high-risk clinics and can be an invaluable resource. The socioeconomic and psychosocial ramifications of an inherited syndrome can be challenging and require multidisciplinary strategies to protect the patients' confidentiality and help them make an informed decision. In all individuals deemed at risk of developing CRC, counseling, educa-

tion, multidisciplinary prevention strategies, and screening are essential.[21]

Dietary recommendations to prevent CRC are another area of active research. Nurses must take the initiative to stay informed, even though the information may seem constantly contradictory. For further information about the importance of screening and prevention, the reader is referred to Chapters 2 and 3.

Finally, we are all at risk of developing cancer of the colon and rectum and, as such, should pay attention to the recommendations to decrease that risk (Figure 1.2).

References

1. Greenlee RT, Murray T, Bolden S, et al. Cancer statistics 2000. CA Cancer J Clin. 2000; 50(1): 7–33.
2. Rudy DR, Zdon MJ. Update on colorectal cancer. Am Fam Physician. 2000; 61(6):1759–1770.
3. Gorman C. Katie's crusade. Time 2000; March 13:70–76.
4. Coia LR, Ellenhorn JDI, Ayoub JF. Cancer Management: A Multidisciplinary Approach, 4th ed. Available at: www.cancernetwork.com Accessed January 23, 2001.
5. Dadoly AM. Moving into the spotlight. Harvard Pilgrim Health Care Your Health. 2000; (Fall): 8–12.
6. Chase JL, Hoff PMG, Pazdur R. Management of colorectal cancer. In: Berg DT, Chase JL, Clanton MS, et al., eds. Disease Management of Colorectal Cancer. Pittsburgh, PA: Oncology Education Services, 1998: 8–34.
7. Schatzkin AG. Colon and rectum. In: Harras A, Edwards BK, Blot WJ, et al., eds. Cancer Rates and Risks, 4th ed. NIH Pub. No. 96-691. Bethesda, MD: National Cancer Institute, 1996: 129–135.
8. Redmond K, ed. A Nurses' Guide to Colorectal Cancer. Brussels, Belgium: European Oncology Nursing Society and AstraZeneca UK Limited, 2000.
9. Coppola D, Karl RC. Pathology of early colonic neoplasia: Clinical and pathologic features of precursor lesions and minimal carcinomas. Cancer Control: Journal of the Moffitt Cancer Center. 1998; 4(2):160–166.
10. Gregorcyk SG. Colorectal cancer incidence may be rising in younger people. Oncology News International 2000; 9(11). Available at: http://www.cancernetwork.com/ Accessed January 23, 2001.
11. Jessup JM, McGinnis LS, Steele GD, et al. The National Cancer Data Base report on colon cancer. Cancer. 1996; 78:918–926.
12. Engelking C. Profiling colorectal cancer: Nature and scope of the disease. Dev Supportive Cancer Care. 1997; 1(2):1–40.
13. Sargent D, Goldberg R, MacDonald J, et al. Adjuvant chemotherapy for colon cancer is beneficial without significantly increased toxicity in elderly patients: Results from 3351 patient meta-analysis. Proc Am Soc Clin Oncol. 2000; 19:933 (abstr).
14. Saltz LB, Cox JV, Blanke C, et al., for the Irinotecan Study Group. Irinotecan plus fluorouracil and leucovorin for metastatic colorectal cancer. N Engl J Med. 2000; 343(13):905–914.
15. Grobovsky L, Kaplon M, Krozer-Hamati A, et al. Features of cancer in frail elderly patients (≥ 85 years of age). Proc Am Soc Clin Oncol. 2000; 19:2469 (abstr).
16. Saddler DA, Ellis C. Colorectal cancer. Semin Oncol Nurs. 1999; 15(1):58–69.
17. Miller BA, Kolonel LN, Bernstein L, et al., eds. Racial/Ethnic Patterns of Cancer in the United States 1988–1992. NIH Pub. No. 96-4104. Bethesda, MD: National Cancer Institute, 1996.
18. Reuters News. Colorectal cancer mortality higher among blacks and the uninsured. Available at: http://oncology.medscape.com/reuters/prof/2000/11/11.06/20001103epid002.html Accessed November 15, 2000.
19. Houlston RS, Murday V, Harocopos C, et al. Screening and genetic counseling for relatives of patients with colorectal cancer in a family cancer clinic. BMJ. 1990; 301(6748):366–368.
20. Olsen SJ, Zawacki K. Hereditary colorectal cancer. Nurs Clin North Am. 2000; 35(3):671–685.
21. Hereditary colon cancer. Available at: www3.mdanderson.org/depts/hcc Accessed January 21, 2001.

22. Glaser E, Grogan L. Molecular genetics of gastrointestinal malignancies. Semin Oncol Nurs. 1999; 15(1):3–9.

23. Read TE. Colorectal cancer: Risk factors and recommendations for early detection. Am Fam Physician. June 1999. Available at: http://www.findarticles.com/cf_0/m3225/11_59/55391765/print.jhtml Accessed January 7, 2001.

24. Laken SJ, Petersen GM, Gruber SB, et al. Familial colorectal cancer in Ashkenazim due to a hypermutable tract in APC. Nat Genet. 1997; 17(1):79–83.

25. Woodage T, King SM, Wacholder S, et al. The APC I1307K allele and cancer risk in a community-based study of Ashkenazi Jews. Nat Genet. 1998; 20(1):62–65.

26. Gryfe R, Di Nicola N, Lal G, et al. Inherited colorectal polyposis and cancer risk of the APC I1307K polymorphism. Am J Hum Genet. 1999; 64(2):378–384.

27. Rozen P, Shomrat R, Strul H, et al. Prevalence of the I1307K APC gene variant in Israeli Jews of differing ethnic origin and risk for colorectal cancer. Gastroenterology. 1999; 116(1):54–57.

28. Clifford C, Ballard-Barbash R, Lanza E, et al. Diet and cancer risk. In: Harras A, Edwards BK, Blot WJ, et al., eds. Cancer Rates and Risks, 4th ed. NIH Pub. No. 96-691. Bethesda, MD: National Cancer Institute, 1996: 73–76.

29. Giovannucci E, Willett WC. Dietary factors and risk of colon cancer. Ann Med. 1994; 26: 443–452.

30. Fuchs CS, Giovannucci EL, Colditz GA, et al., Dietary fiber and the risk of colorectal cancer and adenoma in women. N Engl J Med. 1999; 340(3):169–176.

31. Blot WJ. Alcohol. In: Harras A, Edwards BK, Blot WJ, et al., eds. Cancer Rates and Risks, 4th ed. NIH Pub. No. 96-691. Bethesda, MD: National Cancer Institute, 1996: 61–63.

32. Shopland DR. Cigarette smoking as a cause of cancer. In: Harras A, Edwards BK, Blot WJ, et al., eds. Cancer Rates and Risks, 4th ed. NIH Pub. No. 96-691. Bethesda, MD: National Cancer Institute, 1996: 67–72.

33. Giovannucci E, Martinez ME. Tobacco, colorectal cancer, and adenomas: A review of the evidence. J Natl Cancer Inst. 1996; 88: 1717–1730.

34. Slattery ML, Curtin K, Anderson K, et al. Associations between cigarette smoking, lifestyle factors, and microsatellite instability in colon tumors. J Natl Cancer Inst. 2000; 92:1831–1836.

35. Neugut AI, Terry MB. Cigarette smoking and microsatellite instability: Causal pathway or marker-defined subset of colon tumors? J Natl Cancer Inst. 2000; 92:1791–1793.

36. Reuters News. Obesity to increased risk of colon cancer mortality, especially in men. Available at: http://oncology.medscape.com/reuters/prof/2000/11/11.08/20001107epid003.html Accessed November 15, 2000.

37. Giovannucci E, Ascherio A, Rimm EB, et al. Physical activity, obesity, and risk for colon cancer and adenoma in men. Ann Intern Med. 1995; 122:327–334.

38. Giovannucci E, Colditz GA, Stampfer MJ, et al. Physical activity, obesity, and risk for colorectal adenoma in women. Cancer Causes Control, 1996; 7:253–263.

39. Slattery ML, Edwards SL, Boucher KM, et al. Lifestyle and colon cancer: An assessment of factors associated with risk. Am J Epidemiol. 1999; 150:869–877. Available at: http://oncology.medscape.com/reuters/prof/1999/10/10.15/ep10159a.html

40. Colorectal cancer incidence and death rates by gender and race/ethnicity, 1990–1997. Available at: http://seer.cancer.gov/Publications/ReportCard/ArticleDataPoints/AllFigures.pdf

CHAPTER 2 | # Colorectal Cancer Prevention and Detection: Detectable, Treatable, and Curable

Denise A. Delollo, RN, OCN

Introduction

Screening for a disease can be justified when (1) a disease is common and associated with serious morbidity or mortality; (2) screening tests are sufficiently accurate in detecting early-stage disease; (3) screening tests are acceptable to patients and are feasible in general clinical practice; (4) treatment after detection by screening has been shown to improve prognosis relative to treatment after usual diagnosis; and (5) evidence exists that the potential benefits outweigh the potential harms and costs of the screening.[1] Colorectal cancer (CRC) is the second leading cause of cancer-related deaths and the third most commonly diagnosed cancer in the United States. In the year 2000 approximately 130,200 individuals were diagnosed with CRC, and over 56,000 died of this disease.[2] CRC, if caught in the early stages, has a 90% cure rate. This chapter focuses on screening methods, risk factors, barriers to screening, guidelines for screening, and the nurse's role in prevention and detection.

CRC is a silent disease, with individuals not having symptoms until in its later stages. With a widespread campaign of early screening, it is estimated that more than 30,000 lives could be saved.[3] It is a misconception that CRC is a man's disease, when in fact it affects men and women equally. African Americans and Hispanics are usually diagnosed in the later stages of this disease, thus having a higher mortality rate than Caucasians. The cause of CRC is unknown, but it usually develops from polyps. Lifestyles, environmental issues, and genetic predisposition are felt to be factors contributing to the development of the disease. CRC progresses in stages, stage I being 95% curable and stage IV having about a 3% probability of cure. Since CRC has a long preclinical phase, easily accessible diagnostic testing and early detection improve survival. Research has shown that appropriate screening and early treatment can reduce the mortality rate from this disease. Polyps and early-stage CRCs are usually asymptomatic with a high cure rate, but the lesions that are large enough to cause symptoms have a worse prognosis. This demonstrates a need to screen asymptomatic individuals (individuals without symptoms).

What Is a Screening?

Cancer screenings are set up to test individuals who are healthy and not experiencing any symptoms (asymptomatic), but who are at risk for developing cancer; this is also called early detection. *Screening guidelines* are formed from data showing that cancer occurs in a particular age group with or without a family history and with certain preexisting conditions that could become cancerous. This identifies a *target* population that may have certain characteristics which make them appropriate for screening. *Screening tests* are used to detect a particular cancer. After doing an accurate risk assessment, the appropriate screening tests are chosen.

Cancer Risk Assessment

Cancer risk assessments are a key component of all three levels of cancer prevention. An accurate risk assessment is needed before the correct method of prevention is determined. *Risk factor* is a trait or characteristic associated with a statistical and increased likelihood of developing a particular cancer. After these risks

are identified, the appropriate prevention/detection methods are chosen. Risk can be measured in several ways. One is *absolute risk*, which is the measure of cancer incidence in the general population (e.g., the average risk). This gives us the specific data that determine the chance of getting a certain cancer (e.g., 80 new cases of cancer per 100,000 people annually) or lifetime risk of getting cancer (1 in 8 women will get breast cancer in her lifetime). *Relative risk* compares an individual's risk for developing a particular cancer. For instance, a woman with no known risk factors for breast cancer may be compared with a woman who has several risk factors for breast cancer. *Attributable risk* is the amount of disease in a population that could be prevented by alteration of a risk factor (e.g., tobacco use, alcohol consumption).[4]

Cancer Prevention

How can one prevent cancer? One, by identifying risk factors and two, by changing the behaviors that are attributed to the particular cancer (Table 2.1). With more inventive pro-

Table 2.1   Preventive Measures

- Get a screening test, starting at age 50.
- Eat a low-fat diet, with less red meat.
- Take a multivitamin with folate every day.
- Exercise at least 30 minutes a day.
- Maintain ideal body weight.
- Limit alcohol intake to less than 1 drink a day.
- Eat 3–5 servings of vegetables or fruits each day.
- Take an aspirin regularly (only with your doctor's approval).
- For women, taking birth control pills and/or post-menopausal hormones may be preventative.

Source: Adapted from Your cancer risk: Colon cancer fact sheet. Available at: http://www.yourcancerrisk.harvard.edu Accessed November 20, 2000.

grams currently available for prevention and detection, it is still very difficult to get an individual to change a behavior, as many factors are involved. For instance, increased knowledge about risk factors may help one change a behavior, or one may not have the ability to change a behavior due to lack of resources. Positive reinforcement is needed to continue behavior changes. By eating a low-fat diet with lots of vegetables and exercising regularly, you are decreasing your risk of cancer; also, avoiding alcohol and tobacco decreases your risk of cancer. Taking an aspirin a day improves cardiac function, and there are studies underway to determine whether taking an aspirin or an antiinflammatory agent every day decreases the risk of CRC.[5]

What does prevention mean in regard to cancer? *Primary cancer prevention* is reducing the risk of cancer by avoidance of a known carcinogen before the diagnosis of cancer. This includes the avoidance of tobacco, alcohol, dietary fat, ultraviolet light, asbestos, radon, and chemical exposure. *Secondary prevention* is the promotion of smoking cessation, dietary changes, and chemopreventative agents presumed to act as promoters of cell growth.[6] For example, if a woman is in the high-risk group for breast cancer, she may be placed on a chemoprevention trial to determine whether this drug will prevent her from getting cancer in the future. *Chemoprevention* is defined as the use of specific natural or synthetic agents that reverse or suppress the progression of premalignancy to invasive malignancy. *Tertiary prevention* consists of removing, arresting, and reversing a premalignant lesion to prevent recurrence or progression to cancer—for example, removing a polyp that has the capability to turn cancerous before it does so. Also, it is preventing the recurrence of cancer once a cancer diagnosis has been made. Secondary prevention through screening seems to be the way of the future. Its importance has grown since the

discovery of cancer genes and tumor markers, which make it easier than before to identify people with increased risk of developing certain types of cancers.[7]

Who Is at Risk?

In the United States, we consume a diet high in animal fat and low in vegetables, fruit, and fiber. In addition, Americans have a tendency toward very little or no exercise, and thus a propensity toward obesity. This puts people in the United States at high risk for developing CRC. For the average person, the primary factor related to the development of CRC is just being aged 50 or over. The incidence of CRC increases with age. Factors associated with an above averaged or high-risk group include a personal or family history of CRC or adenomatous polyps and those with long-standing chronic ulcerative colitis. Those with hereditary factors (familial adenomatous polyposis [FAP] or hereditary nonpolyposis colorectal cancer [HNPCC]) are at high risk as well for developing the disease. Approximately 70% to 80% of new CRC cases are from average-risk individuals, approximately 15% to 20% are from moderate-risk individuals, and 5% to 10% are from high-risk individuals (Figure 2.1).[1]

Who Should Be Screened?

All men and women over the age of 50, regardless of race or ethnic background, should be screened for CRC; this would be considered an average-risk individual. These individuals have no other risk factor than age, but approximately 75% of colorectal malignancies occur in this average-risk group. Moderate-risk individuals are those with a personal history of CRC or a family history of adenomatous polyps or inflammatory bowel disease (ulcerative colitis or Crohn's disease). Women with a family history of breast, ovarian, or endometrial cancer are

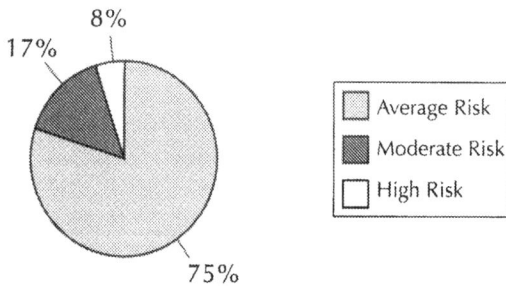

Figure 2.1   Approximate percentage of colorectal cancer found in U.S. population.

Source: Data from Winawer S, Fletcher R, Miller L, et al. Colorectal screening: Clinical guidelines and rationale. Gastroenterology. 1997; 112:594–641.

also at an increased risk of developing CRC and may need to be screened before the age of 50. This moderate-risk group accounts for 20% to 30% of colorectal malignancies. Those individuals with hereditary factors such as FAP or HNPCC are at high risk and may develop CRC at young ages. These individuals should be screened earlier than usual. Only about 5% of colorectal malignancies are associated with individuals in the high-risk group. It is important for individuals to share their family history and risk factors with their primary care provider so a true level of risk can be ascertained.[9]

Screening Performance

Before getting into screening methods, we need to understand screening performance. The goal of any screening test is to determine whether an individual has the disease; the sensitivity of the screening test usually determines whether there is any benefit from screening. *Sensitivity*, in preventative medicine, is a measure of the reliability of a screening test based on the proportion of people with a specific disease who react positively to the test (the higher the sensitivity of the test, the fewer the false negatives). This contrasts with *specificity*, which is the pro-

portion of people free of the disease who react negatively to the test (the higher the specificity, the fewer the false positives). Though these are theoretically independent variables, most screening tests are designed such that if the sensitivity is increased, the specificity is reduced and the number of false positives may rise to wasteful proportions.[10] Usually a false-positive result ends with the patient requiring further testing, which can be costly and does have some risks for the individual. *Positive predictive value* refers to the portion of persons with a positive result who do have the disease. *Negative predictive value* refers to the proportion of persons with a negative result who do not have the disease. The *efficacy* is the impact of the screening test under ideal conditions. *Effectiveness* is the impact of the screening test under typical conditions.[11] *Reliability* is the same result upon retesting.

Screening Methods

Current screening methods are used to detect and remove precancerous polyps and can detect the CRC if the disease starts to develop. At present, there are five principal screening tools in use to detect CRC. The two tests that have data supporting their efficacy are the fecal occult blood test (FOBT) and sigmoidoscopy. The other screening tools are the digital rectal exam (DRE), double contrast barium enema (DCBE), and colonoscopy. Limitations of screening evaluations are noted in Figure 2.2. There are studies underway to determine the efficacy of the remaining tests. Patients who are offered these exams should be well informed of the complications and false positives that occur with them.

Digital Rectal Examination

DRE is a relatively painless, simple examination that can detect many rectal cancers. This

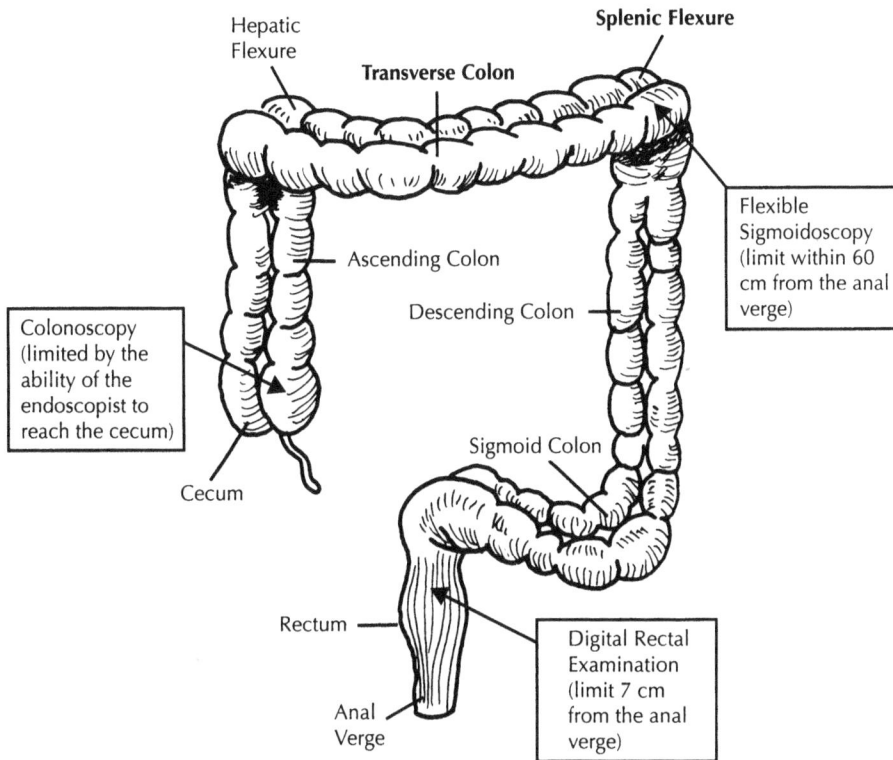

Hepatic
Flexure

Splenic Flexure

Transverse Colon

Flexible
Sigmoidoscopy
(limit within 60
cm from the anal
verge)

Ascending Colon

Descending Colon

Colonoscopy
(limited by the
ability of the
endoscopist to
reach the cecum)

Sigmoid Colon

Cecum

Rectum

Digital Rectal
Examination
(limit 7 cm
from the anal
verge)

Anal
Verge

Figure 2.2   Limitations of screening evaluations for colorectal cancer.

Source: Data from Ellis C, Saddler D. Colorectal cancer. In: Yarbro CH, Frogge MH, Goodman M, et al., eds. Cancer Nursing Principles and Practice, 5th ed. Boston, MA: Jones and Bartlett Publishers; 2000: 1117–1137.

can be done in the physician's office and needs no preparation. Rectosigmoid cancers have a shorter dwell time than colon cancers. Fewer than 10% of these tumors are within the reach of the examiner's digit, but the DRE has only a 5% to 10% sensitivity for CRC.[1] For this reason, this method should not be used as the only screening tool. There are no data that suggest the DRE decreases the mortality rate of rectal cancer.

Fecal Occult Blood Testing

FOBT detects blood in the stool and has been found to be effective in screening the asymp-tomatic patient and can reduce the mortality rate significantly. This is a noninvasive test, with the sampling of stool obtained from three consecutive bowel movements in a patient who has not ingested red meat, aspirin, turnips, horseradish, vitamin C, or antiinflammatory drugs for 2 days prior to testing. The advantages of this test are that it is fairly inexpensive, and the compliance rate is better with this test than with one more invasive; still, compliance is an issue. One disadvantage is that CRCs often do not bleed until the later stages. The bleeding of a lesion or polyp may be intermittent, so it may not show up at the time of testing. The most commonly used version of the guaiac-based test is the Hemoccult II Test, which has a sensitivity for detecting CRC of 72% to 78% and a specificity of 98%. Rehydrating the stool specimen on the slide prior to testing can enhance this sensitivity, but this manipulation is associated with a decrease in the specificity to 90% to 92%. HemeSensa, like the rehydrated Hemoccult II, allows an increased sensitivity but at the expense of a decreased specificity.[12] Patients are asked to take stool specimens on three consecutive bowel movements; if the specimen card is not brought in quickly, it can affect the outcome of the true test. There are new FOBT tests based on the immunochemical detection of hemoglobin, but there are not sufficient data at this time to discard the more commonly used tests.

Sigmoidoscopy

Sigmoidoscopy is a screening tool that offers more advantages than the FOBT kit. It is usually recommended for average-risk, asymptomatic patients with a negative FOBT. It allows visualization of the rectum and lower part of the colon. This test is usually done in a doctor's office, and patients do not need to be sedated. It does, however, require several cleansing enemas to the lower colon a few hours before the test. Patients should be well informed of the possible complication of this test, which is perforation of the bowel. A rigid sigmoidoscope is 30 cm in length but is not used as often as the flexible sigmoidoscope, which is 60 cm in length and has a better view of the larger part of the lower bowel. Patients are positioned on their left side with knees to their chest. The end of the sigmoidoscope, after being well lubricated, is inserted into the anus. The insertion of the tube may be uncomfortable and patients may feel as though they need to move their bowels at the beginning of insertion of the tube, but this passes. During the procedure, patients may also experience cramping as air is inserted into the bowel to allow the physician a better

view of the colon. A biopsy can be taken, if needed, for polyps less than 1 cm. For polyps greater than 1 cm, the polyp usually is left alone and patients then undergo a colonoscopy, as there is an increased risk of malignancy in larger sized polyps as well as the possibility of additional polyps in other areas of the colon not reached by the sigmoidoscope. Suction is used to remove stool or secretions in the bowel for a better view of the colonic lining. This procedure varies in time, depending on the proficiency of the practitioner doing the exam.

After the procedure, patients may experience some flatus, and if a biopsy was taken, some blood may be noted in the stool. Patients can go back to their regular activities right after the procedure. Randomized, controlled trials have not proved that sigmoidoscopy reduces the mortality rate for CRC, although case control studies have shown a benefit. The Prostate, Lung, Colon, and Ovary Trial, which is being supported by the National Cancer Institute (NCI), is currently evaluating the effectiveness of flexible sigmoidoscopy in a randomized, controlled setting; however, mortality data are not expected to become available until 2008.[13]

Double Contrast Barium Enema

A barium enema can be performed in two ways: as a single contrast study using barium alone, which reveals filling defects; or as a double contrast barium enema (DCBE), in which air is instilled into the colon after the barium has been removed. DCBE is preferred over a single contrast exam for screening; the double contrast provides better delineation of polyps. Bowel preparation is achieved with low-residue diet, laxatives, and enemas during the 24 hours preceding the examination. Patients are encouraged to drink fluids to avoid dehydration. The double contrast barium enema takes about 20 to 30 minutes and can be performed without sedation.[11] Patients may be given an antispasmodic during the procedure, but no sedation is required. Patients usually lie prone, with a soft tube 2 cm in diameter inserted 3 to 5 cm into the rectum as the liquid barium is instilled. The barium's progress is then monitored by fluoroscopy as the patient changes position, that is, rolls to the left, then to the right, and then tilted to a standing position to fill the colon as far as the cecum. Air is instilled to assist the progress of the barium through the bowel and to provide a double contrast examination. This can cause some discomfort, especially if the air is instilled too quickly. Radiographs of the bowel are then taken, outlining the colon. Patients can leave the hospital after the exam. They usually will pass barium for a few days and may experience some constipation. A laxative may be prescribed to prevent impaction of the barium.

Interfering factors for this exam include an inadequate bowel preparation, which impairs the quality of the x-ray film. Barium swallow performed within several days before a barium enema impairs the quality of subsequent x-ray films. Also, the inability of patients to retain the barium enema causes an incomplete test.[14]

DCBE has not been assessed adequately in a screening population. There is information available concerning its detection rates of polyps and cancer, but the individuals were symptomatic. The sensitivity for DCBE is 50% to 80% for polyps smaller than 1 cm, 70% to 90% for those larger than 1 cm, and 55% to 85% for Dukes' stage A and B cancers.[1] The benefit from this test is that it can pick up polyps less than 1 cm. The disadvantage of this test is that it offers evaluation but does not offer therapeutic capabilities. Thus, if a lesion is seen, it cannot be biopsied; therefore, a colonoscopy will be needed, putting the patient through yet another procedure.

Colonoscopy

Colonoscopy offers complete visualization of the colon, with therapeutic ability. It requires full-bowel preparation with either an oral cathartic solution or laxatives and enemas. Because this is an invasive procedure, patients who are at high risk for endocarditis will need antibiotic prophylaxis. Patients are on a clear liquid diet for 48 hours prior to the exam. They are given either 10 oz of magnesium citrate or 1 gallon of Go-Lytely. They are instructed to drink the entire laxative; a clean colon is a must for this exam. When these patients go to the hospital the next morning, they may receive an intramuscular or intravenous injection of a sedative of the doctors' choosing. This sedative is given for three reasons: the discomfort caused by the colon being distended with air, the length of the colonoscope, and the duration of the procedure. Again, patients should be well informed of any possible complications of the test. Consent forms are usually obtained with a sigmoidoscopy and colonoscopy.

The scope is lubricated when inserted into the anus. Patients may feel the need to defecate, but this feeling passes. Patients will lie on their left side with their knees flexed, just as in a sigmoidoscopy. The scope is advanced through the rectum into the sigmoid to the descending sigmoid junction. The scope then passes through the splenic flexure; it is advanced through the transverse colon, through the hepatic flexure, and into the ascending colon and cecum. During the exam, suction may be used to remove blood or excessive secretions that obscure vision. Biopsy forceps or a cytology brush may be passed through a channel in the colonoscope to obtain specimens for histologic and cytologic exams. Patients are monitored for side effects from sedation and for signs of bowel perforation: malaise, bleeding, abdominal pain and distention, fever, and mucopurulent drainage. The doctor should be notified immediately if any of these symptoms occur. When patients are alert and vital signs are stable and there are no signs or symptoms of perforation, they then can be discharged home. After the procedure, patients may resume their usual diets. Patients may pass large amounts of flatus. If a polyp was removed, patients must be warned that there may be some blood in their stools. The ability of colonoscopy to reduce deaths from CRC has been demonstrated indirectly through studies showing that the detection and removal of polyps reduces the incidence of CRC, and the detection of early cancers lowers the mortality rate for this malignancy.[13]

Screening Recommendations

In 1995 a group convened by the U.S. Agency for Health Care Policy and Research (AHCPR) looked at the issue of screening recommendations.[9] This group of experts came from several professional organizations, including the American College of Gastroenterology, the American Gastroenterological Association, the American Society of Colon and Rectal Surgeons, the American Society of Gastrointestinal Endoscopy, and the Society of American Gastrointestinal Endoscopic Surgeons. Their charge was to evaluate the available data on CRC and to develop recommendations for clinical practice guidelines. They researched material on colorectal screening from 1966 to 1994.[15] After 2 years of reviewing this information, in 1997 they put forward their recommendations for colorectal guidelines. The American Cancer Society (ACS) and the Crohn's and Colitis Foundation of America have endorsed these recommendations for CRC screening guidelines. The recommendations are outlined in Table 2.2.

Summary of Screening Guidelines

The following is a summary of the data from Table 2.2[16]:

- *Average-risk individuals:* Annual FOBT, flexible sigmoidoscopy every 5 years, a dou-

ble contrast barium enema every 5 to 10 years, or a colonoscopy every 10 years. The recommendations for average-risk individuals with a positive test on any FOBT sample is an accurate examination of the entire colon and rectum by colonoscopy. An alternative is DCBE, preferably with flexible sigmoidoscopy.

- *Recommendations for people at increased risk for CRC:* Individuals with close relatives (sibling, parent, or child) with CRC or an adenomatous polyp should be offered the same options as the average-risk individual but at the age of *40*. If the close relative was diagnosed with CRC before age 55 or an adenomatous polyp by the age of 60, then special efforts should be made to ensure that screening takes place starting at an age prior to that diagnosis.

- *Recommendations for people with FAP:* These individuals should receive genetic counseling and consider genetic testing to see whether they are gene carriers. A negative genetic test result rules out FAP only if an affected family member has an identified mutation. Gene carriers or people with indeterminate cases should be offered flexible sigmoidoscopy every 12 months starting at puberty to see whether they are expressing the gene. If polyposis is present, they will eventually need to undergo a colectomy, and thus should start to consider the risks and benefits of this procedure.

- *Recommendations for people with a family history of HNPCC:* Individuals with cancers diagnosed in multiple close relatives and across several generations, especially when the cancers occurred at a young age, should receive genetic counseling and consider genetic testing for HNPCC. They should be offered an examination of the entire colon every 1 to 2 years starting between the ages of 20 to 30 years, increasing to every year after the age of 40.

Table 2.2 Colorectal Cancer Screening: Evidence-Based Summary AHCPR, 1997[9]

Average Risk (asymptomatic, age 50)	Increased Risk (age 40)	Individuals with FAP	Individuals with HNPCC	Adenomatous Polyps	History of CRC	Inflammatory Bowel Disease
Annual FOBT	Should be offered same options as average-risk, but begin at age 40	Genetic counseling and testing	Genetic counseling and testing	Exam of the colon every 3 years after initial exam	If no preoperative exam of the colon was done, then exam should be at one year of resection	Surveillance colonoscopy
Flexible sigmoidoscopy every 5 years		Flexible sigmoidoscopy, starting at puberty, every year	Exam of the entire colon every 1–2 years ages 20–30 and every year after age 40	If normal follow-up, can go 5 years to next exam		
FOBT and flexible sigmoidoscopy every 5 years					If preoperative exam is normal, then exam should be offered in 3 years and then, if normal, every 5 years	
DCBE every 5 to 10 years						
Colonoscopy every 10 years						
Positive results from FOBT should have the entire colon reviewed by colonoscopy						
Alternative: DCBE, preferably with flexible sigmoidoscopy						

AHCPR, Agency for Health Care Policy and Research; FAP, familial adenomatous polyposis; HNPCC, hereditary nonpolyposis colorectal cancer; CRC, colorectal cancer; FOBT, fecal occult blood testing; DCBE, double contrast barium enema.

Source: From Colorectal cancer screening. Summary, evidence report: Number 1. AHCPR Publication No. 97-0302. Rockville, MD: Agency for Health Care Policy and Research, 1997, with permission.

- *Recommendations for people with a history of adenomatous polyps* (i.e., polyps that were numerous or large [> 1 cm diameter]): These polyps should be removed at colonoscopy, with a repeat examination of the colon every 3 years after the initial examination. The interval between subsequent examinations depends on the type of polyps that were detected. If the first follow-up is normal or only a single, small, tubular adenoma is found, the next examination can be in 5 years. In special circumstances (e.g., polyps with invasive cancer, large sessile adenomas, or numerous adenomas), a shorter interval may be necessary, according to the judgment of the clinician and the wishes of the patient.
- *Recommendations for people with a history of CRC* that has been resected with curative intent (but who did not undergo a complete, adequate colonoscopic examination preoperatively): A complete examination of the colon within 1 year after resection. If this or a complete preoperative examination is normal, subsequent examination should be offered after 3 years and then, if normal, every 5 years.
- *Recommendation for people with inflammatory bowel disease* (long-standing extensive inflammatory disease): surveillance colonoscopy, looking for dysplasia as a marker for CRC risk. The extent and duration of the disease are factors used to determine when or if a colectomy should be considered.

The ACS also has screening guidelines and recommendations. The only difference between the AHCPR recommendations and the ACS guidelines is that the ACS does not include FOBT as an isolated option, but rather only in combination with sigmoidoscopy.[17] At the present time, the ACS is revising their guidelines, which will be published sometime in 2001.

In July of 2000, the NCI published an article entitled, "Conquering Colorectal Cancer: A Blue Print for the Future."[18] The NCI's Colorectal Cancer Progress Review Group assessed what is known about CRC and made recommendations on improving research efforts against the disease. The report consists of two sets of recommendations: One is aimed at questions of scientific priority, and the other is aimed at overarching and resource issues. The scientific questions address the biology of colorectal neoplasm development and the etiology of how they arise (i.e., lifestyles, genetics, diet, and endogenous factors). For prevention, the NCI is defining pathways for nutritional and chemo-preventative interventions. Research into early detection strategies for implementing current screening method recommendations, evaluation of new modalities before they are used, and the development of newer modalities and markers for CRC early detection are being evaluated. The report also fostered uniform delivery of accepted treatments and development of new regimens for locoregional disease. Lastly, they addressed the need for follow-up care after treatment is given. Overarching and resources recommendations were to identify those individuals who were predisposed to CRC and determine how genetic screening interventions affect morbidity and mortality and quality of life, in order to address counseling issues.

Controversies in Colorectal Cancer

At present, there is some controversy over which screening methods to use for CRC. The FOBT kit can yield false-negative and false-positive results. There have been three randomized trials studying the FOBT kit, and the outcomes have shown that it has reduced the mortality rate by approximately 30% to 40%. While there was a reduction in mortality, overall survival was not improved. This may be due to comorbidity of other diseases in screening aged adults. Although the FOBT kit is useful in detecting blood in the stool, it does not detect tumors in the rectosigmoid colon. As stated earlier, polyps or cancerous lesions may bleed intermittently and may not be picked up when doing an FOBT. There is controversy over which slide kit to use. The suggested false-positive results with the FOBT kit may be due to using nonhydrated hemoccult. Studies suggest using rehydrated hemoccult or one of the newer guaiac or hemoglobin immunoassay tests is similar, in that they pick up blood but have an improved sensitivity and specificity, reducing the rate of false positives.[19]

Sigmoidoscopy detects lesions in the left colon and is better at detecting small polyps than is the FOBT. Sigmoidoscopy detects 50% to 60% of cancer and polyps, with fewer false positives. However, sigmoidoscopies do not examine the entire colon and have a low sensitivity for picking up adenomas of less than 1 cm. Some studies suggest that with age there is an increase in adenomas proximal to the sigmoid junction to the descending colon. If this is the case, this is beyond the reach of the sigmoidoscope. Sigmoidoscopy has been compared with doing a screening mammogram on only one breast. Therefore, colonoscopy would be the choice for screening exam, as it examines the whole colon.

At present, colonoscopies are expensive, ranging from $400 to $1,600. As stated, colonoscopies view the entire colon and have therapeutic capabilities, but the risks are higher for complications and patients need to be sedated. In addition, if colonoscopy were to become the national screening standard, there may not be enough endoscopists to perform the procedure. Considering these facts, there is controversy as to using this exam for the average-risk individual without symptoms, but with a positive FOBT a view of the entire colon should be performed. Alternatively, the primary provider may order a DCBE with a flexible sigmoidos-

copy instead of a colonoscopy as a low-cost alternative to the patient. There is consensus as to patients with a cancer or polyp larger than 1 cm, who should be referred for colonoscopy, and those patients having only hyperplastic polyps, which need no further evaluation. There is controversy, however, as to how to manage the adenomas smaller than 1 cm. There are limited studies that suggest that adenomas smaller than 1 cm have less than a 1% risk of more advanced lesions, but an adenoma smaller than 1 cm or one that contains villous elements has a 10% risk of more advanced lesions. Most polyps found on sigmoidoscopies are less than 1 cm; this would reduce the need for referring for a colonoscopy, therefore reducing the screening costs considerably.[11]

Although it appears that no single test is adequate for CRC screening, when used in combination these modalities can be very effective in detecting early-stage disease.

Cost Effectiveness of Screening

The cost effectiveness of screening for CRC continues to be debated. Because recommendations for screening should balance cost restraints, the exact age at which screening should be implemented is based on a variety of considerations, including statistical data and cost-benefit analyses.[20] Estimating a cost of screening for colorectal cancer is difficult and complex because a positive result on initial screening may lead to further testing and continued screening for patients with negative results. The most recent study prepared by the Office of Technology Assessment of the U.S. Congress evaluated all screening modalities, including FOBT, sigmoidoscopy, DCBE, and colonoscopy.[21] The agency built a model to predict the average additional lifetime costs and years of life saved for a population of 100,000 individuals aged 50 years who followed a specific screening strategy for the rest of their lives.[22]

This study indicated that colorectal screening for the average-risk person would cost $15,000 to $20,000 per year of a life saved, which is very cost effective, considering that the federal government deems $40,000 per year of life saved to be cost effective.[21,22] The results showed that every screening technique analyzed was cost effective when compared with the mammography benchmark ($37,000 per year of life saved); none of the methodologies costs more than $20,000 per year of life saved. Flexible sigmoidoscopy every 5 years costs $12,000 per life saved; sigmoidoscopy every 10 years was even more cost effective, at $8,000 for each year of life saved. DCBE every 4 years was $13,000 per year of life saved.[22]

What is year per life saved? This number divides total life-years gained by net lives saved to obtain the estimated increase lifespan for each individual with a prevented CRC death. Years per life saved range from a low of 7.3 to a high of 9.2, indicating that preventing a CRC death may increase an individual's lifespan by approximately 8 years.[1] These cost-effective models take into account age, mortality, compliance, screening intervals, false positives with the tests, and costs of the tests. These models, at present, show that screening with the current modalities shows a reduction in CRC mortality.

New on the Horizon

New tests are under investigation at the present time. One is the new virtual colonoscopy. This is a screening method that uses magnetic resonance imaging (MRI) or computerized tomography (CT) scan to make a computer-generated, three-dimensional image of the colon. This is being done in a few centers across the United States. It is still considered experimental and is not currently covered by most insurance providers. Patients must still undergo complete colon preparation and have air introduced into the colon; thus, there is discomfort with this exam. However, it is not an invasive procedure, as is standard colonoscopy. The test is accomplished quickly, and sedation is not needed. Studies are under way to determine the efficacy of this examination, as there are some negative aspects to virtual colonoscopy: It tends to miss large polyps, particularly if they are flat and on the right side of the colon. Moreover, if a polyp is found, patients must still undergo a standard colonoscopy to biopsy or remove the polyp, thus requiring an additional bowel preparation and procedure. For now, standard colonoscopy is the recommended test.[23]

Researchers are also trying to perfect a test to detect gene abnormalities in the stool. DNA is contained in cells that are continuously shed from precancerous polyps and cancerous tumors within the colon. By examining patients' stools in a laboratory, DNA can be detected. No special diet, medication restrictions, or enemas or bowel preparations are required.[24] This will make compliance much easier for the patient. One drawback of this test is that the cancer may be so small it may not be detected by current methods.

Another method for the future utilizes a gene that can indicate how aggressive a CRC may be. This is called the pituitary-tumor transforming gene (PTTG1). This gene tends to be expressed in more aggressive tumors and growths. It is hoped that this tendency will be able to determine which tumors might spread and which polyps may turn cancerous. It may be a marker for aggressive CRC in the future.[25]

Aspirin and nonsteroidal antiinflammatory drugs have been found to inhibit cyclooxygenase-2 (COX-2). This enzyme is necessary for the formation of blood vessels that feed cancerous tumors. An overexpression of COX-2 has been induced by growth factors, oncogenes, and tumor promoters, and has been observed in colon cancer.[26] Interestingly, COX-2 is not overexpressed in normal tissue. Aspirin impacts two different COX enzymes: COX-2, as noted, and COX-1. COX-1 appears to be involved in heart disease and can cause some negative side effects, such as gastrointestinal distress and bleeding. Inhibitors of COX-2 block prostaglandin pathways in tumor cells and lead to reversal of dysplasia and other precancerous events. Three trials are under way with sulindac, Exisulind, and celecoxib, which appear to enhance programmed cell death in precancer and cancerous cells. Chemoprevention trials to reduce a person's risk of developing cancer are also ongoing. In addition to the nonsteroidals, studies are being done on folic acid, calcium, fiber supplements, and vitamin E and their role in preventing CRC. These compounds show promise in high-risk groups, though there is no evidence yet as to their ability to prevent cancer in the general population.[27] Additional information about chemoprevention and dietary modifications can be found in Chapter 3. Further research into the genetics of CRCs will lead to better drugs and therapies in the future and, one hopes, reduce the barriers of colorectal screening.

Barriers to Screening

There are many barriers to colorectal screening: emotional, financial, practical, cultural, and even professional. First is the emotional hurdle. Bodily functions are not a normal topic of conversation. Although discussing breast cancer now is commonplace, the reluctance of even some health professionals to discuss the colon keeps many persons from getting help.

Second, many health plans do not cover CRC screening, or they reimburse only a small percentage of the cost. Many individuals over 50 are on a fixed income and cannot afford the cost of screening examinations. Prior to 1998, Medicare covered screening only for those individuals at high risk for the disease.

Third, the tests themselves are uncomfortable and embarrassing. Patients fear the examinations as well as the potential results. Many patients are not well informed about the tests, and if the result is positive, they do not understand, or are not fully told, what happens next. Some cultures are fearful of the medical community and thus either stay away or do not heed the physicians' recommendations. Written material for colorectal screening tends to be in English, some in Spanish, but it may not be specific enough for some cultures, and they may not relate to this particular disease or test.

Finally, there may be a lack of awareness on the primary care physicians' part as to colorectal screening guidelines. They may not know current protocols for CRC screening and may assume that a guaiac in the office, performed on the glove used in a rectal exam, constitutes an FOBT.[28] Many physicians feel they lack the time and staff to explain the screening tests to patients during routine clinic visits. Many offices do not have a system in place to prompt the physician when a screening is due.[29]

If a positive result is noted with the FOBT, many patients are not referred for the appropriate follow-up test. If the primary care physician does refer the patient to a gastroenterologist, there may be several delays: Patients may need approval from their health plans; it may take at least a week, if not two, to obtain a consult; then there is another delay to schedule an endoscopy. As a result, the patient may be waiting up to 4 to 6 weeks for follow-up testing; this may even be longer in some cases.

Fortunately, education programs are underway for patients, primary care physicians, and managed care organizations. These programs are designed to increase awareness of the impact of CRC and of the value of screening and surveillance. Following the cases of several well-known persons, the news media have substantially increased the attention given to this topic. And new tests are being developed that may be less uncomfortable for the patient.

The Role of Nurses in Education and Prevention

Nurses play a major role in prevention and detection of cancer disease. They are the people who have the most contact with patients. The most important tool in prevention and detection of CRC is the risk assessment form, which needs to be filled out completely and accurately. This begins the role of nurses in educating patients on epidemiology, risk factors, and signs and symptoms of the disease. Nurses can inform patients of screening clinics and the importance of early detection, especially in relation to CRC. From the assessment form, nurses may make the appropriate referral to counselors and for genetic testing. If patients are appropriate for chemoprevention trial, this information may be gleaned from the risk assessment forms as well. Education on prevention and detection is the *key*. The more informed patients are about their health, the more likely they are to take responsibility for their well-being. Cancer control is focusing on wellness and prevention and detection, which will eventually decrease the morbidity and mortality of cancer.[4] The role of nurses is not limited only to education and the development of screening programs. Nurse practitioners are performing screening sigmoidoscopies in gastrointestinal clinics all across the United States. They are taking an active role in primary and secondary prevention.

As a community outreach nurse, one of my responsibilities is screening programs. Recently, I was involved in a large-scale colorectal screening program. Our hospital collaborated with Eckerd Drug Company, Impact Health, and our local TV station. Impact Health provided the Colocare drop-in FOBT kit. These kits were sold at 36 Eckerd Drug stores in their pharmacy departments. In addition, CRC guidelines were available on the counters, and a large number of pharmacy assistants met with me to answer questions about CRC in general and the Colocare test specifically. The tests were sold for $1 each (to prevent throw-aways), and 20% of each sale was given to The National Colorectal Cancer Research Alliance (NCCRA), which was founded by Katie Couric, Lilly Tartikoff, and the Entertainment Industry Foundation.

We first introduced our screening program during an early-morning TV interview with our local health reporter. She interviewed the director of our cancer care program, the inpatient nurse manager on the oncology floor, and me. Because all of us are oncology nurses, she discussed how important the oncology nurse is to the community and our role in educating the public on CRC. For the next 3 days, we had a colorectal hotline set up at our hospital. The hotline number was displayed on TV during a series of pretaped interviews with patients. The health reporter also interviewed us live from the hotline, with our hotline number repeatedly flashed on the TV screen.

The patient interview series started with an interview of a 38-year-old woman who was diagnosed at age 34, a single parent with 4 children, a postal carrier who was diagnosed with CRC when in his 40s, and a young man with a history of FAP. The reporter also interviewed a gastric surgeon, a gastroenterologist, and a medical oncologist. A colorectal surgery was taped, as well as a colonoscopy. The series was done over 4 weeks, with the interviews the first 3 days of March and then one a day for the next 2 weeks, with one follow-up in early April.

After the initial 3 days, the hotline was operational one evening a week for the next 2 weeks. We received a total of 324 calls. The questions ranged from "What are the symptoms?" to "Why won't my provider refer me for a colonoscopy?" It was a great opportunity to educate the public on CRC. We also had a mechanism in place to refer patients with no insurance or who needed a primary physician to our community referral line, where they could speak with a social worker to get the help they needed. Eckerd Drugs sold approximately 18,000 kits, and $3,000 dollars was given to the NCCRA Foundation. Out of 18,000 kits sold, 2,000 cards were returned, and from those cards, 98 were positive. Of those 98 who did see their physician, many were given the FOBT kit again, some were referred to a gastroenterologist for a colonoscopy, and many were diagnosed with hemorrhoids. One case of CRC was found (a Dukes stage C), in addition to 4 adenomatous polyps and one Barrett's esophagus. Moreover, we felt that we were able to educate a large adult audience. Early detection does improve survival, and we as healthcare providers need to continue to educate the public on the positive outcomes of early detection and prevention of CRC.

Conclusion

Until recently, CRC has not received a lot of publicity. March 2000 was the first National Colorectal Awareness month. CRC is now receiving public attention from the media, especially in light of Katie Couric's efforts to increase public awareness due to the death of her husband from the disease. It is hoped that this will spur energy and money into prevention programs and screening methods. In addition, Katie's "live" colonoscopy this year was a step toward alleviating the fear associated with having one performed. The keys are education and awareness. With all the attention on CRC, it is also hoped that the public will be more receptive toward screening and prevention methods. Because CRC has a long preclinical phase and the screening tools have been found to be adequate, no one need die of this disease any longer. An article published in *Primary Care and Cancer* noted that some patients seek care only when faced with acute or emergency situations.[29] Others are more well-educated and more demanding. Their focus, as well as their physicians', has increasingly been on preventive care. It is now more important than ever that we use those guidelines dictated by evidence-based medicine to educate our patients and prevent disease.[3] The best prevention against CRC is regular exercise, a low-fat diet high in fiber, and screening on an annual basis. As a community outreach nurse for a cancer care center, I have seen more and more attention focused on prevention and detection. This is definitely the wave of the future, and more and more data are emerging to support the fact that the mortality and morbidity rates will come down with these measures. We need not to be embarrassed any longer, nor die of this disease.

References

1. Winawer S, Fletcher R, Miller L, et al. Colorectal screening: Clinical guidelines and rationale. Gastroenterology. 1997; 112:594–641.
2. American Cancer Society. Cancer Facts and Figures—2000. Atlanta, GA: American Cancer Society.
3. Levin B. Is colorectal cancer screening overlooked? Prim Care Cancer. 2000; 20 (March). Available at: http://intouch.cancernetwork.com/journals/primary/p0003g.htm Accessed on November 3, 2000.
4. Mahon S. Principles of cancer prevention and early detection. Clin J Oncol Nurs. 2000; 4(4): 169–176.

5. Prevention and early detection of colorectal cancer. American Digestive Health Foundation. Available at: http://www.gastro.org/adhf/cc-prev.html Accessed on August 29, 2000.

6. Screening for Colorectal Cancer. Guide to Clinical Preventative Services, 2nd ed. Report of the US Preventative Services Task Force. Baltimore: Williams & Wilkins, 1996. Available at: http://cpmcnet.columbia.edu/texts/gcps/gcps0018.html Accessed November 12, 2000.

7. Caplan LS, Hutton M, Miller DS, et al. Secondary prevention of cancer. Curr Opin Oncol. 1996; 8(5):441–446.

8. Your cancer risk: Colon cancer fact sheet. Available at: http://www.yourcancerrisk.harvard.edu Accessed November 20, 2000.

9. New National Colorectal Cancer Practice Guidelines: Recommended Life Saving Tests. American Gastroenterology Association, 1997. Available at: www.gastro.org/phys-sci/fact-sheets/newguidelines.html Accessed November 16, 2000.

10. The Bantam Medical Dictionary. New York: Laurence Urdang Associates, 1982.

11. Bilhartz L, Croft C. Rational approach to colon cancer screening. In: Bilhartz L, ed. Gastrointestinal Disease in Primary Care. New York, NY: Lippincott Williams & Wilkins, 2000: 119–131.

12. Bretnell T, Nguyen T, Wong E, et al. Colon cancer screening. Available at: http://www.uwgi.org/cme/cmecourseCD/ch_08/ch08txt.htm Accessed November 28, 2000.

13. Read T, Kodnerl I. Colorectal cancer: Risk factors and recommendations for early detection. AAFP. Available at: http://aafp.org/afp/990600ap/3083.html Accessed August 29, 2000.

14. Contrast Radiography. Illustrated Guide to Diagnostic Testing. Springhouse, 1993: 841–843.

15. Read T. Colorectal cancer: Factors and recommendations for early detection. AFP. 1999. Available at: www.findarticles.com/cf_0/m32225/11_59155391765/print.jhtml Accessed November 20, 2000.

16. Colorectal cancer screening. Summary, evidence report: Number 1. AHCPR Publication No. 97-0302. Rockville, MD: Agency for Health Care Policy and Research, January 1997.

17. Rex D. Recommendations for colorectal cancer screening. Prim Care Cancer. 1999; 19(6), (suppl 3). Available at: http://intouch.cancernetwork.com.journals/primary/p9906sup3b.htm Accessed November 20, 2000.

18. National Cancer Institute. Conquering colorectal cancer: A blueprint for the future. Oncol News Int. 2000; 9(7). Available at: http:/intouch.cancernetwork.com/journals/oncnews/n0007nn.htm Accessed November 20, 2000.

19. Ahen D, Lynch K. Colorectal screening in average- and high-risk groups. Adv Intern Med. 2000; 46:71–106.

20. Rosenblaum D, Shiff S. Chemoprevention of colorectal cancer: A practical approach. Prim Care Cancer. 1999; 19(6), (suppl 3). Available at: http://intouch.cancernetwork.com/journals/primary/p9906sup3f.htm Accessed November 20, 2000.

21. Costable J Jr, Weissman G. What the primary-care physician needs to know about sigmoidoscopy. Prim Care Cancer. 1999; 19(6). Available at: http://intouch.cancernetwork.com/journals/primary/p9906sup3c.htm Accessed November 20, 2000.

22. Colorectal cancer screening is cost-effective OTA study shows. Oncology. 1996; 10(5). Available at: http:intouch.cancernetwork.com/journals/oncology/o9605n.htm Accessed August 29, 2000.

23. Virtual colonoscopy techniques feasible in detecting polyps. Oncol News Int. 1996; 5(7). Available at: http://intouch.cancernetwork.com/journals/oncnews/n9607i.htm Accessed November 20, 2000.

24. Taus M. New colon cancer test developed. Newsday. 2000. Available at: http://newsday.com/ap/healthscience/ap545.htm Accessed December 20, 2000.

25. Gene may identify aggressive colon cancer.

Available at: http://www.cancerpage.com/cancernews/cancernews402.htm Accessed November 10, 2000.

26. COX2 inhibitors promising in prevention. Oncol News Int. 1999; 8(7). Available at: http://intouch.cancernetwork.com/journals/oncnews/n9907cc.htm Accessed August 29, 2000.

27. Colorectal research. Available at: http://gi.bsd.uchicago.edu/diseases/colorectandother/colorectal/colorectresearch.html Accessed November 10, 2000.

28. Wolf S. Overcoming barriers to change: Screening for colorectal cancer. AFP. March 15, 2000. Available at: http:/findarticles.com/cf_o/m322516_61/61432856/print.jhtml Accessed November 10, 2000.

29. Primary care physicians and colon cancer screening: Not so easy. Prim Care Cancer. 1999; 16(8). Available at: http://intouch.cancernetwork.com/journals/primary/p9609d.htm Accessed August 29, 2000.

CHAPTER 3 | Prevention Strategies and the Diet Connection

Kathy Christiansen, RN, BSN, OCN

Introduction

"It would be far better to work at the prevention of misery than to multiply places of refuge for the miserable."

—Denis Diderot (1713–1784), 1745

Denis Diderot was a French philosopher of the sixteenth century, and was acclaimed as one of the most powerful writers of his time. As we read his eloquent words, we can understand that the importance of disease prevention was not as recently recognized as we might have believed. As far back as the middle of the 1700s people were writing and promoting disease prevention, and as we begin the twenty-first century it is still an essential piece of our healthcare.

One hundred years ago, cancer was the eighth leading cause of death in the United States. As we start the twenty-first century, heart disease is the number one cause of death, with cancer as the second leading cause of death. Many of the infectious diseases that contributed to Americans' mortality at the start of 1900 have been wiped out completely or, for the most part, controlled. However, as the death rate from small pox, measles, and tuberculosis declined, the proportional impact of cancer grew.[1]

At the same time that we were winning the war against the deadly infectious diseases, great changes were occurring in American lifestyle behaviors, especially tobacco use, diet, and exercise. These changes led to considerable increases in certain types of cancers, such as lung and colorectal, and quickly thrust cancer up into the ranks of deadly diseases. As we moved through the twentieth century, our fight against cancer focused mostly on the treatment of advanced disease, while the overall burden of cancer steadily grew. Even as recently as a few years ago, it was thought that cancer would surpass heart disease as the leading cause of death.

Then, at the end of 1996 came the exciting news of the first-ever sustained decline in overall, age-adjusted cancer mortalities in the United States. Since then, both mortality and incidence rates have decreased progressively with each passing year. Now as we begin the twenty-first century, despite several areas of concern, there is good reason to believe that these declines will continue.

The declines in incidence and mortality rates can be attributed to a number of factors, including the very promising area of cancer prevention. *Cancer prevention* can be defined as all measures that limit the progression of cancer at any time during its course. It is now believed that controlling certain risk factors, such as tobacco use, poor diet, and lack of exercise, might cut cancer incidence and mortality in half during the normal human lifespan.

Colorectal cancer is the second leading cause of cancer deaths in both American men and women. Our risk for colorectal cancer begins to increase after the age of 40 and rises sharply at the ages of 50 to 55. Despite advances in surgical technique and adjuvant therapy, there has been only a modest improvement in survival for patients with advanced neoplasms. It is simple to understand the importance of effective prevention approaches if the morbidity and mortality of colorectal cancer is to be reduced in the twenty-first century.

Colorectal Cancer Prevention

Traditionally, there are three levels of prevention that have been described in nursing literature. *Primary prevention* is the promotion of health strategies and specific protection

recommendations to decrease the vulnerability of a healthy individual or population. *Secondary prevention* defines high-risk individuals or populations, and consists of early diagnosis, early detection, screening, and treatment of all stages of disease. *Tertiary prevention* minimizes morbidity resulting from permanent or irreversible disease by preventing complications.[2]

The conventional definition of *prevention* takes in the entire health continuum, but does not necessarily reflect the growing science of cancer prevention. Generally, cancer prevention has occurred when a change or adjustment of self-care behaviors or exogenous factors results in reduced cancer risk. Using this definition and the principle of carcinogenesis, primary cancer prevention can relate to initiation, secondary cancer prevention to promotion, and tertiary cancer prevention to progression.

Following these definitions, primary colorectal cancer prevention (Table 3.1) would involve the avoidance of exposure to carcinogens, diet changes, and the use of specific chemopreventive agents to limit exposure to carcinogens that initiate carcinogenesis. Examples of primary colorectal cancer prevention might include the adherence to a low-fat, high-fiber diet; minimal or no alcohol consumption; adequate physical activity in proportion to calorie intake; avoidance of solvents, abrasives, and fuel oils; and chemoprevention with antioxidants or NSAIDs.

Secondary colorectal cancer prevention would include the interventions that prevent the process of promotion of carcinogenesis. Examples might be alcohol cessation, weight loss by diet changes and an exercise program, and the use of chemopreventive agents that work on promotion. Cancer screening activities have often been used to describe secondary cancer prevention, but it is hard to imagine preventing a lesion that is already present and is just now detected.

Table 3.1   Examples of Types of Prevention

Type of Prevention	Examples
Primary prevention	Low-fat, high-fiber diet
	Little or no alcohol consumption
	Adequate physical activity in proportion to calorie intake to prevent obesity
	Avoidance of occupational exposures to asbestos, acrylonitrile, ethyl acrylate, synthetic fibers, halogens, printing materials, and fuel oils
	Regular use of antioxidants (vitamins C and E, beta-carotene, selenium, and calcium)
	Regular use of NSAIDs
Secondary prevention	Adapting a low-fat, high-fiber diet or an exercise program to lose weight
	Stopping alcohol consumption
	Regular use of antioxidants
	Regular use of NSAIDs
	For persons not at high risk, beginning at age 50, following the recommended American Cancer Society's colorectal cancer screening guidelines (yearly fecal occult blood test plus digital rectal exam and flexible sigmoidoscopy every 5 years; *or* digital rectal exam and colonoscopy every 10 years; *or* digital rectal exam and double contrast barium enema every 5–10 years)
Tertiary prevention	Removal of an adenomatous polyp by colonoscopy
	Regular use of NSAIDs

Tertiary colorectal prevention might include arresting, removing, or reversing the effects of a premalignant colorectal lesion (with chemotherapy or surgery) to prevent recurrence or progression to cancer.

Chemoprevention Approaches Utilized for Colorectal Cancer

The basis of cancer chemoprevention is to minimize the effects of potential carcinogens, with the ultimate intent of preventing the occurrence of a malignancy. Another definition for *cancer chemoprevention* is a pharmacologic intervention with certain nutrients or other elements to control or reverse carcinogenesis and to prevent the development of invasive cancer. One basic concept that supports cancer chemoprevention is the multistep process of carcinogenesis.[3] The

process of carcinogenesis is characterized by the accumulation of specific genetic and phenotypic alterations that can evolve over a 10- to 20-year period from the first initiating event. The premise of cancer chemoprevention is that one can intervene (and control) at many of the steps in this process and over a many-year period.

Agents that inhibit carcinogenesis generally are classified by the point in the process at which they are effective. For instance, chemopreventive agents could be used to limit or prevent exposure to tumor initiators or promoters. They could also stimulate the inactivation and excretion of potential initiators or promoters. They could block the oncogene expression by inhibiting, modifying, or blocking the activation of proto-oncogenes.[4] Chemopreventive agents could also regain control over cell replication and differentiation by inactivating tumor-suppressor genes. In other words, chemoprevention has the potential for primary, secondary, and tertiary cancer prevention.

Antioxidants

During the promotional phase of carcinogenesis, active oxygen is produced, which can be very damaging to the cellular DNA. Antioxidants, such as vitamins C and E, beta-carotene, and folic acid, have been shown to block this oxidative damage to the cellular DNA. It is for this reason that antioxidants are included in the category of colon cancer chemoprevention.

In some studies looking at colon cancer development and the use of vitamins C and E, there is evidence that a higher intake of vitamin E may decrease the risk of colon cancer, especially in the over age 65 group.[5] In other studies looking at the long-term use of multivitamins with folic acid, it was shown that they might substantially lower the risk of colon cancer, with the primary effect being associated to folic acid.[6] However, there have been other trials that have shown antioxidants to have little or no impact on colorectal cancer prevention.[7]

Aspirin and Nonsteroidal Antiinflammatory Drugs

The mechanism by which aspirin (ASA) and nonsteroidal antiinflammatory drugs (NSAIDs) work as colorectal cancer chemoprevention is not entirely understood. It is thought that prostaglandins play a role because certain of these stimulate cell proliferation and tumor growth and immune response. ASA and NSAIDs are thought to work on prostaglandins by the inhibition of cyclooxygenase (COX), the enzyme involved in the formation of prostaglandins. COX exists in two forms: COX-1, which serves as a "housekeeping" enzyme and is made throughout the gastrointestinal tract, and COX-2, which is primarily inducible and appears to play a role in inflammation and tumor promotion. If

prostaglandin synthesis is inhibited, then this may result in a suppression of cell proliferation, as well as the stimulation of an immune response.[8] Both of these processes could be beneficial in the prevention of colorectal cancer.

This hypothesis is supported by findings from basic research and observational epidemiologic studies. First, experimental studies in animals indicate that NSAIDs can prevent chemically induced colorectal cancer. Second, patients with rheumatoid arthritis who use NSAIDs on a regular basis appear to have a decreased incidence of colorectal cancers. Third, several intervention trials demonstrate that the NSAID sulindac can cause dramatic regression of colon polyps in patients with the hereditary colorectal cancer syndrome, familial adenomatous polyposis (FAP). Although sulindac has been reported to cause both regression and suppression of colon polyps in patients with FAP and Gardner's syndrome, the Food and Drug Administration (FDA) has not approved this chemopreventive indication for sulindac.

In the data from the Physicians' Health Study, there was a strong association between regular, long-term use of ASA and a decreased death rate from colorectal cancer. Another study conducted by the American Cancer Society established reduction in the mortality rate of colorectal cancer for those participants who used ASA on a regular basis. In some trials, "regular ASA use" is described as two times per week.

The use of the NSAIDs in colorectal cancer prevention has been, unfortunately, restricted by the frequency of NSAID-induced complications. The gastrointestinal (GI) side effects (GI ulceration and peptic ulceration) are thought to be a result of COX-1 inhibition produced by the standard NSAIDs. These GI toxicities and the limited long-term use of standard NSAIDs have led to great interest in the chemopreventive potential of the relatively new generation of NSAIDs, the selective COX-2 inhibitors.

It has been shown that there is a lack of COX-2 expression on the normal mucosa of the colon, but an overexpression of it in colon neoplasms.[9] The use of selective COX-2 inhibitors as colorectal cancer chemopreventive agents is being actively investigated. A trial of the COX-2 inhibitor celecoxib in participants with the hereditary syndrome FAP has been reported to have a significant reduction in the number of colorectal polyps.[10] In late 1999, celecoxib was approved by the FDA as an adjunct to usual care for patients with FAP.

Possible Dietary Factors in Colorectal Cancer Prevention

On a daily basis it is possible to hear or read about the latest vitamin, food, or food additive that has the possibility to have a positive or a negative impact on our health. For most of humans' time, our diet and its role in our health have had an important influence in our lives. The current fast-paced world of drive-through, convenient fast foods might occasionally resent its influence. However, we are not the first of humankind to begrudge the influence of diet on our health. In 1678, François, Duc de La Rochefoucauld wrote in his *Sentences et Maximes Morales*, "To safeguard one's health at the cost of too strict a diet is a tiresome illness indeed." Even with the readily available supply of fruits and vegetables, U.S. culture seems to prefer the high-calorie, high-fat "cheeseburger and fries."

Not unlike the conditions of heart disease or diabetes, there is thought that the development of colorectal cancer can be influenced by our dietary intake. And, just as in those diseases, the role of diet in its prevention can be confusing, and at times, controversial. The following is a summary of some of the factors that have been presented as influential in colorectal cancer progression.

Dietary Fat

Once we have ingested the dietary fats in our diet, they are broken down into fatty acids that are able to pass into the bloodstream. Fatty acids are categorized as either saturated or unsaturated. Saturated fats are derived mostly from animal sources, such as meat and cheese, whereas the sources of unsaturated fats tend to be from plant or vegetable sources. The typical Western (American) diet consists of dietary fat, making up 40% to 50% of the daily food calories.

In the past couple of decades, reduction of dietary fat has been at the center of cancer prevention efforts. The National Academy of Sciences review of diet, nutrition, and cancer in 1982 had as its primary recommendation the reduction in dietary fat to 30% of daily calorie intake.[11] The relation of dietary fat to cancer incidence first got attention in the 1970s as the large international differences in cancer incidences were noted and appeared to be strongly associated with dietary fat consumption. The populations of the Western Hemisphere had higher incidences of breast, colon, prostate, and endometrium cancers, and, as was noted previously, their diets were rich in dietary fat. Complementing these correlational observations, it was also noted that populations that migrated from areas of low-incidence cancer rates to the Western Hemisphere adopted the higher-incidence rates of their new environment. Although these observational studies had limitations, several animal studies also made the area of dietary fat intake a convincing suspect.

Although the mechanism between a high-fat diet and colorectal cancer development is not yet established, bile acids as a possible carcinogen have been suggested. An increased bile acid concentration in the intestinal tract goes together with a high-fat diet, because bile acids are released from the gallbladder after fat ingestion. The intensity of bile acids in the colon is greatly influenced by the amount and type of fat in the diet.[12] The possible mechanism of action of bile salts in colorectal carcinogenesis is unknown, although it has been suggested that it is mediated by diacylglycerol.[13] The conversion of dietary phospholipids to diacylglycerol by intestinal bacteria is advanced by a high-fat diet. It is proposed that diacylglycerol enters the epithelial cell of the colon directly, stimulating protein kinase C, which is involved in cell growth and tumor promotion.

Another possible relationship between colorectal cancer and dietary fat intake is the possibility that diets high in meat intake (a source of saturated fats) may contain carcinogens. Cooking meat at high temperatures, such as broiling or frying, may result in a compound, benzo[a]pyrene, which has proved to be carcinogenic in animal studies. Epidemiologic studies of a Swedish population suggest that the association between meat consumption and colorectal cancer risk was highest when the meat surface was heavily browned during frying.[14]

Dietary Fiber

Dietary fiber is a particularly complex mixture, which is generally defined as a group of compounds that are resistant to human digestive enzymes. High-fiber foods include wholegrain products and cereals, vegetables, fruits, and legumes—particularly vegetable and fruit skins, berries, and the bran layers of grains. This group contains both insoluble fiber (typified by bran layers of grain) and soluble fiber (usually legumes).

Ingestion of fiber could alter carcinogenesis in the large bowel by a number of potential means. One direct means by which dietary fiber reduces the risk of colorectal cancer may be absorption of water by insoluble dietary fiber; this increases fecal bulk, diluting the concentration of carcinogens in the feces, and also decreases transit time, which reduces the possi-

bility of interacting with the mucosal cells of the colon. Certain types of fiber may stimulate bacterial fermentation in the intestine, with a subsequent increase in bacterial mass and the production of short-chain fatty acids that may have anticarcinogenic effects. Fiber may also influence the process of bile acid production, which could decrease the growth of colon adenomas.

The evidence on whether dietary fiber plays a protective role in reducing the incidence of colorectal cancer is mixed. Most animal and epidemiologic studies show a protective result of dietary fiber on colon carcinogenesis. However, because dietary fibers vary in composition, it is unlikely that all are equally protective against colorectal cancer. For instance, investigations into the effects of wheat, oat, and corn brans showed that wheat bran was effective in stimulating bacterial fermentation, oat bran had little effect, and corn bran had no effect.[15]

Several studies from different countries have concluded that the intake of fiber-rich foods is related to lower incidences of cancers of both colon and rectum. The studies' results were similar in extent for left- and right-sided colorectal cancers, for gender, and for different age groups.[16] In another prospective study looking at legume intake and the risk of colorectal cancer, it was suggested that eating legumes more than two times per week was more protective than eating legumes just one time per week. Other studies have corroborated these protective effects of dietary fiber.

Despite the evidence of protective effects, results from other large prospective studies, such as the Nurses' Health Study, found no difference in the risk of colorectal cancer with respect to dietary fiber. In another study, the Polyp Prevention Trial, half of the participants were given a standard brochure on healthy eating and the other half had intensive counseling to adopt a low-fat, high-fiber, fruit- and vegetable-enriched eating plan. In the 4 years of the trial, there was no evidence that adopting a low-fat, high-fiber, fruit- and vegetable-enriched diet reduced the recurrence of colorectal polyps.[17] Another study also showed that the addition of a bran-fiber cereal supplement to the daily diet for 3 years provided no evidence of reduction of colorectal polyp recurrence.[18]

Because almost all the available information from prospective studies is based on less than 10 years of follow-up, some researchers believe that further evaluation of the effects of diet earlier in life and at longer intervals of observation is needed. All the same, someone who is interested in reducing the risk of colorectal cancer could, as a practical measure, be instructed to minimize the intake of foods high in animal fat and increase the intake of fruits and vegetables. A high-fiber, low-fat diet is likely to be beneficial not only for prevention of colorectal and other cancers, but also for the prevention of the leading cause of death in the United States, cardiovascular disease.

Micronutrients

The components of food can be broadly classified into a common classic division of macronutrients and micronutrients. Macronutrients include fat and fiber, and their role in colorectal cancer prevention has been discussed previously. Micronutrients are commonly subdivided into vitamins and minerals (Table 3.2). Micronutrients mediate their effect in a variety of strategies, but in general their reason for existing is to prevent damage to the cells either by changing the cellular response or by directly preventing DNA alteration. In performing this, they can affect cancer development.

Two of the mechanisms by which micronu-

Table 3.2 Sources of Micronutrients

Micronutrients	Sources
Vitamins	
Fat-soluble	
Vitamin A	Some vegetables, dairy products, liver, and fish-liver oil
Vitamin E	Vegetable oils, wheat germ, liver, and leafy green vegetables
Vitamin D	Egg yolk, liver, tuna, and fortified milk
Carotenoids (beta-carotene)	Colored vegetables, such as carrots or squash
Water-soluble	
Vitamin B_2 (riboflavin)	Liver, milk, meat, dark green vegetables, whole-grain and enriched cereals, pasta, bread, and mushrooms
Vitamin C (ascorbic acid)	Acidic fruits and vegetables
Vitamin B_6 (pyridoxine)	Whole (but not enriched) grains, cereals, bread, liver, avocadoes, spinach, green beans, and bananas
Folic acid	Organ meats, leafy green vegetables, legumes, nuts, and whole grains
Minerals	
Calcium	Milk and milk products, cheese, and tofu
Iron	Lean meats, beans, green leafy vegetables, shellfish, enriched breads and cereals, whole grains
Selenium	Whole grains, meat, and fish; also found in some soils
Copper, zinc	Widespread

trients can affect cancer development are by antioxidation and by enhancing differentiation and growth inhibition. Vitamin E and beta-carotene are considered fat-soluble and function both in a lipid environment and as antioxidants. Vitamin C and selenium are considered water-soluble and work in a water-soluble environment, but are also considered to be antioxidants. Vitamins A and D and calcium are known to be essential for normal growth and differentiation of epithelial tissue.[19]

Calcium can reduce the proliferation of epithelial cells in the colon and rectum by the binding of fatty and bile acids, which results in the formation of insoluble bile salts. One study has shown that a daily calcium supplement in patients at high risk of colorectal cancer decreased the amount of colorectal epithelial cell production. It has also been noted that some colorectal cancer patients tend to have had a lower intake of calcium, and persons with an increased intake of vitamin D and calcium have a decreased risk of colon cancer.[20] Animal studies have suggested a preventive effect in colorectal cancer, but human studies have not been reliable.

As mentioned previously, vitamin C is considered an antioxidant and can protect the colorectal epithelial lining from carcinogenic damage. Even with this information, results from epidemiologic studies using vitamin C are conflicting, with some showing a colorectal cancer preventive benefit and others showing no benefit.

In women, there is noted to be an association between low serum levels of vitamin E and colorectal cancer. However, dietary supplementation of vitamin E has not shown a remarkable advantage.[21]

In a study looking at the impact of a daily supplement of selenium on basal cell or squamous cell skin cancers, it was noted that the participants receiving selenium had lower rates of colorectal cancer also. Other studies looking at selenium and cancer risk have had various outcomes.[22]

Dietary Carcinogens

Dietary carcinogens can suggest a possibly considerable source of increased cancer risk for the general population. The general population probably would credit the source of carcinogens in our food supply to food additives, synthetic pesticides, and an assortment of elements that have contaminated the natural environment. In reality, these sources are estimated to represent less than 1% of the carcinogens in our food. Most dietary carcinogens are made of "natural pesticides" (toxins produced by plants for protection against insects, fungi, and other predators), mycotoxins (secondary metabolites produced by mold in foods), and substances that are produced by food preparation.

Plant foods contain numerous phytochemicals, which are naturally occurring compounds that exhibit varied molecular structures and characterize a range of chemical classes. Many phytochemicals have been found to have cancer-inhibiting properties, but others may increase the risk of cancer. However, only a few of the possible carcinogens produced by plant foods have been tested. The cabbage plant contains 40 natural pesticides, but only a very few have been tested for their ability to be carcinogenic. It is complicated to estimate dietary exposure to natural pesticides, and research in this area has been difficult.

Mycotoxins might result because of contamination of crops, such as peanuts, cottonseed, corn, wheat, barley, and other cereals. This contamination is common and is influenced by temperature conditions, harvesting practices, insect infestation, and moisture levels in the field and in storage. Some mycotoxins are potent animal carcinogens and are presumed to contribute to human cancer risk. Assessing dietary exposure to mycotoxins has been a problem, and most epidemiologic studies to date have only shown an association between mycotoxins and liver or esophageal cancers.

The dietary carcinogens that are produced by food preparation and preservation are heterocyclic aromatic amines (HAAs), which are formed during frying, grilling, and charring high-protein foods; polycyclic aromatic hydrocarbons (PAHs), formed during broiling and smoking foods; and n-nitroso compounds (NOCs), formed in salted and pickled foods and in foods cured with nitrate or nitrite. As mentioned earlier, it is thought that carcinogens produced by cooking meat at high temperatures may be associated with colorectal cancer risk. To minimize this risk, it might be safer to select lower temperature cooking techniques when preparing meat.

Continuing research needs to be done to understand the complex interactions between all the dietary factors that might have an effect on the development of colorectal cancer. Although there is still some work to be done in proving that dietary change can prevent colorectal cancer, there remains a great deal of evidence that adopting a diet low in animal fat, high in whole grains, and rich in vegetables and fruit can improve one's overall health and reduce the risk of chronic disease, including several common cancers.[23]

Relationship of Lifestyle Factors and Colorectal Cancer Prevention

Physical Activity and Body Weight

A sedentary lifestyle has been associated with colorectal cancer risk. In addition, being very overweight also may increase a person's risk of colorectal cancer. An international study was done, looking at the incidence of persons of Chinese heritage in China and western North America. It was noted that men who were employed in more sedentary occupations in both continents had an elevated risk of colorectal cancer.[24]

It might also be that the association between colorectal cancer risk and saturated fat is stronger among those with a sedentary lifestyle, as opposed to those with a more active lifestyle. Men with a bigger body mass, which might be related to physical inactivity, had a greater incidence of colorectal cancer in a study that was done in Sweden.[25] The American Cancer Society has recommended getting at least 30 minutes of exercise on a regular basis, and achieving and maintaining a healthy weight. These healthful practices could be very beneficial in not only the prevention of colorectal cancer, but also many other diseases.

In the past several decades, Americans have been falling away from these healthy practices. Urbanization and the development of the technology boom have contributed to the sedentary lifestyle. Televisions, remote controls, portable phones, digital phones, computers, and computer games have contributed to a change in how Americans have spent their leisure time during the past 50 years. Americans are also intrigued with high-fat convenience foods, and the advertisement and promotion of these high-calorie foods has permeated almost every part of U.S. culture. Unhealthy eating, along with minimal physical activity, is having an impact on the rising numbers of diet-related illnesses, such as diabetes and coronary artery disease, and may impact the incidence of colorectal cancer in the future.

In the most recent survey of U.S. diet done by the Department of Agriculture, it was shown that two-thirds of adults in the United States believe that it is important to eat a diet filled with fruits and vegetables. However, there has actually been little increase in the consumption of fruits and vegetables in the past 30 years. There has been a 40% increase in the consumption of bread, cereal, rice, and pasta in the past

30 years, but less than one-third of U.S. adults believe that a diet that includes grain products is important. Although the amount of fat consumed in the U.S. diet has decreased from 40% in the late 1970s to 33% in the mid 1990s, only one-third of U.S. adults met the goal of 30% or less recommended by most nutritionists.[26]

It might be that by balancing energy expenditure with caloric intake, physical activity is able to help protect against colorectal cancer. Animal studies and epidemiologic studies have supported that an imbalance between caloric intake and output can lead to becoming overweight and obese, and increased colorectal cancer risk. Physical activity stimulates movement through the colon, which, in doing so, could reduce the length of time that the lining of the colon is exposed to possible carcinogens.

Alcohol Consumption

There might be an association of colorectal cancer with alcohol consumption. However, as with other risk factors, results have been mixed in the evidence provided by studies. It is thought that alcohol may act to stimulate the proliferation of the mucosal cells of the colon lining. It may also activate the possible carcinogens in the colon, as well as provide a source of unabsorbed carcinogens that are able to reach the distal large bowel. A French study, looking at the impact of diet and the adenoma–carcinoma sequence, found that alcohol could act at the promotional phase of the progression of an adenoma to carcinoma.[27]

Practical Application

It has been suggested that about one-third of the approximately 500,000 deaths that occur in the United States each year because of cancer could be related to cigarette smoking. Another third is due to dietary factors. Therefore, for the majority of Americans that do not smoke, the most modifiable cancer risks are dietary intake and physical activity. Although genetics is a factor in cancer development, it does not work alone. Lifestyle factors such as physical activity, cigarette smoking, and dietary choices can change the risk of cancer at all stages of its development.[28]

It is possible to lower the risk of developing colorectal cancer by managing the risk factors that can be controlled, such as diet and physical activity (Table 3.3). It has been shown that it is important to limit the intake of high-fat foods and to eat plenty of fruits, vegetables, and whole grain foods; and to get even small amounts of exercise on a regular basis has been shown to be helpful.[29]

Role of Clinical Trials in Colorectal Cancer Prevention

Cancer clinical trials are research studies to determine the value of cancer treatment or cancer prevention. The two key elements of research are that (1) conclusions are supported by results rather than plausible reasoning, and (2) the research is planned out and conducted under controlled conditions in order to provide conclusive answers to well-defined questions.

Clinical trials require very careful planning. The first result of the planning process is a written protocol, which is the blueprint of the study. The protocol needs to describe the treatment and evaluation process for a well-defined group of participants. It also needs to define the specific questions to be answered by the study and to directly justify that the numbers of participants and the nature of the controls will be adequate to answer these questions.

There are a series of orderly steps that are involved in the clinical research of a new drug or treatment. These steps, or phases, protect the

Table 3.3   Examples of Practical Prevention Strategies

Prevention Strategy	Examples
Try to eat more foods that are from plant sources.	Eat five or more servings of fruits and vegetables a day.
	Eat foods each day from other plant sources, such as grain products, cereals, bread, pasta, or legumes.
Try to control or reduce high-fat foods in your diet, especially those from animal sources.	Limit intake of meats, especially high-fat meats, such as red meats.
	Select foods low in fat. (Even if a food is labeled as low-fat, it may remain high in calories.)
Try to eliminate or control alcohol intake.	If drinking alcohol, avoid beer and strong spirits, as they may contain nitrosamines, which can be carcinogenic in the colon.
Try to be physically active on most days.	Thirty minutes of moderately active exercise each day is recommended.
	Examples of moderately active exercise are walking briskly for 30 minutes, gardening, yardwork, jogging, dancing, housework, or calisthenics.
Try to maintain a healthy weight.	Stay within recommended healthy weight ranges.
	Consume more healthy foods, such as fruits, grains, vegetables, and beans.
	Limit serving sizes, especially of high-fat foods.

Source: From Willett WC. Goals for nutrition in the year 2000. CA Cancer J Clin. 1999; 49:331–352.

participants and result in reliable information about the drug or treatment. Clinical trials are usually classified into one of three phases: *Phase I trials* look at the safety and toxicity profiles of a new drug or treatment, and usually only involve a small number of participants; *Phase II trials*, which usually focus on a specific cancer, continue to look at the safety of the drug or treatment, and begin to evaluate its efficacy; *Phase III trials*, which usually involve large numbers of participants, examine how a new drug or treatment, or a new combination of drugs or treatments, compare with the standard treatment.

Cancer treatment trials research new cancer treatment approaches, such as a new chemotherapy agent, a new combination or administration schedule of chemotherapy agents, new approaches to surgery or radiation therapy, or new methods of cancer treatment, like gene therapy.

In cancer prevention trials, new strategies are examined that researchers believe may lower the risk of cancer in specific populations. The research involves investigating the best methods to prevent cancer in people who have never had cancer or a recurrence in people who have already been diagnosed with cancer. Cancer prevention clinical trials generally involve two types that study the ways of reducing the risk of cancer. There are the *action* studies, which focus on exploring whether actions participants take, such as exercising more or changing their diet, can prevent cancer. The other type is *agent* studies, which examine whether taking certain medications, vitamins, or food supplements (or a combination) can prevent cancer (Table 3.4).

The Development of Cancer Chemoprevention Trials

In cancer chemoprevention trials, people are assigned by chance, often by a computer, to either receive the study agent (the *intervention* group) or not (the *control* group). This process is called *randomization*, and is used to prevent bias in the trial. The control group in a cancer chemoprevention trial will receive either an agent already proven to prevent the specific cancer, or a placebo (a sugar pill). The studies may be either a single-blind study, in which the participant is not told whether she/he is in the intervention group or the control group; or

double-blind study, in which neither the participant nor the participant's doctor knows which group the participant is in.

The participants in chemoprevention trials are usually selected for the study because they have a higher risk for a particular cancer than the general population. In order to be eligible to participate in the trial, they must meet certain criteria. The eligibility criteria generally include age, family cancer history, exposure to specific carcinogens, and other identified risk factors to the specific cancer being studied.

Other factors that need to be considered when developing a cancer chemoprevention trial include the total number of participants in the trial, the duration of the trial, and the endpoints of the trial. The endpoints of a cancer chemoprevention trial may include death, diagnosis of cancer, or reaching the target of an established biologic marker.

Table 3.4   Comparison of Cancer Treatment Trials and Cancer Prevention Trials

Cancer Treatment Trials	Cancer Prevention Trials
The *objective* is to decrease cancer morbidity/mortality and increase cancer remission/cure.	The *objective* is to decrease cancer incidence/mortality, prevent second cancer, and prevent or improve cancer risk markers.
Participants have a confirmed diagnosis of cancer.	*Participants* do not have cancer and could be from the general population, from a high-risk population, people with precancerous lesions, or disease-free cancer survivors.
The *study agent* has moderate to severe toxicity, which is acceptable.	The *study agent* has no to moderate toxicity, which is acceptable.
The *design* of the study protocol may be simple, therapy vs. placebo, therapy A vs. therapy B, or therapy A vs. therapy B vs. therapy C.	The *design* of the study protocol may be simple, intervention vs. placebo, intervention A vs. intervention B vs. intervention AB vs. placebo, or multiple simultaneous interventions.
It usually *involves* a small number of participants (hundreds).	It usually *involves* a large number of participants (thousands).
Length of study may be short for aggressive cancers and longer for adjuvant or slower growing cancers.	*Length* of study may require up to 5 to 10 years (or more) of intervention and then follow-up.
Participants' compliance is easier to maintain because it is physician-dependent.	*Participants' compliance* may be difficult to maintain because it is participant-dependent.

Recruitment to and Enrollment in Cancer Chemoprevention Trials

Recruitment to cancer chemoprevention trials requires much cost, time, and effort. It is simple to find people at general population risk, but more complicated to find people at high risk for a certain cancer. To further complicate recruitment, of all the eligible individuals for a chemoprevention study, approximately only 10% to 25% will decide to enroll in the study.

Study participants for cancer chemoprevention trials come from a variety of sources. These may be referrals from physicians who provide care for the specific patient population, screening clinics, high-risk assessment clinics, or approved public advertisement. Because of patient confidentiality protections, study personnel must be careful in using tumor registries or pathology databases in recruitment efforts.

Some of the barriers to chemoprevention trial recruitment could be the study's eligibility/ineligibility criteria, learning the potential side effects of the study agent, and the possibility of being assigned to the placebo arm. Additionally, if the study involves an easily accessible agent, such as an over-the-counter vitamin or mineral, the participant might elect not to join the study, but instead follow the prescribed therapy on his or her own.

Once written, informed consent has been obtained from participants, they are enrolled in the chemoprevention trial; they are randomly assigned to either the intervention group or the control group. Once this has occurred, study personnel are responsible for protecting the safety of the participant. This includes the early identification of toxicities and the careful observation of the prescribed follow-up monitoring.

Adherence to the assigned therapy is also crucial to the success of the chemoprevention trial. Most chemoprevention trials last several years (5–10), and, if at all possible, will also include a long-term follow-up after completion of the intervention. Participants in chemoprevention trials that deal with a lifestyle change, such as eating a certain diet, may have more difficulties than participants in a chemoprevention trial that involves a study agent. To promote compliance, study personnel need to develop a relationship with each participant that promotes honesty and trust. They also need to be cognizant of the continually developing media and scientific information in the area of cancer prevention, and be aware of alternative therapies, as well as the latest health fads.[30]

Colorectal Cancer Prevention Trials

Clinical trials looking at colorectal cancer prevention have generally been divided into two categories: (1) chemoprevention and (2) diet and nutrition. Currently, there is a colorectal cancer prevention trial looking at the use of celecoxib for the prevention of new colorectal adenomas in persons who have previously had a colon polyp removed. There is also a study looking at the effect of high-dose folic acid for persons who have had a colon polyp removed, compared with a control group with no intervention; and a trial looking at the effect of three plant compounds versus sulindac on the colonic mucosa. The three plant compounds are circumin (the main ingredient in the spice, turmeric), rutin (which is obtained from leaves of the buckwheat plant), and quercetin (which can be found in onions, apples, green tea, and black tea, and is sometimes referred to as a phytoestrogen).[31]

Through past colorectal prevention clinical trials, we have learned about the impact of dietary fat and fiber on the development of colorectal cancer. We know that routinely taking an aspirin or an NSAID has decreased the further development of adenomas that can progress to carcinomas. It has been shown that physical activity and body weight might be associated with colorectal cancer risk. Much of our current information about colorectal cancer prevention is derived from the many individuals who generously agreed to participate in a clinical trial in order to further our knowledge of cancer and to have an impact on cancer incidence in future generations.

Prevention for High-Risk Individuals

There are several risk factors that researchers have discovered that increase a person's chance of developing colorectal cancer (Table 3.5). These include family history of colorectal cancer, personal history of colorectal cancer, personal history of intestinal polyps, personal history of inflammatory bowel disease, familial or hereditary colorectal cancer syndromes, aging, diet and obesity, and physical inactivity. Management of lifestyle factors has been discussed previously.

Individuals with a first-degree relative with colorectal cancer have approximately twice the risk of the general population of developing adenomatous polyps. Some physicians recommend that all individuals with colorectal cancer have an evaluation of their family cancer history. Persons with a family history suggesting a colorectal cancer syndrome might want to consider genetic counseling and genetic testing.

Individuals with a first-degree relative with colorectal cancer diagnosed younger than age 60, or individuals with two or more first-degree relatives diagnosed at any age should begin their colorectal cancer screening early. They should start having a total colon examination (TCE) by colonoscopy or double contrast barium enema by age 40, or 10 years before the youngest relative was diagnosed. The TCE should be repeated at least every 5 years.

Individuals with a personal history of colorectal cancer, who have had a colon resection with the intent of cure, should have a TCE within 1 year of resection. If examination is normal, then a TCE should be repeated within 3 years. If it is still normal within 3 years, the TCE can be repeated in 5 years.

People who have a history of adenomatous polyps need to have further colorectal cancer screening based on the size and number of polyps found at initial diagnosis. If they had a single polyp and it was less than 1 cm in size, they will need to have a TCE within 3 years of initial polyp removal. If that examination is normal, they can begin general population colorectal screening guidelines. If the individuals had an initial polyp greater than 1 cm, or they had multiple polyps of any size, they will need to have a TCE within 3 years of initial polyp removal. If that examination is normal, they will need to have a TCE repeated every 5 years.

In persons with ulcerative colitis, the risk of developing colorectal cancer is five to ten times higher than in the general population. Individuals with inflammatory bowel disease should begin colorectal screening at least 8 years after their entire colon is affected, and 12 to 15 years after the start of left-sided colitis. They will need to have colonoscopies with biopsies every 1 to 2 years.

In families with a known history of FAP, it is suggested that screening and surveillance begin at an early age. Once the family member has reached puberty, he or she will need to begin screening with endoscopy every 1 to 2 years. If appropriate, the family member could be referred to a genetic counselor to consider genetic testing. If he or she were to test positive, the option of colectomy could be presented.[32]

A new option for individuals with FAP is chemoprevention using specific or nonspecific COX-2 inhibitors, such as celecoxib or sulindac, respectively. The FDA has approved celecoxib for polyp prevention in FAP, based on evidence from a clinical trial. Celecoxib re-

Table 3.5 Moderate- to High-Risk Factors for Colorectal Cancer

Risk Factor	Explanation
Family history of colorectal cancer	Colorectal cancer seems to run in some families. For example, there is an inherited tendency to develop colorectal cancer among some Jews of Eastern European descent.
Personal history of colorectal cancer	Although a colorectal cancer has been completely removed, new cancers may develop in other areas of the colon and rectum.
Personal history of intestinal polyps	Some types of intestinal polyps do not seem to increase the risk of colorectal cancer. Other types, such as adenomatous polyps, do increase the risk of colorectal cancer, especially if they are large or there are many of them.
Personal history of inflammatory bowel disease (ulcerative colitis or Crohn's colitis)	With these conditions, the colon is inflamed over a long period of time and may have ulcers in its lining. This increases the risk of colon cancer.
Familial (or hereditary) colorectal cancer syndrome	The following conditions make it more likely that a family could develop cancer:
	Familial adenomatous polyposis (FAP) and its variants: Individuals that have inherited FAP typically develop hundreds of polyps in the colon and rectum. If preventive surgery is not done, cancer nearly always develops in one or more of these polyps when the person is between the ages of 30 and 50. Some variants of FAP can also cause benign tumors of the skin, soft connective tissue, and bones.
	Hereditary nonpolyposis colon cancer (HNPCC) and its variants: Individuals that inherit HNPCC can develop colorectal cancer at a young age without first having had many polyps. Females who inherit HNPCC also have an increased risk of developing endometrial cancer.
Age	About 9 out of 10 individuals who develop colorectal cancer are over age 50.

Source: From Risk factors for colorectal cancer. Available at: http://www3.cancer.org Accessed November 12, 2000.

duced the number of polyps in patients with FAP by 20%; however, it is not known whether this will translate into reductions in colorectal cancer incidence or mortality, or improvements in quality of life. At the present time, it is not clear how to incorporate COX-2 inhibitors into the management of persons with FAP.[33,34]

Families with a known history of hereditary

nonpolyposis colon cancer (HNPCC) also need to begin screening and surveillance early. Once the family member has reached age 21, he or she needs to begin having colonoscopies every 2 years. Genetic counseling and testing could also be considered for this family member, if appropriate. If the genetic test is positive, this person will need to continue the screening colonoscopies every 2 years until the age of 40, and then have an annual colonoscopy. Because many of the HNPCCs occur on the right side of the colon, using sigmoidoscopy as a screening test is not effective. It is also critical to maintain the frequency of the screening, as the progression from adenoma to carcinoma can be rapid.

Women of HNPCC families should also be instructed on endometrial cancer screening. Endometrial cancer is the second most common cancer in HNPCC families. Women of HNPCC families need to report any abnormal or postmenopausal bleeding. Although routine screening for endometrial cancer has not been shown to be effective in the general population, it has been recommended that it be considered for women who are members of HNPCC families. It has been suggested that they have transvaginal ultrasound or endometrial biopsy annually, starting between the ages of 25 and 35 years.[35]

Little is known about the effects of NSAIDs on the development of polyps in families with HNPCC. There is currently a clinical trial looking at the effect of the COX-2 inhibitor, celecoxib, in individuals that are known carriers of HNPCC, and if it should prove to be significant, there will, no doubt, be more to follow.

There is not much information on whether lifestyle factors, such as diet and physical activity, are protective in people who are known to have an hereditary colon cancer syndrome. In one study, physical activity and low-fiber intake were significantly related to cancer risk in people with no family history of colorectal cancer, but no relationship was shown in people with a family history.[36]

Summary

As we progress into the twenty-first century and its many anticipated medical advancements, it is very likely that the field of oncology will move from its treatment-oriented model to a prevention-oriented model. There will be more value placed on intervening before the beginning or promotion of carcinogenesis, rather than later, when the process cannot be halted or slowed down.

Nurses, and especially oncology nurses, will be able to continue to play a vital role in colorectal cancer prevention. They will still be able to identify individuals at high risk and perform the valuable service of patient education about cancer prevention. There will also be the opportunity to do effective cancer risk assessment and prevention counseling, and the chance to promote the available cancer prevention clinical trials.

Oncology nurses will need to be prepared with a beneficial foundation of the process of cancer prevention. By being actively involved and knowledgeable about the rapidly changing field of cancer prevention, oncology nurses will have the opportunity to influence the interventions and outcomes of cancer prevention now and in the years to come. Another French philosopher, and one of the most important writers of the twentieth century, wrote about the impact of our current efforts on future generations.

"Real generosity towards the future lies in giving all to the present."
—Albert Camus (1913–1960), 1951

References

1. Seffrin JR. An endgame for cancer. CA Cancer J Clin. 2000; 50:4–5.
2. Loescher LJ. Dynamics of cancer prevention. In: Groenwald SL, Frogge MH, Goodman M, Yarbro C, eds. Cancer Nursing: Principles and

Practice. Sudbury, MA: Jones and Bartlett, 1997: 95.

3. Mayne ST, Lippman SM. Cancer prevention: Chemopreventive agents. In: DeVita VT Jr, Frogge MH, Goodman M, Yarbro C, eds. Cancer: Principles & Practice of Oncology. Philadelphia, PA: Lippincott-Raven, 1997: 585.

4. Loescher LJ. Dynamics of cancer prevention. In: Groenwald SL, Frogge MH, Goodman M, Yarbro C, eds. Cancer Nursing: Principles and Practice. Sudbury, MA: Jones and Bartlett, 1997: 98.

5. Bostick RM, Potter JD, McKenzie DR, et al. Reduced risk of colon cancer with high intake of vitamin E: The Iowa Women's Health Study. Cancer Res. 1993; 53:4230–4237.

6. Giovanucci E, Stampfer MJ, Colditz GA, et al. Multivitamin use, folate, and colon cancer in women in the Nurses' Health Study. Ann Intern Med. 1998; 129:517–524.

7. Ahnen DJ. Primary preventive measures for colorectal cancer. Presented at Ninth Annual Oncology Update for Primary Care, Omaha, NE, September 15, 2000.

8. Lee IM, Hennekens CH, Buring JE. Cancer prevention: Use of aspirin and other nonsteroidal antiinflammatory drugs and the risk of cancer development. In: DeVita VT Jr, Rosenberg SA, Hellman S, eds. Cancer: Principles & Practice of Oncology. Philadelphia, PA: Lippincott-Raven, 1997: 599.

9. Ahnen DJ. Primary preventive measures for colorectal cancer. Presented at Ninth Annual Oncology Update for Primary Care, Omaha, NE, September 15, 2000.

10. Steinbach G, Lynch PM, Phillips RK, et al. The effect of celecoxib, a cyclooxygenase-2 inhibitor, in familial adenomatous polyposis. N Engl J Med. 2000; 342:1946–1952.

11. Willett WC. Cancer prevention: Diet and risk reduction. In: DeVita VT Jr, Rosenberg SA, Hellman S, eds. Cancer: Principles & Practice of Oncology. Philadelphia, PA: Lippincott-Raven, 1997: 559.

12. Reddy BS, Engle A, Simi B, et al. Effect of dietary fiber on colonic bacterial enzymes and bile acids in relation to colon cancer. Gastroenterology. 1992; 102:1475–1482.

13. Morotomi M, Guillem JG, LoGerfo P, et al. Production of diacylglycerol, an activator of protein kinase C, by human intestinal microflora. Cancer Res. 1990; 50:3595–3599.

14. Cohen AM, Minsky BD, Schilsky RL. Cancer of the colon. In: DeVita VT Jr, Rosenberg SA, Hellman S, eds. Cancer: Principles & Practice of Oncology. Philadelphia, PA: Lippincott-Raven, 1997: 1146.

15. Greenwald P. Cancer prevention: Dietary fiber. In: DeVita VT Jr, Rosenberg SA, Hellman S, eds. Cancer: Principles & Practice of Oncology. Philadelphia, PA: Lippincott-Raven, 1997: 569.

16. Howe GR, Bentino E, Castelleto R, et al. Dietary intake of fiber and decreased risk of cancers of the colon and rectum: Evidence from the combined analysis of 13 case-control studies. J Natl Cancer Inst. 1992; 84:1887–1896.

17. Schatzkin A, Lanza E, Corle D, et al. Lack of effect of a low-fat, high-fiber diet on the recurrence of colorectal adenomas. Polyp prevention trial study. N Engl J Med. 2000; 342: 1149–1155.

18. Alberts DS, Martinez ME, Roe DJ, et al. Lack of effect of a high-fiber cereal supplement on the recurrence of colorectal adenomas. N Engl J Med. 2000; 342:1156–1162.

19. Meyskens FL. Cancer prevention: Micronutrients. In: DeVita VT Jr, Rosenberg SA, Hellman S, eds. Cancer: Principles & Practice of Oncology. Philadelphia, PA: Lippincott-Raven, 1997: 573–576.

20. Bostick RM, Potter JD, Fosdick L, et al. Calcium and colorectal epithelial cell proliferation: A preliminary randomized, double-blinded, placebo-controlled clinical trial. J Natl Cancer Inst. 1993; 85:132–141.

21. Cohen AM, Minsky BD, Schilsky RL. Cancer of the colon. In: DeVita VT Jr, Rosenberg SA, Hellman S, eds. Cancer: Principles & Practice of Oncology. Philadelphia, PA: Lippincott-Raven, 1997: 1147.

22. Clark LC, Combs GF Jr, Turnbull BW, et al. Effects of selenium supplementation for cancer prevention in patients with carcinoma of the skin. JAMA. 1997; 276:1957–1963.

23. Greenwald P. Cancer prevention: Dietary carcinogens. In: DeVita VT Jr, Rosenberg SA, Hellman S, eds. Cancer: Principles & Practice of Oncology. Philadelphia, PA: Lippincott-Raven, 1997: 579–583.

24. Whittemore AS, Wu-Williams AH, Lee M, et al. Diet, physical activity, and colorectal cancer among Chinese in North America and China. J Natl Cancer Inst. 1990; 882:915–926.

25. Gerhardsson de Verdier M, Hagman U, Steineck G, et al. Diet, body mass and colorectal cancer: A case-referent study in Stockholm. Int J Cancer. 1990; 46:832–838.

26. Cancer Prevention & Early Detection Facts & Figures 2000. American Cancer Society Publication No. 8600.00-R. Atlanta, GA: American Cancer Society, 2000: 12–13.

27. Boutron MC, Faivre J. Diet and the adenoma–carcinoma sequence. Eur J Cancer Prev. 1998; 2:95–98.

28. McGinnis JM, Foege WH. Actual causes of death in the United States. JAMA. 1993; 270: 2207–2212.

29. US Department of Health and Human Services. Healthy People 2000: National Health. Promotion and Disease Prevention Objectives. DHHS (PHS) Publication No. 91-50212. Washington, DC: Government Printing Office, 1990.

30. Loescher LJ. Dynamics of cancer prevention. In: Groenwald SL, Frogge MH, Goodman M, Yarbro C, eds. Cancer Nursing: Principles and Practice. Sudbury, MA: Jones and Bartlett, 1997: 101–105.

31. Open colon cancer prevention trials. Available at: http://cancertrials.nci.nih.gov Accessed November 11, 2000.

32. Byers T, Levin B, Rothenberger D, et al. American Cancer Society guidelines for screening and surveillance for early detection of colorectal polyps and cancer: Update 1991. CA Cancer J Clin. 1997; 47:154–160.

33. Giardiello FM, Hamilton SR, Krush AJ, et al. Treatment of colonic and rectal adenomas with sulindac in familial adenomatous polyposis. N Engl J Med. 1993; 328:1313–1316.

34. Steinbach G, Lynch PM, Phillips RK, et al. The effect of celecoxib, a cyclooxygenase-2 inhibitor, in familial adenomatous polyposis. N Engl J Med. 2000; 342:1946–1952.

35. Burke W, Petersen G, Lynch P, et al. Recommendations for follow-up care of individuals with an inherited predisposition to cancer. I. Hereditary nonpolyposis colon cancer. Cancer Genetics Studies Consortium. JAMA. 1997; 277:915–919.

36. La Vecchia C, Gallus S, Talamini R, et al. Interaction between selected environmental factors and familial propensity for colon cancer. Eur J Cancer Prev. 1999; 8:147–150.

37. Willett WC. Goals for nutrition in the year 2000. CA Cancer J Clin. 1999; 49:331–352.

38. Risk factors for colorectal cancer. Available at: http://www3.cancer.org Accessed November 12, 2000.

CHAPTER 4

Cellular Characteristics, Pathophysiology, and Disease Manifestations of Colorectal Cancer

Joyce P. Griffin-Sobel, RN, PhD, AOCN, CS

Introduction

Twenty years ago, cancer research changed dramatically with the identification of cellular oncogenes and the recognition that cancer is a genetic disease. This shifted research from carcinogens to oncogenes and tumor-suppressor genes, genes that regulate cell division, differentiation, and development. This chapter discusses some of the genetic risk factors in colorectal carcinogenesis and tumor biology, pathophysiology of progression and metastases, and disease manifestations.

Genetic Causes of Tumorigenesis

There is an intricate system for maintaining a delicate balance between cell proliferation and cell death. Cell division, proliferation, and differentiation are strictly regulated under normal conditions. When a need arises in an organ or tissue for new cells, as in repair of damage, previously nondividing cells, resting cells, are rapidly triggered to reenter the division cycle. Resting cells must be turned on for division and proliferation, and turned off after proliferation is completed. Cellular control mechanisms that regulate cell birth and death require social control genes.[1,2]

Growth Factors

Different combinations of protein growth factors, an example of which is interleukin-2 (IL-2), regulate proliferation. Growth factors are highly specific proteins that stimulate cell growth and differentiation. They must interact with highly specific receptors, resulting in transmission of a signal to a cell nucleus, where genes are turned on or off.[1,2]

Overproduction of several growth factors has been implicated in cancer development. Any disruption in the balance between cell proliferation and cell death can result in tumor formation. Virtually every cell in the body has the potential to form tumors. Cancer is an accumulation of mutations that result from multiple events acting together and occurring through many series of pathways.[1] Tumors originate from a cell proliferating abnormally when various genetic changes accumulate. Genetic alterations can be a spontaneous error occurring during the cell cycle, infections, or environmental causes, which can lead to chromosomal damage.[3]

Oncogenes

Oncogenes, which are the excessively active versions of normal cellular genes called protooncogenes, are the genes that encode proteins whose action positively promotes cell proliferation (Figure 4.1). Oncogenes can be overexpressed through amplification, in which the number of copies of a gene increases. As tumor cells progress, they gain the ability to amplify genes as they lose cell cycle control. HER/2Neu often has amplified gene sequences, which may be related to tumor progression. Large numbers of components provide many targets for oncogene activation. Cancers result from aberrant activation of multiple oncogenes. K-RAS oncogenes are found mutated in cancers of the colon, lung, and 90% of pancreas.[1]

Tumor-Suppressor Genes

Tumor-suppressor genes are those that normally suppress or negatively regulate cell proliferation. They typically suppress oncogenes. Examples of tumor suppressor genes include *p53, APC*, the adenomatous polyposis

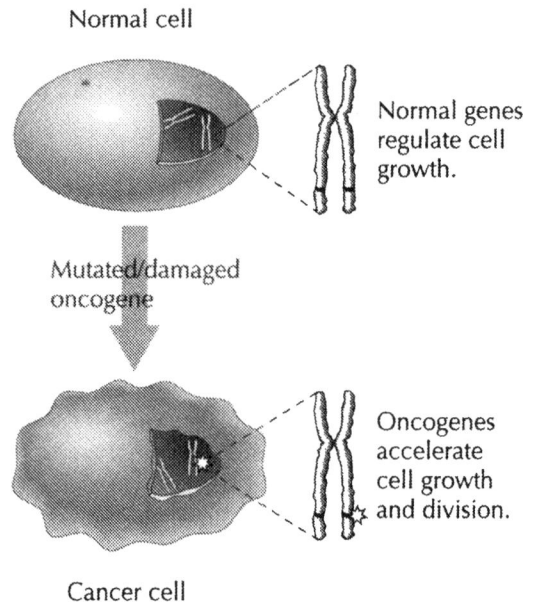

Figure 4.1   Normal genes and oncogenes.

coli gene, and *DCC*, deleted in the colon cancer gene. It is only when multiple oncogenes are aberrantly activated and tumor-suppressor genes are lost or mutated that a malignancy forms.[3]

The *p53* tumor-suppressor gene is the most commonly mutated gene in human cancers, with at least 50% of tumors having abnormal *p53* genes. Loss of *p53* function during tumorigenesis can result in both inappropriate progression through the cell cycle after DNA damage and survival of a cell that might otherwise have been destined to die. Therefore, this causes increased genetic instability and decreased apoptosis, or programmed cell death, contributing to malignant transformation. Some tumors also develop other mechanisms of inactivating *p53*. It is inactivated in 75% of colorectal cases.[1,3]

Genetic Alterations

Multiple genetic alterations have been well characterized in colorectal cancer, including expression of oncogenes *ras, myc, src*; inactivation or deletion of tumor suppressor genes *DCC, p53*, and *APC*; and deletions from chromosomes 1 and 22. One probable schema is the following (Figure 4.2): Loss of the *APC* gene, the earliest identified event in the development of colon cancer and usually the initiating factor, leads to transformation of normal epithelial tissue lining the gut to hyperproliferative tissue, which leads to activation of the *Kras* oncogene and loss of *DCC*, leading to a benign adenoma and loss of the *p53* gene, leading to malignancy.[1–3]

Colorectal cancer usually starts as a benign polyp that progresses to malignancy in about 10 years, the window of opportunity for early detection. The normal colonic mucosa begins to hyperproliferate and an adenoma forms, which gradually becomes more dysplastic and becomes a carcinoma in situ, and on to an invasive cancer.[3]

Cellular Mechanisms in Carcinogenesis

Cancer cells often have a number of phenotypic abnormalities, including loss of differentiation, increased invasiveness, and decreased drug sensitivity. Dysregulation of cell cycle control is found in almost all cancer cells. Usually, there is a lack of normal control responses to the signals that cause the cell to stop growing. The transformation of a normal cell to a tumor cell appears to depend on mutations in genes that normally control cell cycle progression, thus leading to loss of these regulatory cell growth signals. Growth abnormalities of tumor cells result from both too little of the tumor-suppressor action and too much of the oncogene-accelerator action. Also, malignant cells can develop and increase their numbers through defects in apoptosis, or programmed cell death. Apoptosis normally occurs in re-

sponse to some stimuli, such as irradiation, chemotherapy, and viral infection. Loss of apoptosis signals may be a critical mutational event in tumorigenesis.[1,3]

Tumor Metastasis

Metastasis is a complex process. It requires a number of essential steps, including progressive proliferation of neoplastic cells; angiogenesis, the development of a vasculature; penetration of normal vessels; and evasion of host defenses (Figure 4.3 on page 57).

Growth and survival of cells are dependent on an adequate supply of growth factors and removal of toxins. For a tumor to grow, an adequate blood supply must develop. Any expansion of a tumor beyond 2 mm in diameter requires development of a blood supply. This is the process of angiogenesis. Tumor cells release factors that induce an angiogenic response (i.e., angiogenic factors). This is called the *angiogenic switch*. Various substances are released by both tumor and host cells that initiate angiogenesis, including vascular endothelial growth factor (VEGF), epidermal growth factor (EGF), and interleukin-8 (IL-8). Tumor cells produce positive angiogenic factors such as VEGF, which promotes growth and chemotaxis of endothelial cells and which is overexpressed in many tumors. Negative regulators of angiogenesis are just as important and include tumor growth factor beta-1 (TGF-B1), alfa-interferon, and angiostatin. TGF-B1 inhibits the proteolysis necessary for formation of sprouts emanating from parent vessels. Angiostatin, a fragment of the plasminogen molecule, generally prevents proliferation of endothelial cells. A balance between accelerant and inhibitory factors determines the extent of angiogenesis, and *p53* and *ras* oncogenes are believed to play a role. The density and rapidity of angiogenesis is thought to be a prognostic indicator, as malignancies are highly vascular, fast growing, and

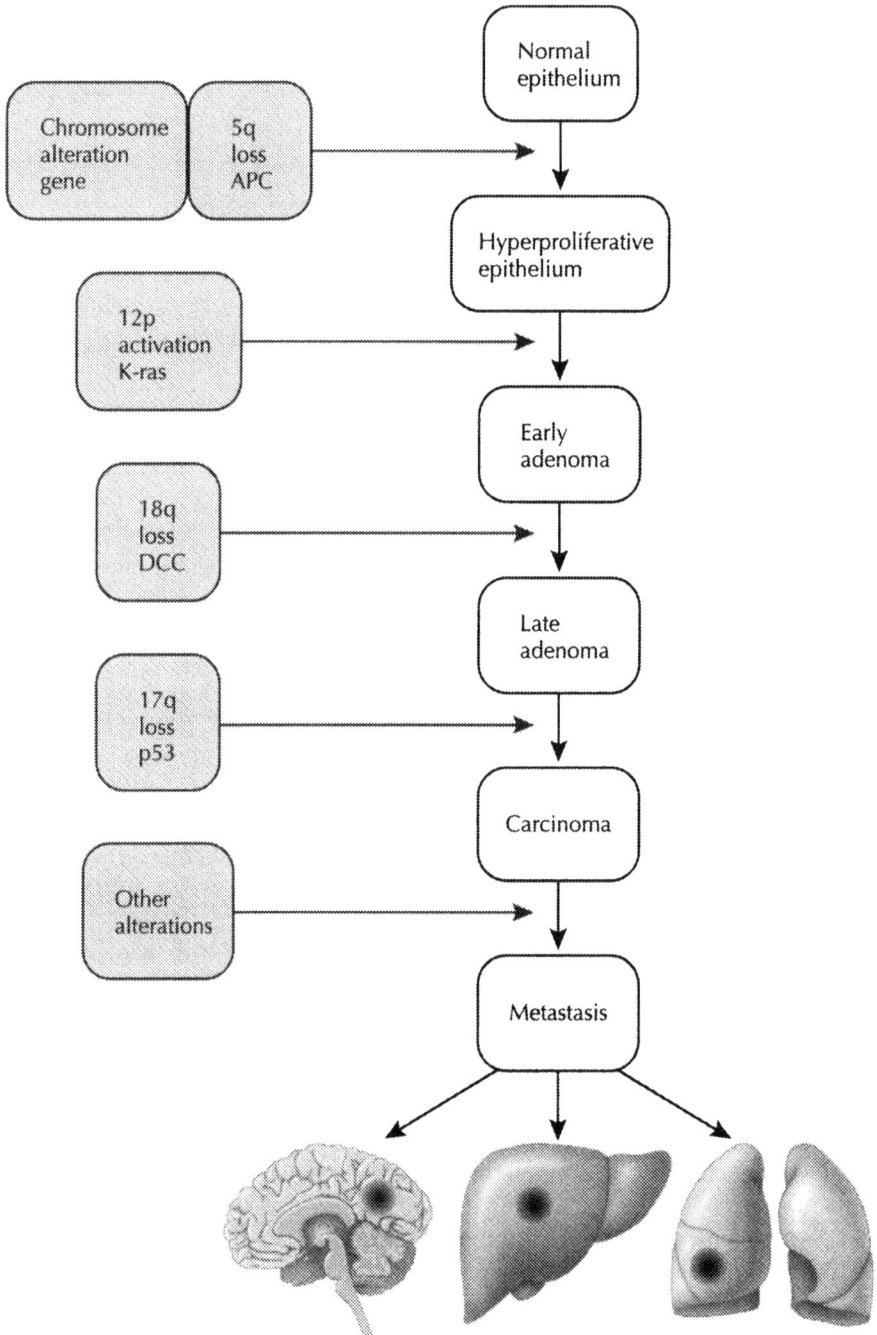

Figure 4.2   A conceptual genetic model for the development of colorectal cancer, illustrating multistep carcinogenesis.

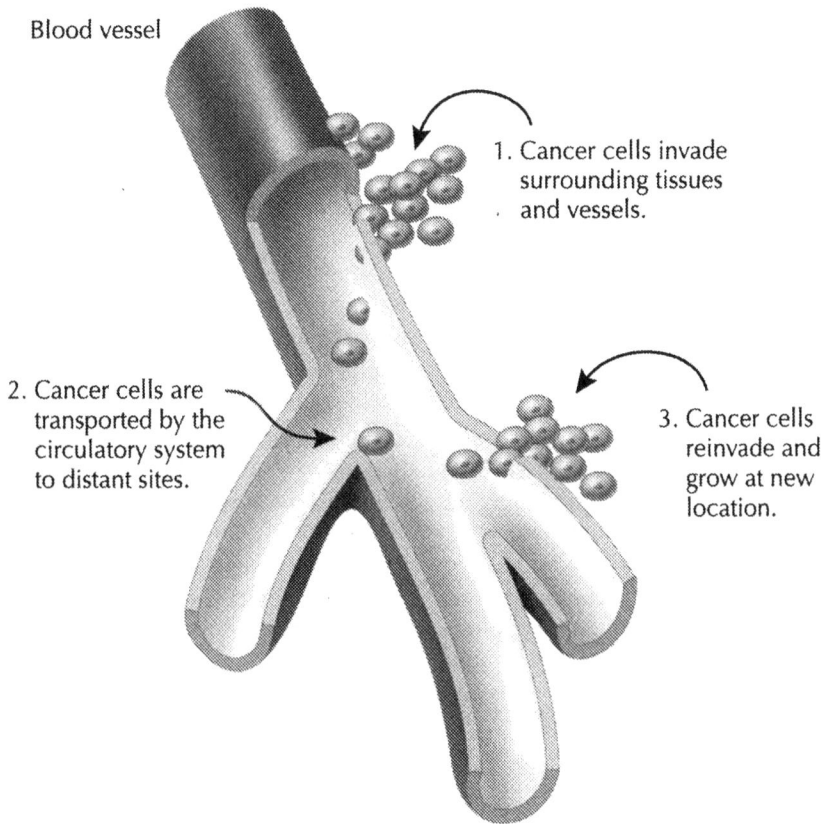

Figure 4.3 Routes of metastasis.
Photo Source: From the National Cancer Institute.

more likely to metastasize. This process is being widely studied for its therapeutic potential (Table 4.1).[1,2]

In order to invade organs, tumor cells must be motile and be able to penetrate basement membranes and the connective tissue extracellular matrix of surrounding blood vessels. Many metastatic tumor cells can produce matrix-degrading enzymes, such as gelatinase and heparinase, which is well correlated with metastatic potential.[1] Cancer cells can invade lymphatics directly or through blood vessels. Lodging of tumor cell emboli in lymph vessels is responsible for lymphatic metastasis. Cells entering the

Table 4.1   Angiogenesis

Angiogenesis Growth Factors	Angiogenesis Inhibitors
VEGF	Angiostatin
EGF	Endostatin
IL-8	VEGF inhibitor
Granulocyte colony-stimulating factor	Platelet factor 4
Tumor necrosis factor-alfa	Interferon-alfa

Source: Adapted from DeVita V, Hellman S, Rosenberg S. Cancer: Principles and Practices of Oncology, 6th ed. Philadelphia, PA: Lippincott-Raven, 2001, 139–141.

circulation are rapidly destroyed by immune surveillance unless they form aggregates. To establish metastases, tumor cells must escape host defenses and lodge in the vasculature. The formation of a fibrin–platelet complex protects tumors cells from destruction and assists in successful attachment to the vascular epithelium.[2] The link between thrombus formation and tumors is well documented. Fibrin deposits and platelet aggregation may protect tumors from host immunity. The increased coagulability seen in cancer patients may be related to high levels of thromboplastin and the production of procoagulants by some tumors.[1,2]

After tumor cells penetrate the vessel wall, they proliferate, often with stimulation by growth factors. Metastasis is successful when cells succeed in angiogenesis, invasion, survival in the circulation, and extravasation into and proliferation in organs (Figure 4.4). Metastatic cells can successfully evade host immune surveillance mechanisms when the host immunity is suppressed.

Colorectal Cancer: Staging and Clinical Manifestations

The colon is made of four layers: the mucosa, the submucosa, the muscularis, and the serosa (Figure 4.5 on page 60). The mucosal and submucosal layers are divided by the muscularis.

Reproduction of cells in the colon takes place in the crypts of Lieberkuhn in the mucosal layer. As new cells are produced, old cells mature, migrate out of the crypt, and shed. Damage to the crypts will affect reproducing cells, and the crypts become prone to errors and to the formation of early adenomas.

Colorectal polyps are closely associated with the development of cancer. A polyp, or papilloma, is a finger-like projection arising from mucosal epithelium. Most are benign. The two major types of neoplastic polyps are pedunculated (stalk) adenomatous polyps and sessile (papillary or villous) adenomas (Figure 4.6 on page 61). Once the adenoma traverses the muscularis, it becomes invasive and malignant. Adenomas can be detected early, and the submucosa may not be penetrated for several years. The larger the polyp, the greater the risk of colon cancer.[1,2]

The large intestine includes the cecum, ascending colon, transverse colon, descending colon, sigmoid colon, and rectum (Figures 4.7 and 4.8 on pages 62 and 63). The liver is the most frequent site of metastatic involvement, due to the anatomy of the portal vein system.[4] Metastases reach the liver by portal vein circulation, lymphatic spread, hepatic arterial circulation, and direct invasion.[1,5] Solitary pulmonary metastases are rare. Other areas of metastases include the brain, bones, kidneys, and adrenals. Rectal cancer is more likely to pro-

Figure 4.4 The metastatic cascade. The multistep cascade begins when genetic events facilitate primary tumor formation. Angiogenesis (vascularization) increases proliferation of the growing tumor. Preceding invasion, there is a decrease in cell–cell contact and adherence to and invasion of the endothelial basement membrane. Once tumor cells have entered the lymphatic system or circulation, they are transported to distant sites. If the tumor cells are successful at evading the immune system, they eventually will arrest in a capillary bed of a distant organ. Establishment of a secondary site will follow once the tumor cells invade the endothelial barrier to gain entrance to the underlying organ tissue bed.

Source: Gribbon J, Loescher LJ. Biology of cancer. In: Yarbro CH, Frogge MH, Goodman M. et al. Cancer Nursing Principles and Practice. 5th ed. Sudbury: Jones and Bartlett, 2000, 31. With permission.

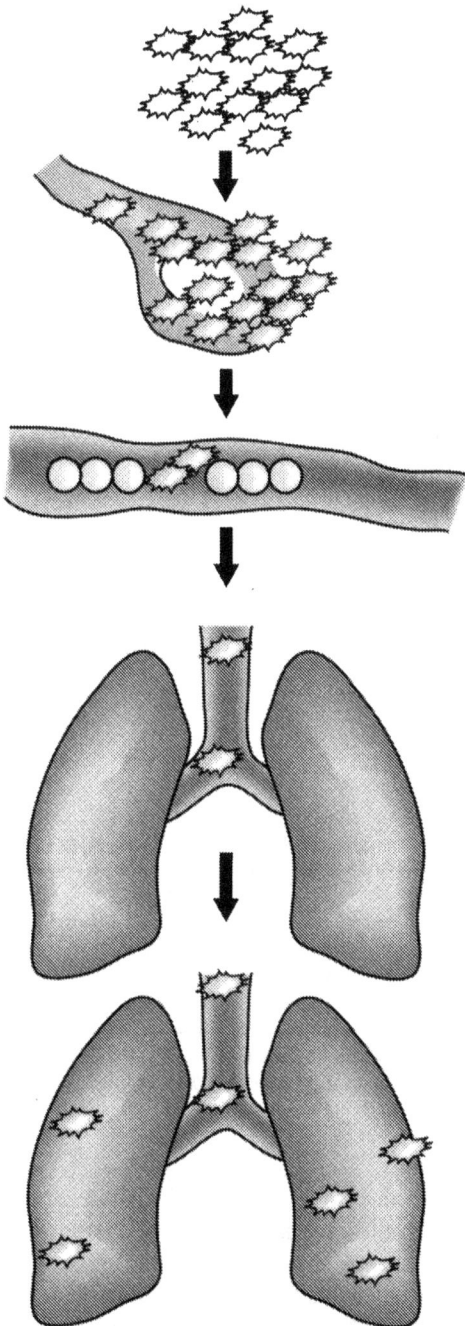

Primary Tumor Forms
• Genetic mutations

Angiogenesis and Invasion
• Decreased cell–cell adhesion
• Detachment from primary tumor and one another
• Adherence to and invasion of basement membrane and endothelial layer
• Invasion of lymphatics

Survival in Circulation
• Transport to distant organs
• Evasion of the immune system

Tumor Cells Arrest in Capillary Bed of Organ
• Adherence to endothelial layer

Establishment of Secondary Tumor
• Invasion of endothelial layer and basement membrane
• Proliferation
• Angiogenesis

| Extent of tumor | No deeper than submucosa | Not through bowel wall | Through bowel wall | Not through bowel wall: lymph node metastases | Through bowel wall: lymph node metastases | Distant metastases |

Mucosa

Muscularis mucosa

Submucosa

Muscularis propria

Serosa

Fat

Lymph nodes

Lung

Liver

Bone

Skin

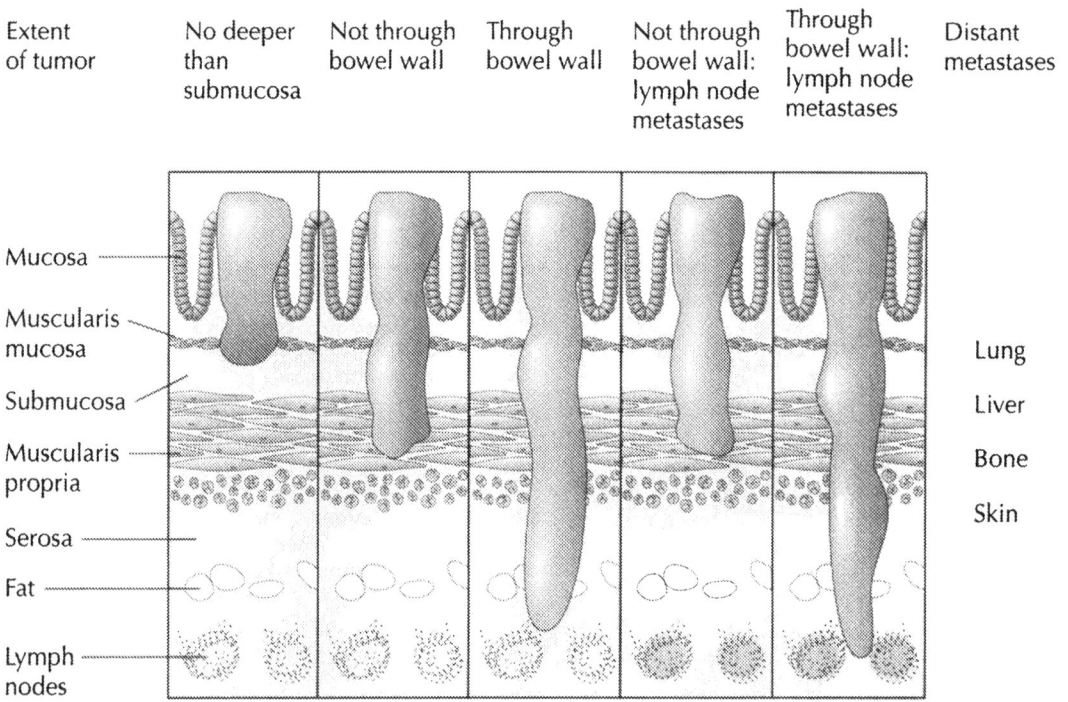

Figure 4.5 Layers of the colon noting tumor penetration.

duce pulmonary metastases because the inferior vena cava is the primary drainage area. Intraperitoneal seeding and carcinomatosis may occur even without lymphatic or visceral spread because of preferential mural growth, or spread through the perineural spaces instead of the circumferential growth seen more commonly in colon cancer.[1]

The most common type of colorectal cancer is adenocarcinoma. More infrequent are carcinoids, lymphomas, sarcomas, and melanomas. There has been a shift from distal to proximal sites of colon cancer (Table 4.2), perhaps due to improved diagnostic techniques and preventive strategies.[1]

Lesions may exhibit different characteristics. Tumors in the ascending colon present as cauliflower-like fungating masses that progress to become ulcerative and necrotic. These are usually well differentiated and have a better prognosis. Tumors in the descending and sigmoid colon present as ulcerative tumors that tend to infiltrate the bowel wall and have a poorer prognosis. Rectosigmoid tumors present as villous, frondlike lesions.[1,6]

Table 4.2 Sites of Colorectal Cancer Incidence

	1986	1992
Cecal/ascending colon	33.9	36.1
Transverse colon	15.8	17.2
Sigmoid colon	36	33.4

Source: Adapted from DeVita V, Hellman S, Rosenberg S. Cancer: Principles and Practices of Oncology, 6th ed. Philadelphia, PA: Lippincott-Raven, 2001, 1218.

Normal colonic mucosa

Pedunculated (stalk) polyp

Sessile polyp

Carcinoma of the colon

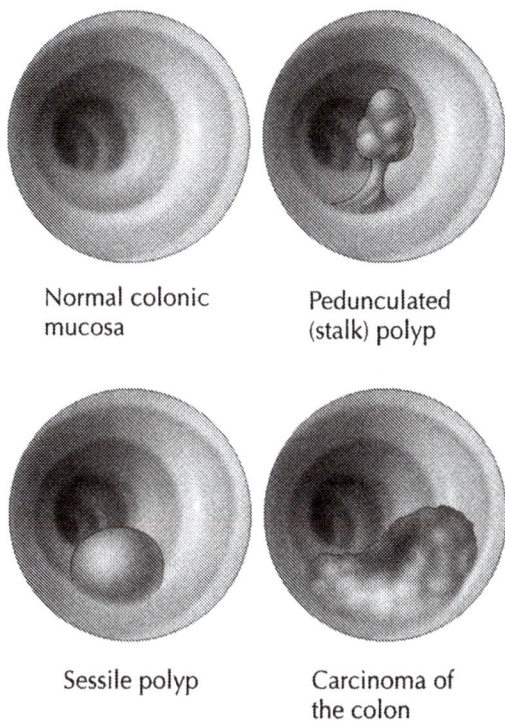

Figure 4.6 Neoplastic polyps: Pedunculated (stalk) and sessile.

Staging

Prognosis is directly related to the stage of disease at time of diagnosis. Stage is determined by depth of penetration of tumor invasion into and through the intestinal wall, the number of regional lymph nodes involved, and the presence of distant metastases. Staging has traditionally been with Dukes' classification, and TNM staging is also widely used (Table 4.3).

Clinical Manifestations

Early cancer is generally asymptomatic. If symptoms exist, they may consist of vague abdominal pain and flatulence, or minor changes in bowel movements, with or without rectal bleeding (Figure 4.9 on page 64). An ascending

Table 4.3   Staging

Stage	TNM Groupings			Dukes' Classification
I	T1/T2	N0	M0	A
II	T3/T4	N0	M0	B
III	Any T	N1,2,3	M0	C
IV	Any T	Any N	M1	D

T, tumor; N, lymph nodes; M, metastatic spread.

colon lesion is usually a large, bulky tumor, and the client may complain of fatigue. Clinical findings may consist of a palpable mass in the right lower quadrant, anemia, and changes in stool. Transverse, descending, and/or sigmoid colon lesions may present with constipation alternating with diarrhea, pain, change in bowel habits, and blood in the stool. Rectal lesions may present with client complaints of rectal fullness, urgency, tenesmus, and pelvic pain.

A complete evaluation for extent and stage of disease is, of course, necessary once a diagnosis of colorectal cancer is made. Laboratory evaluation would include a CBC, chemistry panel, liver enzymes, and carcinoembryonic antigen (CEA). A CEA is a tumor marker, which is overexpressed in adenocarcinomas, especially those of the colon and rectum, but also by cancers such as melanoma, stomach, cervix, breast, and lung. More than 90% of colorectal cancers produce CEA. The level may be elevated in smokers, in those with liver or renal disease, and in inflammatory bowel disease. A correlation does exist between stage of cancer and CEA preoperatively, as well as with prognosis.[7] The ASCO Tumor Marker Panel states that though there is no literature proving an impact of preoperative CEA testing on outcomes such as survival, quality of life, or cost effectiveness, preoperative CEA values are a prognostic factor independent of Dukes' stage and predict a higher rate of recurrence and mortality compared with patients with normal levels.[8]

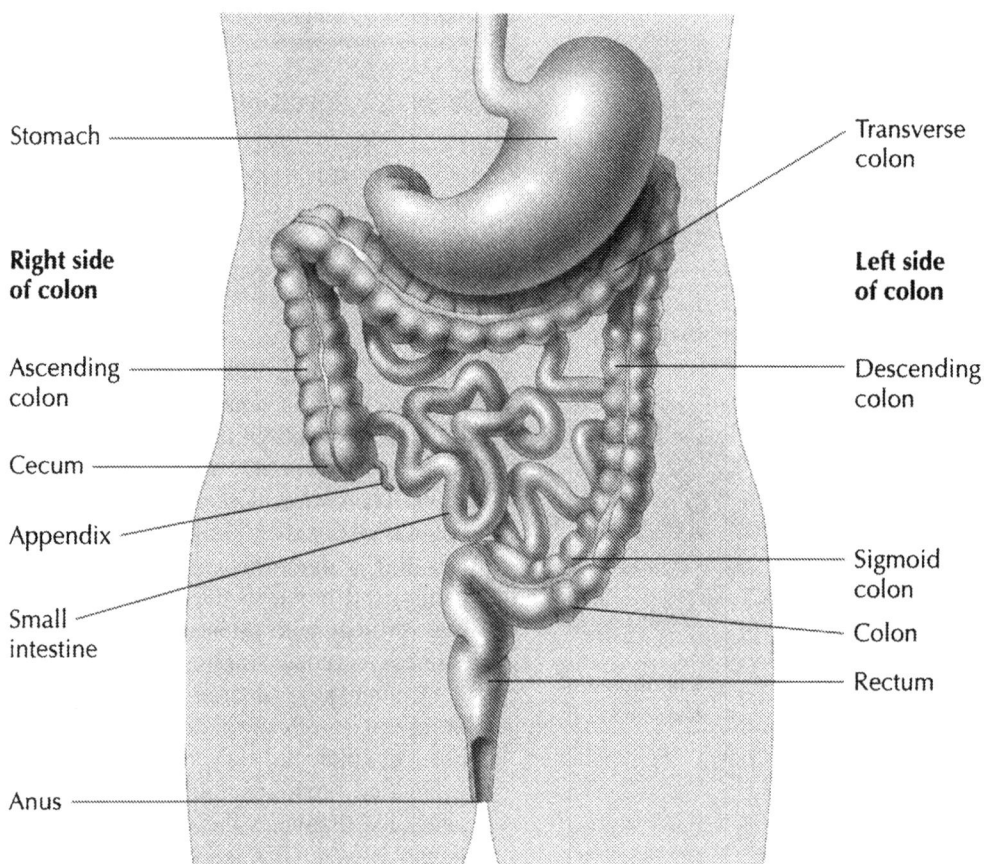

Figure 4.7   Anatomy of the colon.

Source: From the National Cancer Institute.

ASCO guidelines recommend following CEA levels in patients for whom hepatic resections for recurrent disease would be appropriate. CEA does have an important role in managing the clinical course of a patient. The trend, whether up or down, often determines the need for reevaluation. The ASCO Tumor Marker Panel recommends obtaining a baseline CEA before treatment for metastatic disease and every 2 to 3 months during treatment. Most clinicians believe that it is an additional parameter to follow in patients, particularly those at high risk of recurrence, and patients may benefit from the extra vigilance (Table 4.4).

Imaging studies are crucial in the diagnosis and monitoring of advanced disease. The computerized tomograph (CT) is the mainstay of diagnostic imaging, with the spiral, or helical, CT being the most notable recent innovation. The spiral CT eliminates the respiratory motion problem, which can result in a missed lesion. Magnetic resonance imaging (MRI) is particularly useful for the detection of liver metastases. Positron emission tomography (the PET scan) is the only test that does not depict pure anatomy. By administration of a positron-emitting radiopharmaceutical, usually glucose, areas of high metabolism image brightly. In this way,

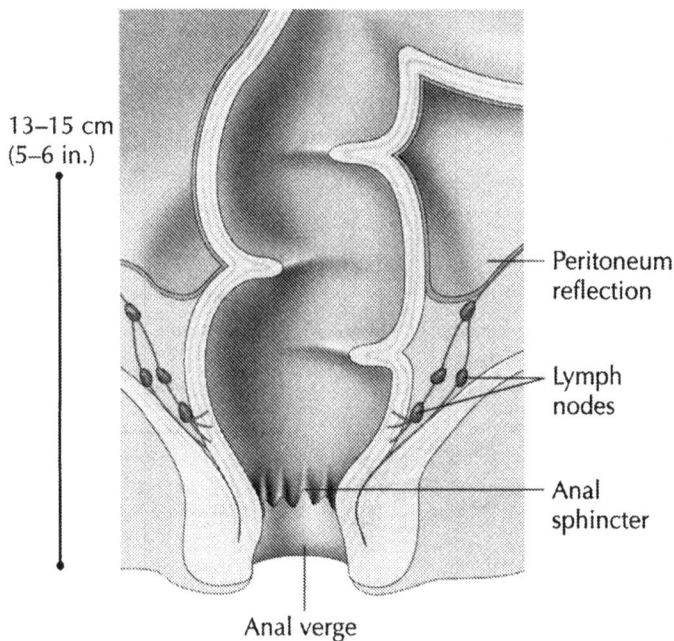

Figure 4.8 Anatomy of the rectum.

13–15 cm
(5–6 in.)

— Peritoneum reflection

— Lymph nodes

— Anal sphincter

Anal verge

Table 4.4   Summary of ASCO Tumor Marker

1. CEA is not recommended for use as a screening test for colorectal cancer.

2. CEA may be ordered preoperatively in patients with colorectal carcinoma if it would assist in staging and surgical treatment planning. Although elevated preoperative CEA (> 5 mg/mL) may correlate with poorer prognosis, data are insufficient to support the use of CEA to determine whether to treat a patient with adjuvant therapy.

3. If resection of liver metastases would be clinically indicated, it is recommended that postoperative serum CEA testing may be performed every 2 to 3 months in patients with stage II or III disease for > 2 years after diagnosis. An elevated CEA, if confirmed by retesting, warrants further evaluation for metastatic disease but does not justify the institution of adjuvant therapy or systemic therapy for presumed metastatic disease.

4. Present data are insufficient to recommend routine use of the serum CEA alone for monitoring response to treatment. If no other simple test is available to indicate a response, CEA should be measured at the start of treatment for metastatic disease, and every 2 to 3 months during active treatment. Two values above baseline are adequate to document progressive disease, even in the absence of corroborating radiographs.

Source: Adapted from ASCO. Clinical practice guidelines for use of tumor markers in breast and colorectal cancers. Classic Paper Curr Comments. 2000; 4(4):974–1009.

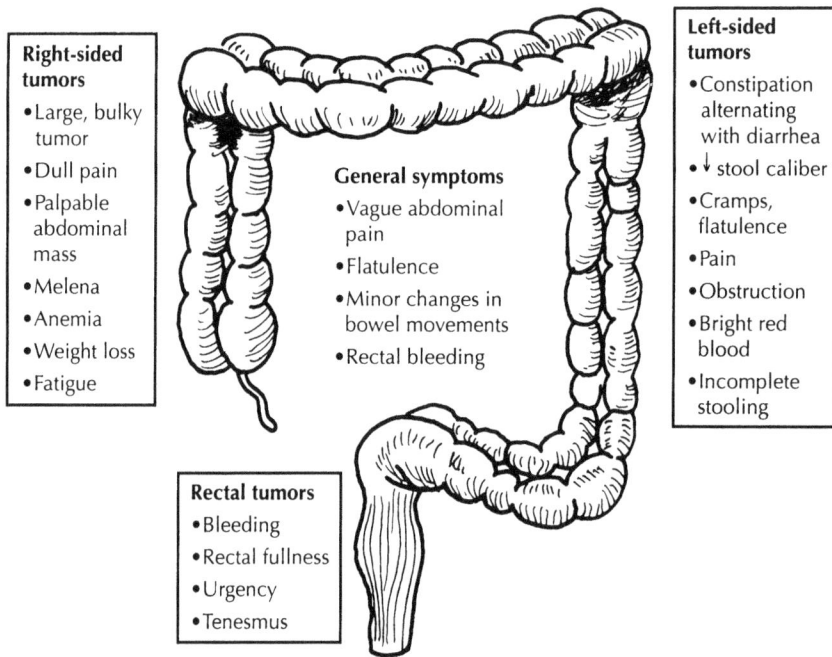

Right-sided tumors
- Large, bulky tumor
- Dull pain
- Palpable abdominal mass
- Melena
- Anemia
- Weight loss
- Fatigue

General symptoms
- Vague abdominal pain
- Flatulence
- Minor changes in bowel movements
- Rectal bleeding

Left-sided tumors
- Constipation alternating with diarrhea
- ↓ stool caliber
- Cramps, flatulence
- Pain
- Obstruction
- Bright red blood
- Incomplete stooling

Rectal tumors
- Bleeding
- Rectal fullness
- Urgency
- Tenesmus

Figure 4.9   Signs and symptoms of colorectal cancer.

tumors can be differentiated from scar or benign lesions.

Summary

In summary, treatment options for colorectal cancer are numerous. However, timely diagnosis and thorough evaluation of extent of disease are imperative. Improved diagnostic and screening techniques increase the likelihood of earlier diagnoses. Education of the public on preventative strategies and screening mechanisms is imperative for all involved in healthcare.

References

1. DeVita V, Hellman S, Rosenberg S. Cancer: Principles and Practices of Oncology, 6th ed. Philadelphia, PA: Lippincott-Raven, 2001.

2. McCance K, Huether S. Pathophysiology: The Biologic Basis for Disease in Adults and Children, 3rd ed. St. Louis, MO: Mosby, 1998.

3. Glaser E, Grogan L. Molecular genetics of GI malignancies. Semin Oncol Nurs. 1999; 15(1): 3–10.

4. Macdonald JS. Cancer chemotherapy and the liver. Clin Liver Dis. 1998; 2(3):631–642.

5. Saddler D, Ellis C. Colorectal cancer. Semin Oncol Nurs. 1999; 15(1):58–69.

6. Curtas S. Diagnosing GI malignancies. Semin Oncol Nurs. 1999; 15(1):10–16.

7. Macdonald JS. Carcinoembryonic antigen screening: Pros and cons. Semin Oncol. 1999; 26(5):556–561.

8. ASCO. Clinical practice guidelines for use of tumor markers in breast and colorectal cancers. Classic Papers Curr Comments. 2000; 4(4): 974–1009.

CHAPTER 5 | # Assessment, Diagnosis, and Staging

Margot R. Sweed, RN, CRNP, CNSN

Neal J. Meropol, MD

Introduction

Colorectal cancer (CRC) is an all too common malignancy affecting both genders and all races. Though approximately 90% of the cases of CRC are diagnosed in people 50 years of age or older, the disease affects all age groups.[1] Therefore, it is important that people, regardless of age, be aware of CRC and its signs and symptoms. Survival depends on one *very* key factor—the extent of disease at the time of diagnosis (Figure 5.1). CRC that is diagnosed early has a more favorable long-term outcome. CRC that is local (i.e., not spread outside the bowel wall) has a 90% 5-year survival.[1] That means that 9 out of 10 people with local CRC will be alive in 5 years. Unfortunately, only about 37% of people are diagnosed with disease that is still confined within the layers of the bowel wall.[1]

For patients whose disease has spread outside the bowel but only has regional involvement of nearby organs or lymph nodes, the 5-year survival drops to 66%. Again, only about 37% of people are diagnosed with regional CRC.[1] Once the disease has spread to distant sites, the 5-year survival rate dramatically drops to 9%. Twenty-five percent of patients present with metastatic disease.[1] Thus, it is crucial that this disease be diagnosed early. This chapter discusses the clinical presentation, signs and symptoms, assessment, diagnosis, and staging of the patient with colon or rectal cancer.

Clinical Presentation

Most, if not all, CRCs develop from a polyp on the inner surface of the bowel that was not

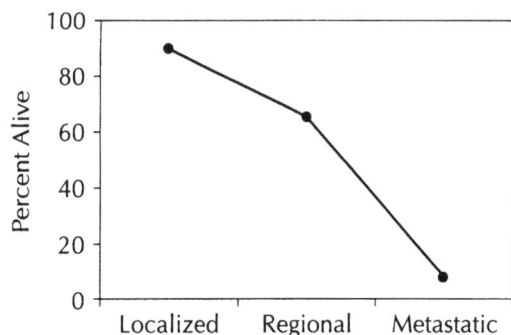

Figure 5.1 Five-year survival based on extent of disease.

Source: Adapted from Greenlee RT, Murray T, Bolden S, et al. Cancer statistics. CA Cancer J Clin. 2000; 50:7–23.

found and removed. The malignant polyp continued to grow and developed into a tumor mass that spread through some or all of the bowel wall. Once outside the wall, the tumor cells can invade nearby organs, lymph nodes, and blood vessels, and can thus spread to distant sites within the body. Approximately 75% of tumors develop in the left side of the colon (i.e., descending, rectosigmoid, and rectal areas), 15% develop in the right colon (i.e., cecum and ascending colon), and 10% develop in the transverse colon.[2] The location of the tumor within a specific area of the colon or rectum helps dictate the direction and sites of metastasis. Tumor spread from the ascending or descending colon may involve the retroperitoneal soft tissues, kidney, ureter, or pancreas. The venous system of the colon and proximal rectum drains into the portal system, thereby making the liver the most common site of metastasis. The vascular drainage of the distal rectum passes directly into the inferior vena cava. Consequently, distal rectal cancers commonly metastasize to the lung.[3] Other sites of metastatic disease that could lead to clinical presentation are lymph nodes, bone, and peritoneum.

In order to make the diagnosis of CRC, it must be suspected. That is, there must be some abnormal sign or symptom experienced by the patient. In addition to the outward spread of cancer cells through the layers of the colon, the tumor may also grow inward, decreasing the size of the lumen. CRC tumors often do not cause symptoms until they are advanced, thus blocking the flow of stool, develop into a palpable mass, or metastasize to other organs. The signs and symptoms frequently associated with CRC are the following:

- Bright red blood with bowel movements
- Stools that are tarry black or have mucus
- Change in bowel habits (e.g., constipation, diarrhea, or alternation between the two, lasting more than a few days)
- Change in size or shape of the stool (e.g., ribbon-like or narrower stools)
- Difficulty having a bowel movement
- Feeling of incomplete stooling
- Stomach or abdominal discomfort, cramping, or pain
- Abdominal bloating or distention
- Unusual and/or continuing fatigue
- Jaundice

Even when symptoms are present, they are often minor, ignored, or misinterpreted as being caused by other conditions. Bright red bleeding, a warning sign of CRC, is also common with hemorrhoids; thus, patients and physicians often delay evaluation of this symptom. Common intestinal viruses or specific foods can cause abdominal cramping, pain, or gas. Other bowel conditions, such as ulcers or inflammation of the colon, can also cause abdominal pain and changes in bowel habits. Signs and symptoms of CRC can be generalized based on the location of the tumor within the colon (i.e., right-sided tumors vs. left-sided tumors) (Figure 5.2). The colon is a flexible tube, and the materials that pass through it start as liquid in the right colon and end as a solid material once

Transverse colon
- changes in bowel habits
- blood in the stool

Right side of the colon (cecum and ascending colon)
- vague pain
- palpable abdominal mass
- melena
- anemia
- weight loss
- anorexia

Left side of the colon (descending and rectosigmoid colon)
- abdominal pain
- changes in bowel habits
- ↓ stool caliber
- cramps, flatulence
- obstruction
- bright red blood on stooling
- incomplete stooling

Rectal tumors
- gross bleeding
- pain
- tenesmus
- incomplete stooling
- constipation

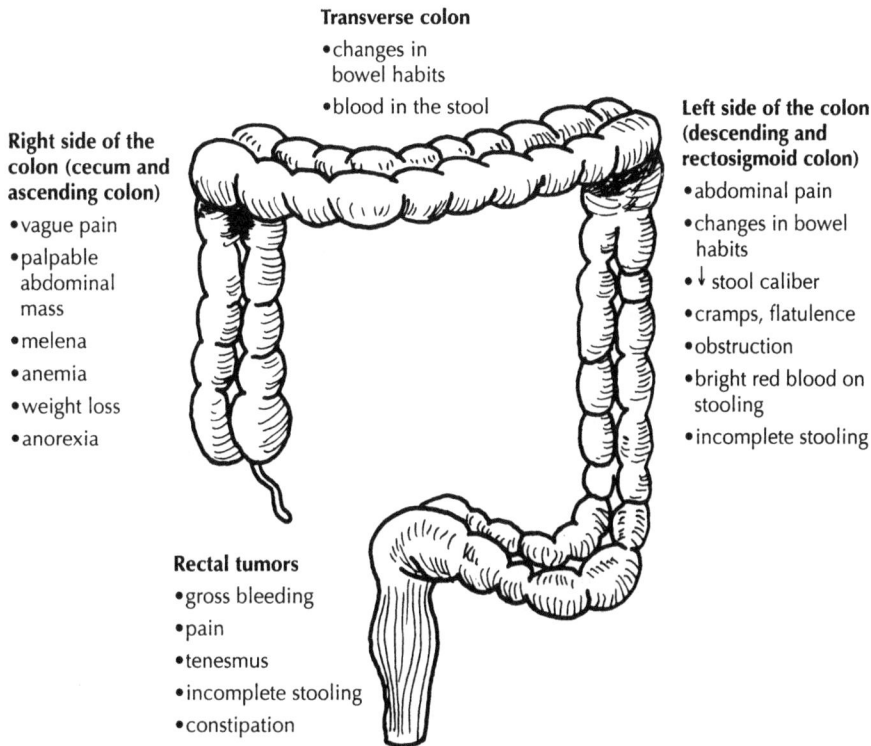

Figure 5.2   Signs and symptoms of colorectal cancer.

it reaches the rectum. For these reasons, tumors in the right colon often exhibit different symptoms and at a later stage than tumors in the left colon. Metastases to the liver may present with hepatomegally and/or a knobby, irregular surface. Once suspected, a complete general history and manual physical examination are initiated to rule out or detect a primary tumor in the colon or rectum or a site of metastasis.

History

A comprehensive history, including social history, history of smoking or alcohol consumption, prior surgical and medical history, and individual and family risks for CRC should be obtained. Inflammatory bowel disease, a personal or family history of cancer, especially colorectal, uterine, ovarian, ureter, bladder, or other cancers associated with hereditary nonpolyposis CRC, in particular, are important. The history should include the age at which the affected family member was diagnosed. This may suggest whether there might be a hereditary or familial pattern of CRC as opposed to a sporadic cancer history (Table 5.1).

A review of symptoms is important to ascertain as many details as possible about whether there are any early or late signs of malignancy. Patients with early disease may have no complaints or have nonspecific abdominal discomfort such as flatulence, abdominal fullness or cramps, and bloating. It is important to note that, for many patients, the abdominal com-

Table 5.1   The History: Questions to Ask

- How old are you?
- How would you describe your ethnic background or race?
- Is there a personal or family history of polyps?
- Do you have a history of ulcerative colitis, diverticulitis, or Crohn's disease?
- Have you ever been told you have hemorrhoids or anal fissures?
- Have you ever had blood in your stools?
- Have you ever had a problem emptying your bowels?
- Is there a family history of colon or rectal cancer? (Include extended family)
- Is there a personal or family history of endometrial, ovarian, gastric, or urinary tract malignancy?
- How old was the person at the time of the cancer diagnosis for colon or rectal cancer and other malignancies?
- Has there been a change in your bowel habits?
- Do you smoke or have you smoked cigarettes, cigars, etc?
- How would you describe your intake of alcohol?

plaints are vague. Characteristic complaints of abdominal pain may be colicky or gnawing in nature. Anorexia may be present with or without nausea. Changes in stool color, pattern, caliber, and habit may be present. Complaints of tenesmus (incomplete evacuation) are classic for rectal malignancy. Unfortunately, individuals frequently attribute persistent bloody smears on toilet tissue to hemorrhoids. Even young adults presenting with rectal bleeding require endoscopic evaluation. Fatigue and unexplained weight loss may be present without anemia. The symptoms of pregnancy, such as constipation, abdominal discomfort, rectal bleeding, and anemia, can obscure a CRC. Reports of pruritus or a history of thrombosis are a red flag for liver involvement and underlying malignancy.

Information gathered from the history will guide the physical examination and imaging tests, and help determine the differential diagnoses. For example, if the history has provided information suspicious for a tumor in the ascending colon, the evaluation will be different than if a rectal tumor is suspected.

Physical Examination

In a patient suspected of colorectal malignancy, a complete physical examination with attention to lymph nodes, breasts, abdomen, and rectum is performed in order to detect the primary lesion or a metastatic site of disease. General examination of the patient is undertaken to assess for signs such as temporal or masseter wasting indicative of severe weight loss or abdominal distention suggestive of ascites. Careful attention is paid to the examination of the abdomen, assessing for masses, areas of tenderness, and signs of bowel perforation. Auscultation of the abdomen can provide important information about the status of the bowels. Hypermotility, or high-pitched bowel sounds, may indicate a partial bowel obstruction, while weak or absent bowel sounds are representative of loss of bowel motion and probable complete bowel obstruction. Tumor masses may be palpable anywhere along the colon but are common with cancers located in the right side of the colon. Perforation of the colon may be acute or chronic. Acute perforation may have a similar presentation to that of appendicitis or diverticulitis, with pain, fever, and a palpable mass. Chronic perforation with fistula formation into the bladder can result from a sigmoid colon lesion and lead to recurrent urinary tract infections and gross hematuria. Complaints of pain in the right flank, right posterior chest, or right upper quadrant may represent liver metastasis that presents synchronously in 10% to 15% of individuals. Even without complaints, palpation of the liver is always important, because hepatomegaly may still be present in an otherwise asymptomatic individual. Other signs of hepatic involvement include scleral icterus, which may be present before the skin appears jaundiced and herald biliary obstruction. A rectal mass may be palpated during a digital rectal exam, which should also include palpation of the prostate in males.[3] A pelvic exam should be performed in women with complaints of pelvic pain, because ovarian metastasis or metastatic disease in the cul-de-sac may be easily palpable. A neurologic exam may uncover suspicious metastatic brain disease or ensuing spinal cord compression.

Other systemic physical findings may aid in the diagnosis of CRC. Metastasis at the umbilicus (Sister Joseph nodules) occurs particularly with carcinoma of the pancreas, stomach, colon, and ovary. Peutz-Jeghers syndrome, an inherited autosomal dominant condition consisting of cutaneous and mucosal hyperpigmentation, is associated with gastrointestinal (GI) tract polyposis. Pigmentary changes involve both the skin and mucous membrane. The macules are frequently grouped around the mouth and eyes or may be present on the fingers and palms or widespread on the skin surface.[4,5] Sebaceous skin tumors may be a sign of Muir-Torre syndrome, another hereditary colon cancer.

Paraneoplastic syndromes are disorders of organ function (such as the skin) that occur at a site that is distant from the primary tumor. It is believed that the mechanisms behind these disorders are related to cytokines and hormones produced by the cancer or to immune reactions to the cancer. GI tract malignancies are capable of producing a paraneoplastic phenomena. Dermatologic paraneoplastic manifestations have some of the strongest associations with GI tumors. The following paraneoplastic phenomena have been associated with colorectal malignancy. Acanthosis nigricans (AN), characterized by symmetric, hyperpigmented, velvety skin thickening, is usually found in flexor areas such as neck, axillae, antecubital, popliteal fossae, periumbilical area, and groin. Nonmalignant forms may be associated with insulin resistance, but presence of malignancy occurs in 50% of acquired adult cases. In malignant cases of AN, the onset is abrupt with rapid spread. Dermatomyositis, characterized by dermatitis and inflammation of the muscles, can be associated with colonic or gastric cancers. Hypercalcemia occurs through the production of a parathyroid hormone (PTH)–like activity. It is the most common paraneoplastic phenomenon seen in patients with malignancy. Patients report lethargy, confusion, dehydration, constipation, abdominal pain, nausea, and vomiting. As previously mentioned, hypercoagulability, commonly seen as superficial or deep vein thrombosis with or without pulmonary embolism, is seen with CRC.[6]

Making the Diagnosis

Laboratory Tests

Routine complete blood count (CBC), chemistries, liver function tests, and coagulation assays are ordered initially, as they may aid in the differential diagnosis. Anemia should trigger investigation with a colonoscopy, as most individuals, except menstruating girls and women, are not usually anemic. Liver function tests, such as alkaline phosphatase and gamma-glutamyl-transpeptidase (GGT), offer important data in patients suspected to have CRC. The alkaline phosphatase may be elevated if metastatic disease in the bone is present. Metastatic disease in the liver may produce elevation in GGT. Patients with CRC often have hypercoagulability conditions, as noted previously.[6,7]

Serum carcinoembryonic antigen (CEA) is a glycoprotein that is checked once a diagnosis of CRC is made. This glycoprotein is expressed normally at very low levels by GI mucosal cells in the large intestine. Normal CEA levels are below 2.5 ng/mL for nonsmokers and below 5.0 ng/mL for chronic smokers; therefore, overexpression is suspicious for a malignancy.[8] CEA is not a tumor-specific marker but is a tumor-associated one, as evidenced by the fact that elevated CEA levels may be present in the blood of patients with an array of tumors, such as lung, pancreatic, and stomach cancers. It appears to be particularly overexpressed in adenocarcinomas of the colon and rectum and frequently corresponds to well-differentiated colorectal tumors. Unfortunately, nonmalignant conditions such as liver disease, peptic ulcer disease, ulcerative colitis, and chronic lung disease may also show elevations in some patients. Smoking cigarettes also commonly causes a mild elevation in CEA. Because of the low sensitivity and specificity of this tumor marker, it is not used for colorectal screening in otherwise healthy individuals. In the patient with CRC, the preoperative CEA level correlates with stage and outcome, and is most useful in the early detection of recurrence following potentially curative resection. Elevated preoperative CEA levels commonly return to normal levels 4 to 6 weeks following curative surgery. Therefore, the preoperative determination is crucial to determine whether the primary tumor is CEA-producing, and hence, whether it will be a useful surveillance tool.[9]

Developments in the molecular diagnosis of CRC have led to work trying to identify a practical, noninvasive screening test to detect tumor DNA with specific mutations in stool, for example, mutations in the *RAS* gene.[10] Early molecular diagnosis is still in the research phase and not yet commercially available.[11]

Imaging, Endoscopy, and Preparation

After completing the history and physical examination, the appropriate endoscopic and im-

aging tests can be ordered. The major goal of these tests is to determine the sites and, ultimately, the clinical stage of disease. Endoscopic procedures such as sigmoidoscopy and colonoscopy can be used to diagnose tumors within the bowel, while imaging studies such as computerized tomography (CT) scans can detect sites of distant metastases. The appropriate test is selected based on the location of the suspicious lesion and patient issues. The test must be able to efficiently detect the lesion, be cost effective, yet cause minimal risk and discomfort to the patient.[12] Imaging tests can be very important in otherwise asymptomatic individuals to establish whether there is any extracolonic disease whose presence could change the surgical plan. Common endoscopic procedures and methods of imaging are presented next. Limitations of selected diagnostic methods are illustrated in Figure 5.3. Recommended preparations for both endoscopic procedures and imaging tests are noted in Table 5.2.

Invasive Diagnostic Techniques

BARIUM ENEMA

A double contrast barium enema utilizes radiopaque barium and air instillation into the colon and is better than the single contrast study. The double contrast barium enema improves visualization of smaller tumors and polyps when compared with the single contrast barium enema. Air-contrast barium enemas show efficacy in detecting colon lesions approaching that of colonoscopy; however, evaluation of the rectum with this technique is inferior. In addition, recent data suggest that for patients who have undergone colonoscopic polypectomy, colonoscopic examination is a more sensitive method of surveillance than the double contrast barium enema.[13] In addition, unlike colonoscopy, a barium enema does not afford the option of biopsy or polypectomy. Barium enemas can help with diagnosis, specifically in individuals unable to tolerate endoscopic evaluation.

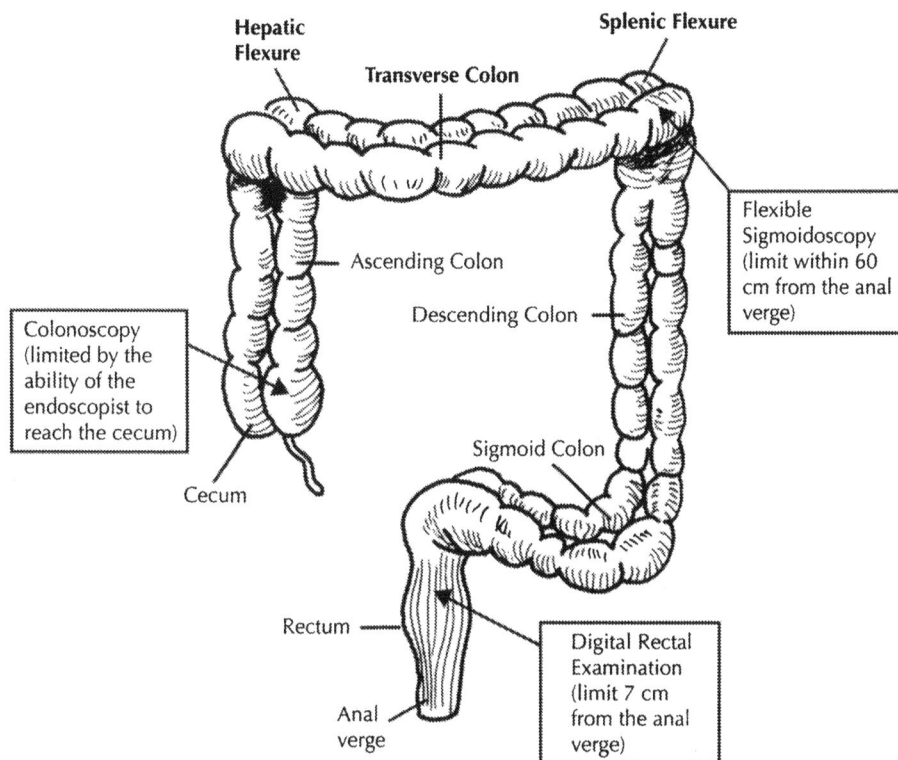

Figure 5.3   Limitations of diagnostic evaluations for colorectal cancer.

Source: Data from Ellis C, Saddler D. Colorectal cancer. In: Yarbro CH, Frogge MH, Goodman M, et al., eds. Cancer Nursing Principles and Practice, 5th ed. Boston, MA: Jones and Bartlett Publishers, 2000: 1117–1137.

Table 5.2   Imaging, Endoscopy, and Preparation

Study	Preparation	Aftercare
Barium enema	Day before, start clear liquids only 5 P.M. night before: 12 oz magnesium citrate 6 P.M. night before: 4 Dulcolax tablets No eating, drinking, smoking day of test Rectal suppository day of test	Drink at least 32 oz liquids within 24 hours after exam. Recommend laxative to facilitate passage of barium
CAT scan (Abdominal and pelvis)	No eating, drinking, or smoking for 3 hours before test. May drink 24 oz of contrast 1 hr prior to exam Frequently, IV iodine contrast Need steroid pre-med for iodine allergy	If IV contrast injected, recommend 32 oz of fluid over next 24 hours
Bone scan	IV injection of a chemical compound, labeled with a small amount of radioactive material	None

(continues)

Table 5.2 *Continued*

Study	Preparation	Aftercare
MRI	For endorectal and pelvis studies: NPO 1 hr before the study. Will get glucagon injection to slow bowel to lessen motion on pictures. Because of strong magnetic field, need to check the following: pacemakers, ear implants, aneurysm clips, other metal, shrapnel, eye exposure to metal shavings, permanent makeup (contains lead). Patient must weigh < 300 lb.	No eating of solid foods for 3 hours if glucagons used. May only drink liquids immediately after glucagon or cramping will occur.
PET scan	Nothing to eat/drink 4 hrs before, except H_2O. Blood sugar must be < 140 mg/mL in order to be accurate. IV injection of radioactively labeled glucose. Entire procedure lasts 2–3 hr.	None
Rectal ultrasound	6 P.M. night before → 1 bottle magnesium citrate Nothing to eat/drink after midnight Take 2 Fleet enemas 30 minutes apart 90 minutes before leaving home	
Sigmoidoscopy	Same as for rectal ultrasound Stop any medications containing aspirin, nonsteroidal antiinflammatory drugs, anticoagulants, Persantine, Ticlid, Plavix for 7 days prior to testing	
Colonoscopy	Clear liquids start breakfast the day before. Evening before, add 1.5 oz Fleet Phospho Soda to 4 oz of any clear liquid. Follow with another 8 oz. Drink a total of 3 more 8-oz glasses of clears before bedtime. *Day of scope:* 1.5 fluid oz Phospho-Soda to 4 oz of clear liquid. Follow with 8 oz liquid. IV conscious sedation is given. Stop any meds containing aspirin, nonsteroidal antiinflammatory drugs, anticoagulants, Persantine, Ticlid, Plavix for 7 days prior.	Need to have someone to drive patient home after conscious sedation.

Source: Courtesy the Fox Chase Cancer Center.

SIGMOIDOSCOPY

Detection of polyps and colorectal malignancy is directly related to the length of the endoscope. The rigid sigmoidoscope, no longer routinely used, which reaches approximately 20 cm, allows visualization to just above the rectosigmoid junction. Flexible sigmoidoscopes may be either 35 cm or 60 cm in length and can reach the proximal end of the sigmoid colon. Advantages of sigmoidoscopy include the lack of sedation needed, less patient discomfort, and less bowel preparation than with colonoscopy. Disadvantages include nonvisualization of the ascending and transverse portions of colon.

Within the United States, *one-third* of CRC are *not* within reach of the sigmoidoscope.[14]

COLONOSCOPY

Colonoscopy visualizes the entire colon and rectum and requires conscious sedation. It may be diagnostic and therapeutic. Biopsy samples, together with removal of polyps, can be performed at time of colonoscopy. Complete bowel preparation, intravenous sedation, and analgesia are used for the procedure. The proximal migration of primary CRC to the right colon makes colonoscopy a preferred screening procedure.

The Food and Drug Administration recently approved the Optical Biopsy System, which is operated through an endoscope that can be used to evaluate polyps less than 1 cm in diameter that would not otherwise be removed. This device utilizes laser light energy to help determine whether or not a small polyp may be malignant[15] (Figure 5.4, see page P-1 of insert).

TRANSRECTAL ULTRASOUND

Transrectal ultrasound is valuable for the preoperative staging of rectal carcinoma. Treatment decisions regarding preoperative versus postoperative adjuvant treatment with chemotherapy and radiation can differ based on clinical staging with ultrasound. Pretreatment ultrasound reportedly is 83% to 88% specific in defining those patients who do not routinely receive adjuvant therapy (T1–T2) from those with T3–T4 tumors. Detection of adenopathy is not as powerful, with only 62% specificity when 7 mm is used as a cut-off for enlarged lymph nodes.[16] Preparation includes an enema, followed by probe placement into the rectum (Figure 5.5, see page P-2 of insert).

Diagnostic Imaging Techniques

CHEST X-RAY

Chest x-ray is appropriate at the time of diagnosis if CT of the chest has not been performed.

Approximately 10% of patients with rectal carcinoma will have lung metastasis at the time of diagnosis.[17] Lung metastases are less common at the time of presentation of colon cancer.

COMPUTERIZED TOMOGRAPHY SCANNING

CT scanning is usually one of the first studies ordered to determine the presence and extent of metastatic or extracolonic disease, particularly in the chest, abdomen, or pelvis. The injection of contrast material before CT scanning increases sensitivity for identification of metastasis. CT is excellent at detecting pulmonary and hepatic metastases. Imaging with a helical (spiral) CT scanner provides greater detail and can be more useful in evaluating metastatic disease. It refers to the acquisition of volumes of CT data rather than individual slices obtained with standard CT. The scanning time is less, thereby decreasing the amount of intravenous contrast utilized[18] (Figures 5.6 and 5.7, see page P-2 of insert). A bone scan should be considered for any persistent bone pain, but it is not performed in all individuals.

CT colonography is a newer technique utilizing volumetric CT data combined with special imaging software. Other terms previously used to describe this technique include *virtual colonoscopy, virtual endoscopy, 3D-endoscopy,* and *CT colography. CT colonography* is now the favored term, and it refers to a CT examination of the fully prepped and air-distended colon. Volumetric CT data in the colon are obtained within a few minutes of scanning and within a total of 15 minutes or less of radiographic examination time. Advanced imaging software combines these data with two-dimensional (2D) and 3D images to assess the colon and rectum.[19] Polyps and tumors are visualized by a virtual "fly-through" of the colon. Patients undergoing this examination still need to undergo colonic cleansing. Colonic insufflation with either air or carbon dioxide is also necessary to distend the large bowel. The apparent benefits of this study include the lack of sedation and internal manipulation with an endoscope. The major disadvantage of CT colonography is the inability to retrieve tissue. This technique is showing some promise, but there is evidence that it is not as good for smaller lesions (< 6 mm).[20] At present, this technique is still undergoing scientific evaluation, and its ultimate role in the diagnosis of CRC remains uncertain.

MAGNETIC RESONANCE IMAGING

Magnetic resonance imaging (MRI) can be useful in detecting recurrent disease. It is a frequent follow-up to questionable abnormalities visualized in the liver on CT exam. MRI is also valuable in preoperative staging, detection of pelvic sidewall and sacral involvement, along with transrectal ultrasound for rectal carcinoma. A major advantage of MRI over CT is the availability of noniodine-based contrast agents if needed for clearer images[14] (Figure 5.8, see page P-3 of insert).

POSITRON EMISSION TOMOGRAPHY

Positron emission tomography (PET) imaging is based on the detection of positrons emitted from radioactive atoms in sugar. Radionuclides are integrated into biomedical tracers that can target and be used to evaluate the metabolism and blood flow of the tumor.[21] PET imaging is a whole-body imaging study that utilizes the increased rate of glycolysis in tumor cells to detect malignancy. The glucose analogue tracer is injected intravenously and becomes trapped in most malignant cells because of the deficiency of glucose-6-phosphatase movement in tumor cells.[22] The role of PET imaging in cancer is not fully defined, but it is approved by many third-party payers to detect CRC recurrence. It may be useful in detection of surgically resectable metastases in liver and lung in the context of elevated CEA levels and no other evidence of disease.[21] It may also help select patients who are not suitable for curative surgery (i.e.,

multiple sites of disease). PET imaging may have limited utility in diabetic patients who do not have optimum glycemic control.

BONE SCANS

Bone scans, which are more sensitive than conventional x-rays, should be considered for any persistent bone pain. Bone scans utilize oral or intravenous ingestion of radioisotope compounds or radiolabeled monoclonal antibodies. The resulting images demonstrate the areas where the isotopes have concentrated, representing sites of abnormal metabolism or malignancy.[5]

Pathology

Treatment planning and determination of prognosis require a careful pathologic diagnosis. In most circumstances, a tissue diagnosis of CRC is obtained prior to definitive treatment planning. This may involve a biopsy obtained from the primary site endoscopically or, less commonly, a biopsy of a metastatic site in an individual with a suspicious colonic mass. In general, biopsy confirmation of metastatic disease is appropriate, given that CRC typically presents in an age group in which other primary malignancies are common. Needle aspirates for cytologic analysis are often adequate for diagnosis of metastatic disease.

In addition to TNM staging (discussion follows), the pathologic evaluation of a CRC specimen should include histopathologic classification (e.g., adenocarcinoma, signet ring cell carcinoma, squamous carcinoma, small cell carcinoma, undifferentiated carcinoma) and histologic grade. The vast majority of CRCs are adenocarcinomas, and moderate differentiation is most common. The presence of poorly differentiated grade and lymphatic or vascular invasion is associated with an inferior prognosis.

Given that adenocarcinomas may arise in

many primary sites (e.g., lung, breast, colon), an extracolonic biopsy yielding "adenocarcinoma" in a context unusual for CRC may not provide a definitive diagnosis. An example of this situation would be lung masses in an individual with stage I CRC several years earlier. Given the high likelihood of cure with the initial presentation, other potential sources of the lung metastases should be sought. In this circumstance, immunohistochemical staining of the metastasis may be helpful. For example, positive expression of estrogen receptors may suggest a breast primary. Likewise, the pattern of cytokeratin expression may suggest an alternate primary site of malignancy.

Staging

Accurate staging of CRC is critical to establishing both prognosis and patient selection for adjuvant therapy (Figure 5.9). In addition, consistent staging approaches permit comparison of outcomes across populations. In general, staging of CRC is based on depth of tumor penetration through the bowel wall, presence or absence of regional lymph node involvement, and presence or absence of distant metastases. In patients without metastatic disease, the number of lymph nodes involved is the most important prognostic indicator. Recent evidence also suggests that the number of lymph nodes removed at surgery may also be prognostic, suggesting that lymph node dissection may be therapeutic as well as prognostic.[23] In contrast to many other malignancies, tumor size is not included in CRC staging. Rather, bowel wall penetration is more prognostic, and hence a major component of staging.

Cuthbert Dukes developed the first staging system in the 1930s. Dukes' system used an A, B, C, classification:

A: penetration into but not through the bowel wall

B: penetration through the bowel wall

C: involvement of regional lymph nodes

This system is simple to use but does not precisely define depth of invasion or number of involved lymph nodes. Subsequent modifications of Dukes' system sought to expand the information contained in a simple staging system. Initial modifications of Dukes' staging system included the Astler-Collier and Gastrointestinal Tumor Study Group (GITSG) systems. In an effort to obtain international consistency, the American Joint Commission on Cancer (AJCC) and the Union Internationale Contra le Cancer (UICC) introduced the TNM (tumor-node-metastasis) classifications, which were modified in 1998 and are now the most widely accepted worldwide. The AJCC/UICC staging system is described in Table 5.3 (page 77).

Predictive Markers and Prognosis

Clinicopathologic prognostic factors described include grade, lymphovascular invasion, and presentation with obstruction. Molecular markers of prognosis are also under investigation (Table 5.4 on page 78). Tumor-suppressor genes are the most commonly mutated class of genes in CRCs. They regulate cell growth by controlling the rate and timing of cell proliferation. *p53* has been identified as a universal tumor-suppressor gene. It is involved in cell cycle control and apoptosis. When it becomes inactivated by mutations, it is an early event in CRC carcinogenesis and portends a poorer prognosis. *p53* mutations are found in approximately 75% of CRCs. The deleted in colon cancer (*DCC*) gene is a tumor-suppressor gene that, when absent, also confers poor prognosis. Thymidine phosphorylase, or platelet-derived endothelial cell growth factor, is an angiogenic enzyme associated with a significantly poorer prognosis.[24] In stage II and stage III rectal cancers, thymidylate synthase (TS) expression was an

Data Form for Cancer Staging

Patient Identification

Name _____

Address _____

Hospital or clinic number _____

Age _____ Sex _____ Race _____

COLON AND RECTUM

Institution identification

Hospital or clinic _____

Address _____

Oncology Record

Anatomic site of cancer _____

Histologic type _____

Grade (G) _____

Date of classification _____

Clin	Path	
		DEFINITIONS

Primary Tumor (T)

Clin	Path		
[ ]	[ ]	TX	Primary tumor cannot be assessed
[ ]	[ ]	T0	No evidence of primary tumor
[ ]	[ ]	Tis	Carcinoma *in situ:* intraepithelial or invasion of lamina propria*
[ ]	[ ]	T1	Tumor invades submucosa
[ ]	[ ]	T2	Tumor invades muscularis propria
[ ]	[ ]	T3	Tumor invades through muscularis propria into subserosa, or into nonperitonealized pericolic or perirectal tissues
[ ]	[ ]	T4	Tumor directly invades other organs or structures, and/or perforates visceral peritoneum**

Tis includes cancer cells confined within the glandular basement membrane (intraepithelial) or lamina propria (intramucosal) with no extension through the muscularis mucosae into the submucosa.

**Direct invasion in T4 includes invasion of other segments of the colorectum by way of the serosa, for example, invasion of the sigmoid colon by a carcinoma of the cecum.*

Regional Lymph Nodes (N)

Clin	Path		
[ ]	[ ]	NX	Regional lymph nodes cannot be assessed
[ ]	[ ]	N0	No regional lymph node metastasis
[ ]	[ ]	N1	Metastasis in 1 to 3 regional lymph nodes
[ ]	[ ]	N2	Metastasis in 4 or more regional lymph nodes

Distant metastasis (M)

Clin	Path		
[ ]	[ ]	MX	Distant metastasis cannot be assessed
[ ]	[ ]	M0	No distant metastasis
[ ]	[ ]	M1	Distant metastasis

Histopathologic Grade (G)

[ ] GX Grade cannot be assessed
[ ] G1 Well differentiated
[ ] G2 Moderately differentiated
[ ] G3 Poorly differentiated
[ ] G4 Undifferentiated

Stage Grouping

Clin	Path					Dukes*
[ ]	[ ]	0	Tis	N0	M0	
[ ]	[ ]	I	T1	N0	M0	A
			T2	N0	M0	
[ ]	[ ]	II	T3	N0	M0	B
			T4	N0	M0	
[ ]	[ ]	III	Any T	N1	M0	C
			Any T	N2	M0	
[ ]	[ ]	IV	Any T	Any N	M1	

*Dukes B is a composite of better (T3 N0 M0) and worse (T4 N0 M0) prognostic groups, as is Dukes C (Any T N1 M0 and Any T N2 M0).

Histopathologic Type

This staging classification applies to carcinomas that arise in the colon, rectum, or appendix. The classification does not apply to sarcomas, lymphomas, or to carcinoid tumors of the large intestine or appendix. Ths histologic types include:

Adenocarcinoma *in situ* *

Adenocarcinoma

Mucinous carcinoma (colloid type) (greater than 50% mucinous carcinoma)

Signet ring cell carcinoma (greater than 50% signet ring cell)

Squamous cell (epidermoid) carcinoma

Adenosquamous carcinoma

Small cell carcinoma

Undifferentiated carcinoma

Carcinoma, NOS

Staged by _____ M.D.

_____ Registrar

Date _____

The terms high grade dysplasia or severe dysplasia may be used as synonyms for in situ adenocarcinoma or in situ carcinoma. These cases should be assigned pTis.

(continues)

Figure 5.9 Data form for cancer staging and anatomic areas of colon and the rectum.

Source: Used with the permission of the American Joint Committee on Cancer (AJCC®), Chicago, Illinois. The original source for this material is the AJCC® Cancer Staging Manual, 5th edition (1997) published by Lippincott-Raven publishers, Philadelphia, Pennsylvania.

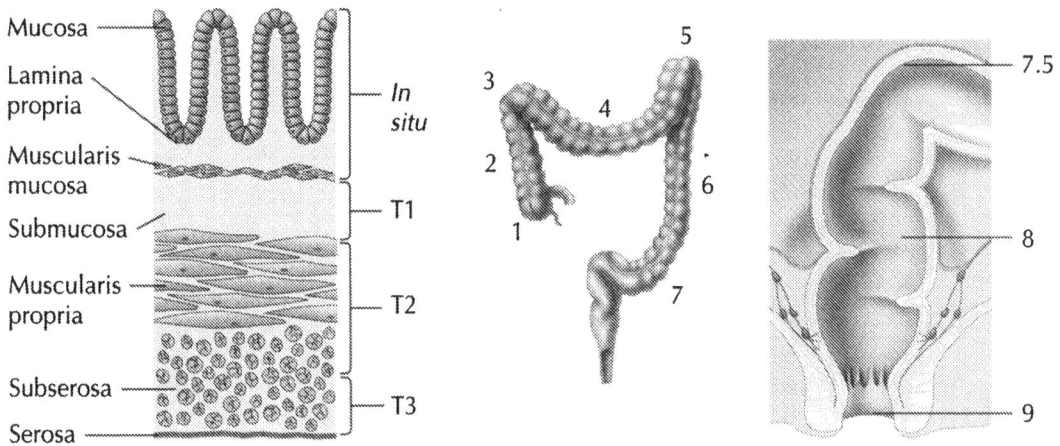

Mucosa

Lamina propria

Muscularis mucosa

Submucosa

Muscularis propria

Subserosa

Serosa

In situ

T1

T2

T3

5
3
4
2
1
6
7

7.5
8
9

For anatomic areas corresponding to numbers, see list below.
Indicate on diagram primary and regional nodes involved.

Anatomic Areas of Colon and Rectum

1. Cecum
2. Ascending colon
3. Hepatic flexure
4. Transverse colon
5. Splenic flexure

6. Descending colon
7. Sigmoid
7.5 Rectosigmoid
8. Rectum
9. Anal canal

Figure 5.9   *Continued*

Table 5.3   Colorectal Cancer Staging

AJCC/UICC	T	N	M	Dukes' System
Stage 0	Tis	N0	M0	—
Stage I	T1	N0	M0	A
	T2	N0	M0	A
Stage II	T3	N0	M0	B
	T4	N0	M0	B
Stage III	Any T	N1	M0	C
	Any T	N2	M0	C
Stage IV	Any T	Any N	M1	—

Source: Used with the permission of the American Joint Committee on Cancer (AJCC®), Chicago, Illinois. The original source for this material is the AJCC® Cancer Staging Manual, 5th edition (1997) published by Lippincott-Raven publishers, Philadelphia, Pennsylvania.

independent predictor of outcome, with low TS expression in tumors associated with the best prognosis.[25] Abnormalities in oncogenes frequently initiate increased cellular proliferation. The most commonly mutated oncogene in human cancer is *RAS*. Mutations involving the oncogene K-*ras* can be found in approximately 50% of CRCs and may be associated with

Table 5.4   Predictive Markers

Poor Prognosis	Better Prognosis
Obstruction	Low TS expression
Mutated *p53*	MSI
Absent *DCC* gene	
Thymidine phosphorylase	
K-*ras* mutation	
Survivin expression	

poorer prognosis. Microsatellite instability (MSI) in tumor DNA is associated with the hereditary nonpolyposis colon cancer (HNPCC) syndrome but is also present in 15% of sporadic CRCs. Recent evidence suggests that microsatellite instability is associated with a better prognosis.

Conflicting data exist with regard to ploidy and prognosis. Cell cycle regulatory gene expression is also correlated with outcome.[26] Flow cytometry can be used to examine biopsy tissue for chromosome pattern and cell division phases. It can ascertain whether there is diploidy (normal chromosome number) or aneuploidy (an abnormal number of chromosomes). Aneuploidy has been associated with poor prognosis in some studies. It is notable that many of these prognostic markers also may predict responsiveness to chemotherapy with 5-fluorouracil.

Nursing Implications

It is incumbent on nurses to know the signs and symptoms of colorectal malignancy. Educating patients, families, and friends to act and seek medical evaluation when these warning signs present will promote earlier detection and higher cure rates for individuals with CRC. Nurses also provide support and teaching through the ordeal of the diagnostic work-up. Fostering communication between the patient

and the medical team goes a long way to help reduce anxiety and assure compliance in this most stressful context.

References

1. Greenlee RT, Murray T, Bolden S, et al. Cancer statistics. CA Cancer J Clin. 2000; 50:7–23.
2. Frank-Stromborg M, Cohen RF. Assessment and interventions for cancer detection. In: Yarbro CH, Frogge MH, Goodman M, et al., eds. Cancer Nursing Principles and Practice, 5th ed. Boston, MA: Jones and Bartlett Publishers, 2000: 150–188.
3. Cohen AM, Minsky BD, Schilsky RL. Cancer of the colon. In: DeVita V, Hellman S, Rosenberg S, eds. Cancer: Principles and Practice of Oncology, 5th ed. Philadelphia, PA: Lippincott-Raven, 1997: 1144–1187.
4. Fitzpatrick TB, Johnson RA, Wolf K, eds. Skin signs of systemic cancers. In: Color Atlas and Synopsis of Clinical Dermatology: Common and Serious Diseases, 3rd ed. New York, NY: McGraw-Hill, 1997: 504–522.
5. Weiss P, O'Rourke M. Cutaneous paraneoplastic syndromes. Clin J Oncol Nurs. 2000; 4: 257–261.
6. Blanke CD, Washington K. Paraneoplastic phenomena associated with gastrointestinal cancer. In: Raghavan D, Brecher ML, Johnson DH, eds. Textbook of Uncommon Cancer, 2nd ed. Chichester, England: John Wiley & Sons, 1999: 469–481.
7. Nicoll D, McPhee S, Chou T, et al. Common laboratory tests: Selection and interpretation. In: Nicoll D, McPhee SJ, Chou TM, et al., eds. Pocket Guide to Diagnostic Tests. Stamford, CT: Appleton & Lange, 1997: 64.
8. Macdonald JS. Carcinoembryonic antigen screening: Pros and cons. Semin Oncol. 1999; 26:556–560.
9. Desch CE, Benson AB, Smith TJ, et al. Recommended colorectal cancer surveillance guide-

lines by the American Society of Clinical Oncology. J Clin Oncol. 1999; 17:1312–1321.

10. Wu S, Hoshino DF, Zhou A, et al. Practical approaches to molecular screening of colon cancer. In: Srivastava S, Lippman S, Hong W, et al., eds. Early Detection of Cancer: Molecular Markers. Armonk, New York: Futura Publishing, 1994: 237–253.

11. Minamoto T, Mai M, Ronai Z. K-*ras* mutation: Early detection in molecular diagnosis and risk assessment of colorectal, pancreas, and lung cancers—A review. Cancer Detect Prev. 2000; 24:1–12.

12. Griffin-Brown J. Diagnostic evaluation, classification, and staging. In: Yarbro CH, Frogge MH, Goodman M, et al., eds. Cancer Nursing Principles and Practice, 5th ed. Boston, MA: Jones and Bartlett Publishers, 2000: 214–239.

13. Winawer S, Stewart E, Zauber A, et al. A comparison of colonoscopy and double contrast barium enema for surveillance after polypectomy. N Engl J Med. 2000; 342:1766–1772.

14. National Comprehensive Cancer Network. Colon and Rectal Cancer treatment Guidelines for Patients. NCCN and ACS. 2000, version 1.

15. FDA approves new device to help distinguish harmless from pre-cancerous growths in colon. Available at: http://apla.org/apla/9501/dehspm .html Accessed November 16, 2000.

16. Heneghan JP, Salem RR, Lange RC, et al. Transrectal sonography in staging rectal carcinoma: The role of gray-scale, colorflow, and Doppler imaging analysis. AJR Am J Roentgenol. 1997; 169:124.

17. Vignati PV, Roberts PL. Preoperative evaluation and postoperative surveillance for patients with colorectal cancer. Surg Clin North Am. 1993; 73:67–84.

18. Schwartz LH. Advances in cross-sectional imaging of colorectal cancer. Semin Oncol. 1999; 26:569–576.

19. Johnson CD, Dachman AH. CT colonography: The next colon screening examination? Radiology. 2000; 216:331–341.

20. Johnson PT, Health DG, Bliss DF, et al. Three-dimensional CT: Real-time interactive volume rendering. AJR Am J Roentgenol. 1996; 167: 581–583.

21. Akhurst T, Larson SM. Positron emission tomography imaging of colorectal cancer. Semin Oncol. 1999; 26:577–583.

22. Whiteford MH, Whiteford HM, Yee LF, et al. Usefulness of FDG-PET scan in the assessment of suspected metastatic or recurrent adenocarcinoma of the colon and rectum. Dis Colon Rectum. 2000; 43:759–766.

23. Le Voyer TE, Sigurdson ER, Hanlon AL, et al. Colon cancer survival is associated with increasing number of lymph nodes removed. A secondary analysis of INT-0089. Proceedings of the American Society of Clinical Oncologists, 2000; 19:925 (abstr).

24. McLeod HL, Murray GI. Tumour markers of prognosis in colorectal cancer. Br J Cancer. 1999; 79:191–203.

25. Johnston PG, Fisher ER, Rockette HE, et al. The role of thymidylate synthase expression in prognosis and outcome of adjuvant chemotherapy in patients with rectal cancer. J Clin Oncol. 1994; 12:2640–2647.

26. Cheng JD, Werness BA, Babb JS, et al. Paradoxical correlations of cyclin-dependent kinase inhibitors p21waf1/cip1 and p27kip1 in metastatic colorectal carcinoma. Clin Cancer Res. 1999; 5:1057–1062.

CHAPTER 6 | Treatment Decision Making

Marilyn Mulay, RN, MS, OCN

Introduction

Surgery has always been the first-line treatment for colorectal cancer (CRC). Chemotherapy and radiation also have been used both in the adjuvant setting and in the setting of advanced disease in most cancer centers. However, because of toxicities associated with cytotoxic therapy, many patients and physicians do not believe that the benefits of treatment outweigh the negative effects.[1] In recent years, each treatment modality has significantly evolved, offering the patient better quality of life while receiving treatment and thereby challenging the medical community to make complicated decisions integrating the best combination of treatment options.

To begin the decision-making process, the physician must consider many factors[2]:

- Is the lesion in the colon or the rectum?
- Is it localized, or has the disease metastasized?
- What are the treatment options?
- What is the availability of new treatments?
- What are the survival benefits of each potential therapy?

- How will the treatment affect the patient's quality of life?
- What are the patient's preferences?

Treatment decisions require input from the patient, who must have relevant information about the proposed therapy, including the likely outcome of the disease and effects of treatment.[3] Clearly, the information explosion has given an individual with CRC access to a wealth of information, all of which can empower the patient, or create an information overload, leaving the patient bewildered and confused. With the diagnosis of CRC, the patient is thrust into a rapid sequence of events and life-altering decisions that have traditionally followed a relatively rigid algorithm (Figure 6.1).

Until a few years ago, the choices at each juncture were well defined, albeit limited. Today, however, although the early sequence of events remains relatively unchanged, the treatment options are vastly different.

Nurses have a significant role in the decision-making process. They are in a unique position to help patients and families sort through the

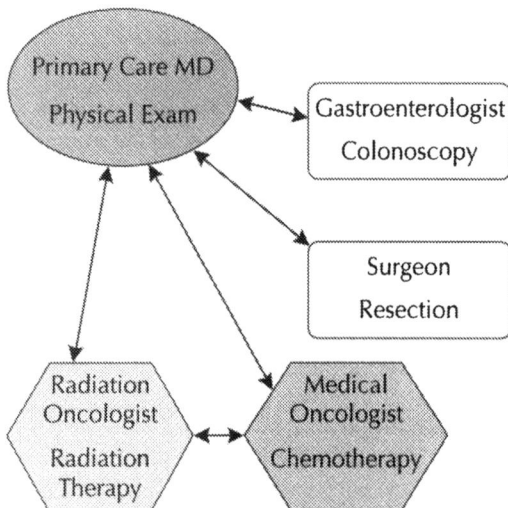

Figure 6.1 Traditional treatment algorithm for colorectal cancer.

emotions and the information to make well-informed and sound decisions. With the large number of healthcare professionals involved in an individual's care, communication and coordination of the treatment plan becomes paramount.[4] As the patient progresses from diagnosis through treatment, the need for information and support changes. Therefore, it is important that nurses understand all possible treatment options.

The Decision Pathway: Colon Cancer

The single most important prognostic feature is the stage of the disease at diagnosis, which is determined by the depth of penetration into the bowel wall, the number of positive lymph nodes, and sites of distant spread.[5] Although several factors, such as age and coexisting medical conditions, contribute to the treatment decision, an understanding of the full extent of the disease is the most critical, and dictates primary treatment.

Defining the Disease

Following a positive biopsy, the patient is typically referred to a surgeon for resection of the malignancy. Unless emergency surgery is needed to relieve an obstruction, a patient should have radiographic evaluation of the chest, abdomen, and pelvis *prior* to surgery in an attempt to define the full scope of disease.

Approximately 25% of newly diagnosed patients will have synchronous lesions outside of the colon or rectum. Recall that small lesions (< 1 cm) may not be visible on computerized tomography (CT) scan; therefore, radiographic scanning may not always show metastatic disease.

Understanding the full scope of the disease prior to the initial surgery is important, because if metastatic disease is found during presurgi-

cal staging, the primary treatment plan may change:

Original Plan	New Plan Because of Metastases
Surgery ⇓ Colon resection	No surgery if widespread disease *or* Concurrent resection of isolated metastasis

A rush to surgery without comprehensive staging can lead to inadequate or inappropriate initial treatment, with potentially disastrous results for the patient.

Tumor Markers

Cancer cells and normal cells affected by cancer cells produce substances or antigens called *tumor markers*. These tumor markers are released into the bloodstream and can be measured. To date, tumor markers are not helpful screening or diagnostic tools, but can be useful in assessing known disease.

In CRC, in addition to the standard laboratory work, complete blood count (CBC), and chemistry panel, the tumor marker carcinoembryonic antigen (CEA) should also be drawn. CEA is not specific to CRC; elevated levels can be found in other gastrointestinal cancers, as well as breast and lung cancers. Not every patient with CRC will have an elevated CEA; therefore, its use to follow disease status must be done with caution. Treatment decisions ideally should not be based on tumor marker values alone, but should be used in conjunction with other diagnostic tools.

Knowing the preoperative CEA level can be valuable. The preoperative CEA level is a good predictor of long-term survivability. The estimated 5-year survival rate of patients with a normal CEA is 60%, as compared with 4% in those patients with an elevated CEA.[6] CEA is considered normal if it is less than 2.5 ng/mL, or less than 10 ng/mL in smokers. Values in excess of these are associated with malignancy. If the CEA level is elevated prior to surgery, expect that it will drop after resection. If the CEA remains elevated postoperatively, it may indicate that there are other still undefined areas of disease requiring further work-up. Some physicians will also draw a carbohydrate cell surface antigen (CA19-9). However, its relationship to CRC is less specific than the CEA.[7,8]

Surgical Staging

During surgical resection of the primary tumor, the surgeon visually and manually explores the abdominal and pelvic cavities. The liver is palpated and peritoneal surfaces are visualized. During the primary resection for colon and rectal cancers, local lymph nodes are removed and analyzed for the presence of microscopic metastasis. With the information from the surgical pathology report, the surgeon makes the final determination of the stage of the disease.

Important Surgical Considerations

Complications of bowel surgery are often related to an inadequate preoperative bowel preparation. Patients are required to maintain a clear liquid diet for a minimum of 2 days, then drink a bitter-tasting solution, and follow a prescribed regimen of oral antibiotics. Even in fully functioning patients, the execution of the bowel preparation is demanding and can leave the patient quite weak.

Assessment of the patient's ability to successfully complete the required bowel preparation is a vital requirement. Nurses must determine whether the patient is able to understand the regimen and is physically capable of managing the preparation at home. Preoperative hospitalization of elderly or frail patients, to achieve a good bowel preparation, may avoid

postoperative complications and prolonged hospitalization requiring more surgery or a delay in further treatment.

Other complications of colorectal surgery can include the following:

- Anastamotic leak
- Intraabdominal abscess
- Staphylococcal enteritis
- Large-bowel obstruction
- Injury to the genitourinary tract
- Sexual dysfunction[9]

Early-Stage Disease

Seventy-five percent of all cases of CRC are diagnosed at an early stage, and the disease is resected with a curative intent.[10] For this patient population, treatment is well defined.

In spite of the variety of systems that are used to define the stages of CRC (as discussed in Chapter 5), the Astler-Coller system is utilized here to help define treatment options (Table 6.1).

CARCINOMA IN SITU

Typically found incidentally during routine colonoscopy, at this stage, carcinoma in situ remains confined to the head of a polyp and can be completely removed by endoscopic polypectomy. Thereafter, an annual colonoscopy should be done to monitor for new sites of disease. New

polyps can be removed during the colonoscopy. According to the widely recognized National Comprehensive Cancer Network (NCCN) guidelines, if the annual colonoscopy is negative, a colonoscopy can then be done every 3 years.[14]

STAGES A AND B₁

If the cancer has spread to the stalk of the polyp or has invaded the bowel wall (stage A), or has invaded the muscularis and serosa (stage B), the affected part of the colon and adjacent lymph nodes must be removed (Figure 6.2). The resection is typically done by exploratory laparotomy, excising the lesion with 2- to 5-cm margins, and creating an anastomosis between healthy tissue.

Performing the resection through a laparoscopic approach has been touted as lessening the patient's discomfort and shortening recov-

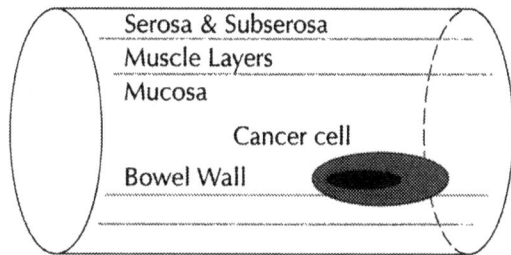

Figure 6.2 Colorectal cancer within the colonic structures.

Table 6.1   Staging Systems for Colorectal Cancer

AJCC/UICC	TNM			Dukes Stage	Astler-Coller
Stage 0	Tis	N0	M0	—	—
Stage I	T1	N0	M0	A	A
	T2	N0	M0	A	B1
Stage II	T3	N0	M0	B	B2
	T4	N0	M0	B	B3
Stage III	T_{any}	N1	M0	C	C1
	T_{any}	N2	M0	C	C2, C3
Stage IV	T_{any}	N_{any}	M1	—	D

ery time. Laparoscopic surgery, however, does not allow the surgeon to fully explore the pelvic cavity. Opponents of this approach believe that the introduction of the laparoscope might cause seeding, or that small lesions may be difficult to identify, resulting in resection of the wrong segment of the bowel.[11] Trials are under way to determine to utility of this approach.

Because the risk of recurrence in stage B_1 cancer is low, it is generally accepted that adjuvant chemotherapy is not necessary.[12] Nonetheless, following resection, vigilant surveillance is important. Eighty percent of patients who have recurrence do so within 2 years of their primary tumor treatment.[13] In addition to an annual colonoscopy, patients should have physical examinations (PEs) every 3 months for the first 2 years that include testing for occult blood and digital rectal exams. If no recurrence is found, the interval for PEs can be lengthened to every 6 months for 3 years, with a colonoscopy every 3 years.[14]

Invasive Disease

When the cancerous lesion extends *through* the bowel wall, the disease is classified as stage B_2. Controversy has surrounded the use of adjuvant therapy for patients with this stage of disease. Features of a patient's disease that may influence the physician's treatment decision about the specific regimens are the following:

- Poorly differentiated disease
- Bowel perforation
- Obstruction
- Positive surgical margins
- Possibly incomplete removal of all disease
- Risk for dissemination of a cancer that penetrates the muscularis[14]

A study, published in 1995 and updated in 1999 by Moertel et al., concluded that patients with stage B_2 who were treated with adjuvant chemotherapy experienced a decreased relapse rate but no improvement in overall survival.[15] Results of several other trials conducted by the National Surgical Adjuvant Breast and Bowel Project (NSABP), also looking at the efficacy of adjuvant chemotherapy in stage B_2 disease, concluded that adjuvant therapy resulted in a definite survival benefit.[16] The NCCN guidelines currently recommend 5-fluorouracil (5-FU) plus leucovorin with or without radiation therapy or adjuvant therapy under the direction of a clinical trial.[14] Patients who have received adjuvant therapy must be restaged at its completion. If there is no evidence of disease, the patient typically follows the same follow-up schedule as other early-stage patients.

Opponents of adjuvant therapy believe that the potential toxicities of combination therapy outweigh the benefit and, therefore, prefer watchful waiting. Periodic PEs with testing for occult blood and serial CEAs *may* be followed as an inexpensive and noninvasive means of watching for recurrence. Radiographic evaluation is done only if the CEA level begins to rise or if the patient becomes symptomatic. However, some practitioners do not believe that serial CEAs are of any benefit and prefer to simply scan the patient at prescribed intervals or wait until the patient develops symptoms.

Disease that has progressed through the bowel and involves regional lymph nodes is classified as stage C. Surgical resection of the primary lesion and the lymph nodes remains the mainstay of treatment. The number of positive lymph nodes and the depth of penetration into the serosa have inverse relationships to survival.[17] That is, patients with a higher number of positive lymph nodes or deeper penetration through the serosa have a shorter length of survival. Stage C is divided into C_1, in which only one to three lymph nodes are involved, and C_2, involving more than three lymph nodes. Regardless of the number of involved lymph nodes, there is general agreement that all patients with stage C disease must have adjuvant therapy.

Since 1990, patients with stage III disease have received 12 months of adjuvant therapy consisting of levamisole and 5-FU. Since that time, multiple studies have been conducted using a variety of 5-FU–based regimens (weekly dosing, daily dosing, and continuous-infusion dosing) with leucovorin, first to find a better regimen and then to determine whether one regimen is superior to the other. Although different regimens work by different mechanisms and produce different toxicities, ultimately, survival was the same with the various 5-FU plus leucovorin recipes.[18] Furthermore, results from recent studies demonstrated two important factors. Adding levamisole to 5-FU and leucovorin did not enhance survival rates.[19] Moreover, when comparing 6 months of 5-FU plus leucovorin adjuvant therapy with 12 months of 5-FU plus levamisole therapy, there was no difference in disease-free survival.[20] These results have brought into question the use of adjuvant therapy containing levamisole. Therefore, the current NCCN recommendation for adjuvant therapy is 6 months of chemotherapy or the combination of 5-FU, leucovorin, and radiation therapy, if there was any perforation.[14]

Some practitioners advocate combining modalities by adding radiation to systemic chemotherapy when treating patients with T4 or N2 disease (see Staging in Chapter 5). Depending on the number of positive lymph nodes and the negative prognostic features noted previously, radiation could be used in any of the ways indicated in Figure 6.3.

After completing adjuvant therapy, to maintain vigilant surveillance for recurrent or new metastatic disease, patients should have a PE with digital rectal examination and CEA every 3 months for 2 years, and then every 6 months for the next 3 years. A colonoscopy should be done 1 year after surgery. If no suspicious polyps are found, the interval between colonosco-

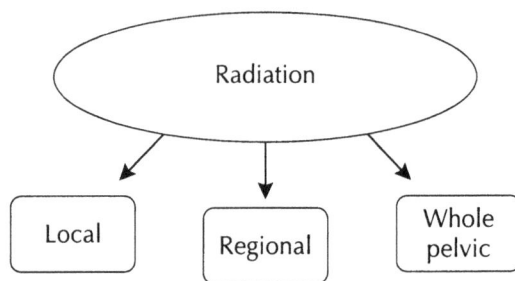

Figure 6.3   Radiation therapy methods.

pies can be extended to 3 years.[48] Recall that not all tumors express CEA and, therefore, CEA levels should not solely dictate treatment decisions. However, any increase in the CEA value above the normal range should prompt radiographic evaluation to rule out disease progression. If the patient becomes symptomatic at any time, a complete work-up should be done immediately. The primary goal of follow-up is to detect recurrent cancer at a curable stage.[11]

Patient Considerations

When adjuvant therapy has been completed, some patients have a psychological separation anxiety from their physician. In spite of the time and travel commitment the patient has made to the therapy, there is a certain comfort in knowing that someone is checking every week to make sure the cancer has not returned. Nurses should bear in mind the bittersweet effect the end of treatment can have on some patients. Referral to a support group of cancer survivors may provide great benefit for these patients.

Conversely, other patients may feel that the end of therapy heralds the final chapter in their cancer experience. This group of patients may simply disappear and refuse to come in for follow-up visits. Nurses must assess into which category each patient falls and counsel the patient appropriately to ensure the necessary surveillance without instilling undue fear.

Metastatic Disease

Disease that has invaded the bowel wall and traveled to distant organs or lymph nodes at initial diagnosis is defined as advanced disease, stage IV. Treatment decision making involves defining which therapy or combination of therapies should be utilized. NCCN recommendations for the treatment of metastatic CRC are shown in Figures 6.4 and 6.5 (pages 88 and 89).

SURGICAL INTERVENTION

At the time of diagnosis, 19% of all patients present with advanced disease.[21] The number and location of metastatic lesions dictate whether the metastases are amenable to surgical intervention. During surgery, a finding of peritoneal metastases or extensive intraabdominal nodal metastases should not deter surgical resection of the primary tumor.[11] If, during presurgical radiographic staging, possible metastatic lesions are seen, the physician may opt for a CT-guided needle biopsy. The pathology will clarify whether these lesions are indeed metastatic disease, benign processes, or, more rarely, another primary cancer.

If, for example, an enlarged ovary is seen on CT, it is extremely important to know whether the patient has CRC with metastasis to the ovary or, instead, a primary ovarian cancer. An error in the initial diagnosis can have devastating results for the patient. Occasionally during surgery, further evaluation of an area is required to fully appreciate metastasis. Intraoperative ultrasonography is sometimes utilized for this purpose.

LIVER METASTASES

Approximately 20% of patients will present with liver metastases at diagnosis; another 20% to 30% will develop liver metastases after their primary treatment.[22] Approximately one-fourth of patients with liver metastases can be treated only with regional therapies directed toward their liver tumors; such therapies can result in a 24% to 38% 5-year survival.[23] Patients with surgically accessible, small (1–2 cm), and fewer than four metastatic lesions in the liver and no other known metastases are candidates for surgical resection, ablation by cryosurgery (freezing), or radiofrequency (heating).[24] Although hepatic resection is believed to provide the best outcome, the overall 5-year survival rate is still low—20% to 40%.[25] Surgical resection or ablative therapy can be done either at the time of the resection of the primary lesion or later, to remove small metastatic deposits after systemic chemotherapy has shrunk the size of the original lesions. Individual lesions may be resected at the time of recurrence.

Combining surgical resection with cryotherapy may convert what was previously believed to be unresectable disease to one that is resectable. Factors influencing the decision to use cryotherapy or radiofrequency ablation are the following:

- No more than four lesions
- Tumors that are less than 5 cm in diameter
- Lesions that are not in close proximity to major vascular structures or bile ducts

Typically, patients with more than four tumors have more, as yet undetectable, hepatic lesions. In such cases, cryotherapy would not be curative. Large lesions or those close to major structures are difficult to safely freeze, heat, or resect.[23] Some surgeons may opt to attempt the procedure on such patients, leaving the final decision to direct visualization of the liver or the intraoperative ultrasound.

Other direct modalities, such as percutaneous acetic acid injection, percutaneous hot saline injection, high-intensity focused ultrasound, interstitial laser photocoagulation,

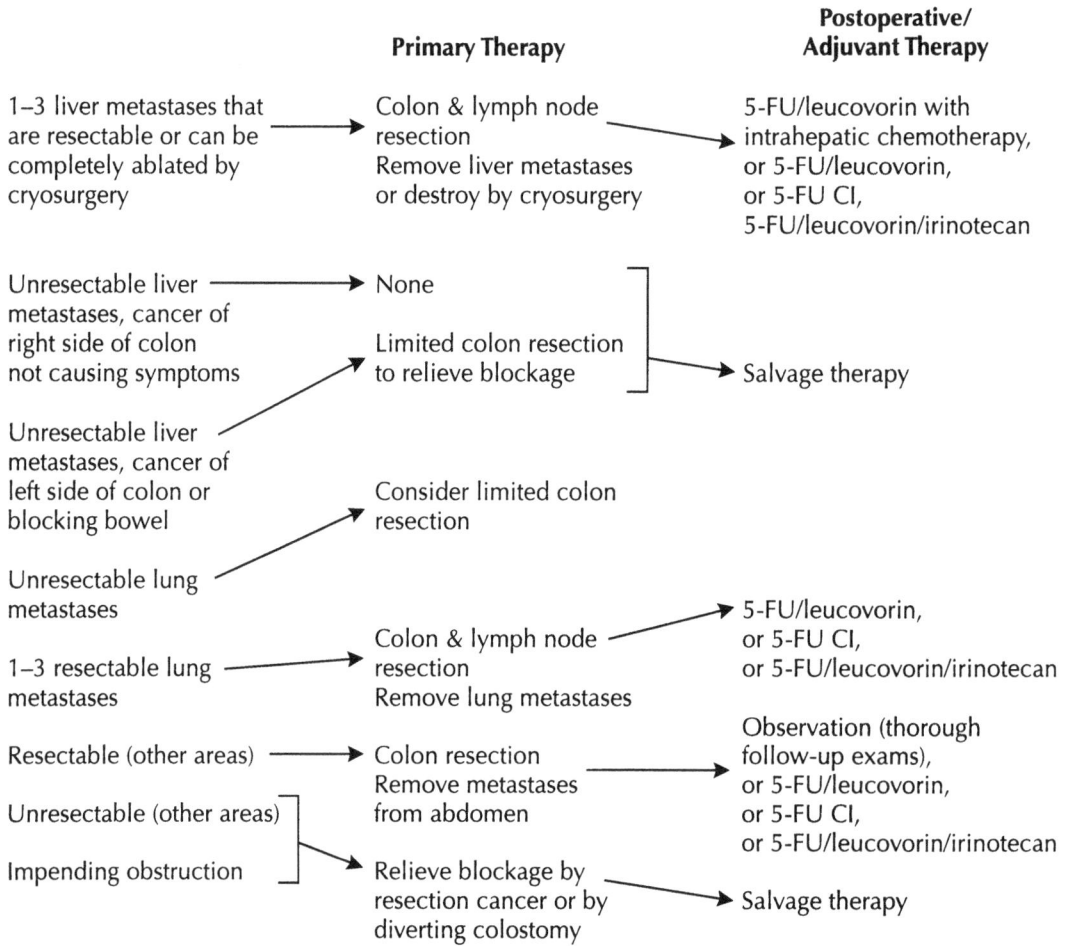

Figure 6.4   NCCN recommendations for primary and postoperative/adjuvant therapies for metastatic colorectal cancer.

Source: Reprinted by permission of the National Comprehensive Cancer Network and the American Cancer Society, Inc.

microwave coagulation therapy, and electrolysis, are being developed, though used in primary hepatoma rather than liver metastases. These methods have not been subjected to clinical trials, and are therefore unproved and not considered the standard of care.[26]

Because liver metastases receive approximately 95% of their blood supply from the hepatic artery, therapy with regional hepatic

arterial chemotherapy is often recommended. This therapy requires surgery to place a pump in the patient's abdominal cavity, with a catheter directly inserted into the hepatic artery. Studies are currently underway, looking at the use of hepatic artery infusion (HAI) after hepatic resection (adjuvant therapy) or as treatment in the setting of unresectable liver lesions.

The use of regional therapy, with or without

**Salvage Therapy of
Recurrent or Metastatic Cancer**

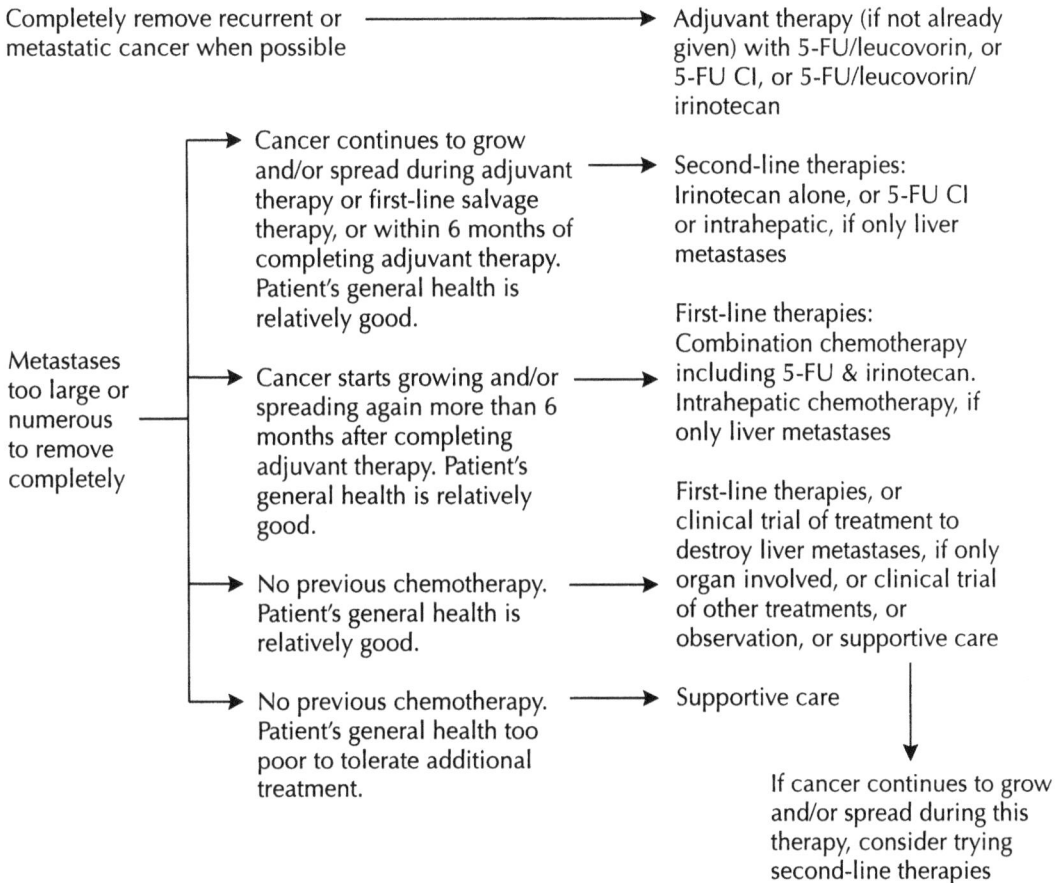

Completely remove recurrent or →→→→→→→ Adjuvant therapy (if not already
metastatic cancer when possible   given) with 5-FU/leucovorin, or
                                                5-FU CI, or 5-FU/leucovorin/
                                                irinotecan

Cancer continues to grow
and/or spread during adjuvant →→→ Second-line therapies:
therapy or first-line salvage   Irinotecan alone, or 5-FU CI
therapy, or within 6 months of   or intrahepatic, if only liver
completing adjuvant therapy.   metastases
Patient's general health is
relatively good.

First-line therapies:
Combination chemotherapy
Metastases   Cancer starts growing and/or →→→ including 5-FU & irinotecan.
too large or   spreading again more than 6   Intrahepatic chemotherapy, if
numerous   months after completing   only liver metastases
to remove   adjuvant therapy. Patient's
completely   general health is relatively
                                    good.

                                                                     First-line therapies, or
                                                                     clinical trial of treatment to
                                                                     destroy liver metastases, if only
                                    No previous chemotherapy. →→→ organ involved, or clinical trial
                                    Patient's general health is   of other treatments, or
                                    relatively good.   observation, or supportive care

                                    No previous chemotherapy. →→→ Supportive care
                                    Patient's general health too
                                    poor to tolerate additional
                                    treatment.   If cancer continues to grow
                                                                                    and/or spread during this
                                                                                    therapy, consider trying
                                                                                    second-line therapies

Figure 6.5   NCCN recommendations for salvage therapy of recurrent or metastatic colorectal cancer.
Source: Reprinted by permission of the National Comprehensive Cancer Network and the American Cancer Society, Inc.

systemic therapy, after hepatic resection is an area of active research, albeit an area with controversial results. A survival benefit for patients who are given adjuvant chemotherapy following hepatic resection has been reported by Kokudo et al.[27] Another study, published in 1999, showed that of 156 patients randomized to treatment with HAI with floxuridine (FUDR) plus intravenous 5-FU or systemic therapy alone following hepatic resection, 86% versus 72%, re-

spectively, were alive at 2 years.[28] Though a survival benefit was noted at 2 years, the overall survival was not statistically significant between the two treatment regimens.

Direct HAI of chemotherapy agents, such as FUDR, has demonstrated improved responses over systemic chemotherapy for patients with isolated unresectable liver disease. Studies are currently underway to evaluate the long-term use of this therapy, which to date has not been proved to positively affect overall survival. The treatment-limiting toxicities are liver toxicity and biliary stenosis.[29]

LUNG METASTASES

CRC is among the most common cancers that metastasize to the lungs. Patients may present with dyspnea, but approximately 85% of the time, patients with lung metastasis are asymptomatic.[30] Patients with surgically accessible, small metastatic lesions in the lungs may be candidates for resection; patients with four or fewer lesions have a better prognosis than individuals with more disease.[31] Patients with lesions confined to only one lung are better candidates for resection than those who have lesions in both lungs. If there are metastatic lesions in both lungs, the likelihood of micrometastases is greater.

Often, the decision about resection of lung metastases revolves around the type of resection—lobectomy versus wedge resection. The latter surgery carries less morbidity and is the preferable approach for disease that is not disseminated throughout the lungs.[32]

OTHER RESECTABLE METASTASES

Similarly, other metastases within the abdominal or pelvic cavity can be resected during the initial surgery. Because approximately 6% of women with CRC have ovarian metastases, some surgeons recommend prophylactic oophorectomy in women who are perimenopausal or postmenopausal.[33] This option should be discussed with female patients prior to the initial surgery.

UNRESECTABLE DISEASE

Patients with metastatic lesions in more than one location (e.g., lung and liver, or peritoneum and liver) typically are not considered surgically resectable. The benefits versus risk ratio must be carefully considered before surgery is chosen as the preferred treatment option. When lesions are present in several areas, the likelihood of other unappreciated lesions or micrometastasis is high. Even if all known lesions are accessible, the surgery is very debilitating and unlikely to be curative. Initiation of systemic chemotherapy is delayed while waiting for the patient to recover, giving potential micrometastasis time to grow unabated. Although the thought of the removal of all known disease is very appealing to the patient, consultation with both the medical *and* the surgical oncologists should be done prior to the final decision. Often, the decision is made to surgically remove the primary lesion to avoid future complications, such as obstruction, while not attempting to remove all sites of disease.[14]

CHEMOTHERAPY

All patients with metastatic disease at the time of diagnosis should have treatment with systemic chemotherapy. Just as in adjuvant therapy, for 40 years 5-FU had been the mainstay of chemotherapy, with many combinations and modulations showing similar survival benefits. In 1996, a new agent, irinotecan, was approved as a second-line therapy for metastatic CRC. Therefore, the common treatment algorithm at that time was a 5-FU–based regimen as the first-line treatment for metastatic disease, followed by a single agent, irinotecan, at the time of disease progression. This algorithm has changed. In a recent phase III study, conducted in the United States and Europe, patients with untreated metastatic disease were randomized to one of three arms:[34]

- 5-FU and leucovorin alone (Mayo Clinic regimen: days 1–5, every month)
- Irinotecan alone (weekly × 4 dosing at 125 mg/m^2 in a 6-week cycle)
- Combination of 5-FU, leucovorin, and irinotecan (weekly × 4 in a 6-week cycle)

Patients on the combination therapy had an increased response rate, a prolonged time to progression, and a longer survival time, without experiencing increased toxicities, compared with patients on the other two arms.[34,35] Consequently, this combination therapy recently received U.S. Food and Drug Administration (FDA) approval as the standard first-line therapy for metastatic CRC. The new algorithm, therefore, is treatment with the combination of irinotecan, 5-FU, and leucovorin at diagnosis of metastatic disease, followed by either a clinical trial investigating a second-line treatment regimen or, potentially, single-agent irinotecan.[14]

Other agents, still under investigation, are being studied as potential first-line treatments. Oxaliplatin, which is approved in Europe for the treatment of CRC, is still under investigation in the United States. The oral drug, capecitabine, which is essentially continuous-infusion 5-FU in pill form, has been approved for use in breast cancer, though many physicians are prescribing it "off-label" for CRC patients. Other exciting novel agents are also under development, such as multitargeted antifolate drugs and angiogenesis inhibitors (see Chapter 10).

Despite the new FDA recommendation, physicians are faced with a difficult treatment decision for patients with newly diagnosed metastatic disease. Some clinicians believe that using the combination of 5-FU, leucovorin, and irinotecan as first-line therapy leaves no FDA-approved treatment options if the patients' disease progresses while on therapy. These physicians may prefer to treat first with 5-FU and leucovorin and then use single-agent irinotecan at the time of disease progression. Conversely, proponents of the combination therapy believe that giving patients aggressive treatment with both drugs as first-line therapy is the best hope for avoiding treatment failure. Clinical trials utilizing novel agents or treatment approaches would then be offered as appropriate at the time of progression.

RADIATION

Radiation has limited use in the primary treatment of advanced colon cancer, but it can be considered for painful lesions that are not responding to chemotherapy. Locoregional radiation may also be recommended for patients whose tumor has perforated into the retroperitoneum, because retrospective studies have shown that the use of radiation improved local control and prolonged disease-free survival.[36]

The use of radiotherapy to the liver is limited due to the poor tolerance for radiation of normal liver tissue. Low doses of radiation—one-half of the dose needed for cell destruction—have been associated with fatal radiation hepatitis.[37]

Metastatic lesions in the bone are sometimes palliated with radiation. Small, isolated brain lesions may be treated with stereotactic surgery. More diffuse brain metastases are typically treated with whole-brain radiation.

COMPLICATIONS OF THERAPY

Patients must be carefully monitored for toxicities of therapy, specifically, myelosuppression, mucositis, and diarrhea. Nurses play an important function in ensuring that patients are knowledgeable about expected side effects and their management.

Physicians are faced with the dilemma of delivering the optimal amount of therapy to achieve the desired goal of therapy without causing severe toxicities. It is impossible to predict how an individual patient will react to therapy. Dose modifications or dosing delays can sometimes help to control side effects.

Small-bowel obstructions can occur as a result of therapy. Patients who present with vomiting, constipation, and/or diarrhea may have an obstruction. Generally, the obstruction will spontaneously resolve by holding treatment and resting the bowel. After recovery, patients can typically resume therapy, but may need a dose reduction.

The most serious of all possible complications is sepsis. Careful monitoring of patients' neutrophil counts and subsequent dose modifications are important to avoid serious problems. Patients must be well educated about febrile neutropenia and encouraged to report such symptoms immediately. Nurses and clinic support staff must understand the need for aggressive management of sepsis with intravenous antibiotics.

Recurrent Disease

Pathologic stage is the most important determinant of risk of recurrence.[38] Approximately 25% of patients who were surgically resected with curative intent will have a recurrence of disease—80% within the first 2 years following their primary treatment.[39,40] Patients may present with new symptoms, a rising CEA, or lesions identified by radiographic examination.

Sometimes, a rising CEA will suggest recurrent disease, but routine CT scans will not demonstrate any lesions. The use of magnetic resonance imaging (MRI) can help to identify illusive lesions. In addition, the use of positron emission tomography (PET) scanning may also identify lesions that are otherwise too small to visualize using conventional methods.

Most frequently, CRC recurs in the liver but may also return locally or at some other distant site. If disease appears to be isolated to a surgically resectable site, hepatectomy or repeat hepatectomy is a potentially curative treatment.[41] If recurrence is less than 6 months after completing adjuvant therapy, the treatment choices are more difficult. It is generally accepted that a recurrence after such a short period of time indicates that the cancer cells developed resistance to the drugs that were previously used.

OTHER OPTIONS

If all FDA-approved treatments have been exhausted, patients face a new set of choices. Some physicians may recommend the use of drugs that have been approved by the FDA for other diagnoses but have not shown specific efficacy in CRC. Depending on the patient's overall performance status, some physicians will recommend stopping aggressive treatment and refer the patient to hospice. The second option is participation in clinical trials, which will be discussed later in this chapter.

CASE STUDY

Dennis Lynch, a 50-year-old white man, presented to his primary care physician with a 3-month history of bloating, chest pressure, and mild fatigue. Because of his strong family history of cardiac disease and his stressful job as an investment broker, however, the initial work-up ruled out coronary artery disease as the cause of the symptoms. Initial blood work, ECG, chest x-ray, and occult blood slides did not reveal any abnormalities. However, the symptoms persisted and Dennis was sent to a gastroenterologist. During the colonoscopy, multiple polyps were found and removed; however, on the far right side of the colon, a fungating lesion, clearly cancerous, was discovered and biopsied.

The next day, Dennis returned for CT of the chest, abdomen, and pelvis, which did not reveal any suspicious lesions. The biopsy of the colonic lesion came back as poorly differentiated adenocarcinoma. During the follow-up visit with the gastroenterologist, Dennis was told that the cancer seemed to be contained and that he should be surgically curable (stage II disease), and that, following 6 months of adjuvant therapy, he could resume his active lifestyle, with quarterly check-ups.

Several weeks later, during the surgery, diffuse peritoneal metastases were found. Five lymph nodes were also removed and biopsied, which were all negative. With the metastatic findings, the final diagnosis was stage IV (Dukes' D) colon cancer.

Dennis had been riding an emotional roller coaster over the previous month: First, thinking that he had life-threatening coronary artery disease, which was, happily, ruled out. Then, the colonoscopy, with the upsetting news of a cancerous lesion; but after the CT scans, Dennis was encouraged to believe that this cancer would simply be a brief interlude in his life. Instead, he was now facing a terminal illness and an unknown future.

While Dennis was still trying to come to terms with the diagnosis, the medical oncologist was discussing the various treatment options: (1) wait and watch; (2) conventional therapy, either single-agent or combination therapy; or (3) clinical trials. The medical oncologist certainly was not recommending the watchful-waiting option. Indeed, he believed that Dennis should be aggressive in seeking treatment using the combination chemotherapy of 5-FU, leucovorin, and irinotecan. Dennis was told that the side effects were manageable and that he should be able to continue to work. He might lose his hair and have intermittent diarrhea, mouth sores, and low blood counts. He would need to be available several hours each week for blood tests and treatment. He was overloaded with information, so the office nurse helped to answer many of his questions and gave him printed material to read and share with his family.

Now, adding to his struggle to accept that a cancer was growing in his body, Dennis needed to decide what to do about treatment. Yes, he definitely wanted to do something about the cancer and prolong his life, but he wasn't planning on letting his entire office in on his private misery. He feared the loss of his job. He also did not want to deal with sympathy or talk about his illness with people who were only business acquaintances. Would he be able to maintain his privacy if he lost his hair? Would he be able to work if he had diarrhea? Would his company demand that he take a leave of absence? Would

his clients lose confidence in him and look for another broker? Maybe if he only took 5-FU and leucovorin he would be able to hide his dilemma, but could he be sacrificing his life?

At work, Dennis confided in his supervisor and a few close friends. He was assured that they would help him, with flexible hours and covering his clients so that he could do whatever he needed to do. One friend, however, could not resist telling him about his wife's cousin who had colon cancer and had an episode of awful diarrhea, couldn't eat, and landed in the hospital with fever and intravenous antibiotics. Another friend brought in some articles about alternative therapies and suggested Dennis would do well to consider them.

Dennis turned to the Internet to seek advice and found information about clinical trials that were testing new drugs. He wondered if this were the best option. Going to a chat room to talk with others who had tried that avenue, he again found ambiguous information. Some people said that they were very excited about the experimental treatment and that it did not cause any serious side effects. The wife of another patient on the same treatment was upset because her husband had died while taking that treatment, and, even though the doctors said it was because his disease had progressed rapidly, she wasn't convinced that the drug had not been at least partly responsible.

The more people Dennis spoke with, the more confused he became. He did not want to bother the medical oncologist, because he knew the doctor was very busy. But he finally did call the office and asked to speak with the nurse. She reviewed each of the therapies, resolved misconceptions, and helped Dennis to organize his priorities.

Dennis finally decided on aggressive combination therapy. He refused to think of himself as a victim of cancer and had decided to make treatment a priority over everything else at the moment. He appreciated the nurse's help in clarifying issues and knew that he had an advocate he could trust.

The Decision Pathway: Rectal Cancer

Patients diagnosed with rectal cancer often assume that surgery will result in a permanent colostomy, with devastating effects on their physical and emotional well-being. Nurses are instrumental in helping patients understand their diagnosis and treatment options and overcome the fear that comes from a lack of information or understanding. In fact, surgical advances have been made in rectal cancer to maintain urinary and sexual functions with low rates of local recurrence and prolonged survival.[42]

Staging

Preoperative determination of the location and extent of disease by physical and radiographic examination is critical to choosing the appropriate approach. In addition to CT scanning, endorectal ultrasound may yield important information about the depth of tumor penetration.[43] For purposes of defining treatment options, rectal cancer is defined by stages I through IV (see Staging in Chapter 5).

Early-Stage Disease

Patients with stage I disease—disease extending into the submucosa or muscularis propria—may be candidates for local excision if the primary tumor is mobile, smaller than 4 cm, and less than 8 cm from the anal verge.[44] If the disease is T1 (extends only to the submucosa), the patient will not need adjuvant therapy. However, if the tumor is classified as T2 (invading the muscularis propria), following the transanal

resection, the patient will be treated with radiation therapy plus chemotherapy.[14]

Patients whose tumor is larger than 4 cm, fixed to the rectal mucosa, or more than 10 cm from the anal verge will need a procedure that gives the surgeon the ability to explore the surgical field—low anterior (LA) resection or abdominoperineal (AP) resection. With the larger field, the surgeon is able to visualize and palpate the abdominal cavity. Just as during a colon resection, regional lymph nodes are removed and sent for analysis. Negative pathology eliminates the need for adjuvant chemotherapy.

By contrast, all patients who present with tumors that have grown through the wall of the rectum (T4) should receive neoadjuvant chemotherapy and radiation to reduce the size of the masses before resection is attempted.[14] If all disease is surgically resected, adjuvant chemotherapy should then be given for at least 6 months.

Regional Disease without Metastases

When patients present with involvement of regional lymph nodes (e.g., T1 or T2, N1 disease, or T3, N0, or N1 disease), the physician is faced with choices between neoadjuvant (preoperative) therapy (Figure 6.6), and adjuvant (postoperative) therapy (Figure 6.7).

The use of intraoperative electron-beam radiation therapy (IOERT) has been studied at a variety of medical centers. During surgery, following preoperative irradiation and infusional chemotherapy, the abdomen is carefully explored to determine whether there are metastases in the liver or peritoneum. If metastatic disease is found, surgery is completed without the use of IOERT. However, if no metastatic disease is found, every effort is made to resect as much disease as possible. Thorough examination of the tumor bed and abdomen is done to identify all high-risk areas and establish the IOERT field.[45]

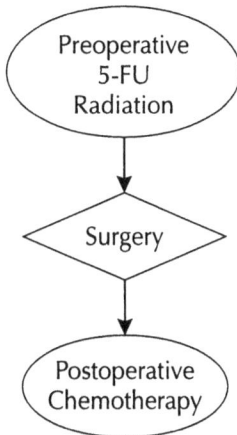

Figure 6.6 Neoadjuvant (preoperative) therapy for rectal cancer.

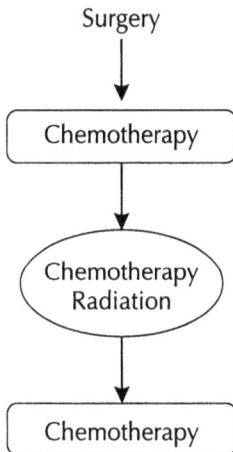

Figure 6.7 Adjuvant (postoperative) therapy for rectal cancer.

Metastatic Disease

RESECTABLE DISEASE

Patients with distant metastases fall into two categories: those whose disease is surgically resectable and those whose disease is unresectable. For patients with node-negative but distant, *resectable* disease, adjuvant chemotherapy

should be given postoperatively.[14] However, for those patients with node-positive and distant, resectable disease, radiation may be added to adjuvant chemotherapy as the best hope against treatment failure. Depending on the location of the tumor and other involved structures, a diverting colostomy may be needed to relieve or avoid a bowel obstruction. The National Comprehensive Cancer Network (NCCN) guidelines recommend that an enterstomal therapist should be consulted preoperatively if a colostomy is a possible surgical outcome.[14]

Complications of skin irritation and possible infection can be avoided with some preoperative planning. The determination of optimal placement of the stoma is best done with the patient in several positions (e.g., standing and lying), helping to identify a site that is away from the patient's normal belt line.

During surgery, every effort is made to conserve sphincter function and avoid a colostomy. In so doing, a significant amount of tumor manipulation may occur, which can result in cell shedding, which can lead to metastases.[11] All patients with metastatic disease must have postoperative chemotherapy. Again, the choice of single agent versus combination chemotherapy is presented. If neoadjuvant radiation was not used, then consideration should be given to adding postoperative radiation to the treatment plan.[45]

UNRESECTABLE DISEASE

Patients with disease that cannot be resected present a greater challenge. Neoadjuvant chemotherapy and/or radiation may be needed to reduce the size of the tumor, converting the patient to one with resectable disease and improving the outcome of surgical resection. Intraoperative photocoagulation is sometimes used to destroy diseased tissue with the use of a laser beam.[14] In addition, these patients may benefit from a combination of different radiotherapeutic approaches, such as external-beam irradiation, interstitial brachytherapy, and intra-cavitary irradiation.

In patients who have unresectable disease or are otherwise unsuitable for radical surgery, cryosurgery should be considered as a palliative treatment.[46] In such situations, cryosurgery may alleviate symptoms caused by a primary lesion or by metastatic disease.

Recurrent Disease

In spite of preoperative irradiation and chemotherapy, many of these patients will experience recurrence. The treatment of recurrent disease is dependent on the location of the recurrence and the patient's prior therapy. If the recurrence is local disease only, it may be amenable to further resection or radiation, if the patient has not received the maximum allowable radiation dose.[47]

If the disease recurrence is metastatic or diffuse, then systemic therapy must be considered. The same decision process used in colon cancer (see pages 85 and 86) should be applied here. Similarly, if all known options have been exhausted, clinical trials and supportive care are the choices.

COMPLICATIONS OF THERAPY

Patients receiving therapy for rectal cancers often experience diarrhea, myelosuppression, skin reactions, and fatigue. Diarrhea and myelosuppression are the most common complications of radiation therapy to the rectum and lower pelvis. Recall that 25% of the patient's bone marrow is in the pelvis, and thus, unless shielded adequately, could be within the radiation field. Therefore, patients receiving whole pelvic radiation are at risk of significant bone marrow store depletion. The use of radiation may, in fact, limit the amount of chemotherapy that the patient can tolerate.

Diarrhea is a complication of both chemotherapy and radiation. Therefore, patients who receive both are at high risk of diarrhea and

need to be monitored closely. Small-bowel obstruction may also be a complication with the combined-modality therapies. Dose modification and dosing delays may help control some of the symptoms, but sometimes radiation must be stopped prior to completing the full course of therapy if side effects put the patient at risk.

Radiation therapy enters the body through the skin. Current radiation techniques aim to decrease the severity of skin reactions by administering the external radiation beam from different angles. However, some degree of skin reaction is common and requires astute symptom management.

Fatigue is also a common side effect of pelvic radiation. The patient must be aware of its possibility, and the nurse must educate the patient and family about possible interventions. (See Chapter 8 for a comprehensive review of radiation therapy in patients with CRC.)

Other Factors Influencing Treatment Decision Making

Age

Patients under the age of 40, diagnosed with CRC, typically have more negative prognostic characteristics than their older counterparts, such as the following:

- Mucoid adenocarcinoma
- Higher rate of lymphatic metastases
- Delay in diagnosis
- Rapid disease progression[14]

However, it has been felt that the younger patient generally has better tolerance to the side effects caused by aggressive therapy, as opposed to the elderly patient, who is more prone to dehydration caused by diarrhea and/or mucositis. Nonetheless, many physicians prefer to begin with aggressive therapy unless a patient is particularly frail. If it is determined that a patient cannot tolerate the side effects, the treatment can be altered to either single-agent therapy or combination therapy at lower dosages. In CRC, in both the adjuvant and metastatic settings, there is growing evidence that elderly patients who have the same characteristics as younger patients (e.g., good performance status, liver function tests close to normal range) experience the same rates and types of toxicities and have the same potential benefit from chemotherapy.[35, 48–50] In a trial recently reported in the *New England Journal of Medicine*, age greater than 65 was associated with a longer time to tumor progression and a trend toward increased survival, regardless of the treatment assignment.[38]

Symptoms

It is unclear whether the presence of symptoms at diagnosis has any bearing on prognosis. For patients who are asymptomatic at diagnosis, the disease may be at an early stage. On the other hand, patients who have had mild symptoms for several months prior to diagnosis may have slow-growing disease. There is no evidence to indicate that either situation helps to define prognosis.

As the physician evaluates the patient for the best treatment option, the presence or absence of symptoms and their duration are generally only significant in their effect on the patient's general health. A patient who is severely anemic due to rectal bleeding or is malnourished due to obstructive symptoms will have less tolerance for treatment side effects. If a patient is able to regain nutritional or hemodynamic equilibrium prior to starting therapy, these factors become nonissues.

Comorbidity

Other medical conditions are only significant if there is some impact on the patient's general health. As long as coexisting conditions are well managed and under good control, they should not affect treatment decisions.

Clinical Trials

Clinical trials are important for defining the safety and efficacy of new treatments. All of the treatments in use today were first tested in clinical trials, and further progress in diagnosis and treatment is dependent on research. Therefore, every patient should be considered a potential candidate for a clinical trial.[51] Clinical research is conducted in four phases, each one designed to answer specific questions.

Phase I clinical trials test new drugs or treatments to determine the correct dose, the toxicity profile of a specific treatment or drug, and how a drug is metabolized. Small numbers of patients with many different diagnoses are given the drug in escalating doses until an unacceptable toxicity is identified. The maximum dose is defined as the highest dose that patients can tolerate without unacceptable side effects.

Typically, phase I trials test experimental drugs for which the only data on efficacy (response rates) and side effects are from laboratory and animal testing. Even if some responses are seen, because the patients have many different diagnoses with different prior therapies, no statistically significant statement can be made about efficacy. In spite of the fact that some new therapies receive a lot of media hype, no scientific information about their use in the treatment in humans is known. Therefore, only patients who have exhausted all therapies with known efficacy or who absolutely refuse conventional therapy should consider participating in phase I trials.

Phase II clinical trials are designed to define efficacy. In this phase of drug testing, entry requirements are typically more specific to achieve a more homogeneous group of participants. For example, one study may require all participants to have untreated metastatic CRC.

All of the patients are given the same dose of the investigational drug on the same schedule. At prescribed intervals, the patients are re-staged. As long as the disease has not grown significantly from the baseline staging, the patient may continue to receive the investigational drug. At the end of the study, the number of patients who have shown a response determines the drug efficacy in that disease. For example, 30 patients with untreated CRC may be enrolled in a study; if 6 patients show an objective response, the drug will be said to have a 20% efficacy.

Phase II clinical trials offer patients a somewhat better chance at receiving effective treatment. Sometimes, drugs being tested in the United States have already been approved in Europe and, therefore, more information may be available about efficacy.

Phase III clinical trials are designed to compare a standard therapy with an investigational therapy. These trials are usually conducted at many clinical centers, sometimes 50 to 100, and enroll several hundred patients. The study typically has two or more treatment arms, and patients are randomly assigned to one arm. For example, a large phase III study was conducted to determine the efficacy in untreated metastatic CRC when patients were treated with 5-FU and leucovorin alone, irinotecan alone, or a combination of 5-FU, leucovorin, and irinotecan. Over 600 patients were enrolled and randomly assigned to one of the three arms. At the time of this study, irinotecan had already received FDA approval as second-line therapy, after patients had failed 5-FU therapy. The results of the study showed that patients who were treated with the combination therapy had a prolonged time to recurrence over either one of the other two arms. As a result of the study, the FDA approved the combination therapy for first-line therapy in April 2000.[39]

It is important to note that all of the cancer patients who participate in clinical trials in the United States receive treatment intended to treat their disease. No placebos are given. Some studies allow patients to cross over to a different arm if their disease progresses or if they experience unacceptable toxicity. However, even if that is not allowed, patients who receive an investigational therapy can withdraw from the clinical trial and go on to receive further therapy. That therapy may either be an FDA-approved treatment or one that is part of another clinical trial.

Only 3% of all patients with cancer participate in clinical trials. Most likely, this is because many patients are unaware of the existence of this treatment option. However, some patients may also fear that they will be treated as a number. The opposite, in fact, is the case. Because clinical trials set forth very rigid requirements for monitoring, patients are carefully followed. Participation in a clinical trial may be the best way to receive an effective treatment years before it is commercially available.

Nurses are in a unique position to educate patients about clinical trials and help them find cancer centers that are participating in research. Clinical trials can offer hope to patients who may be told that there is no other treatment option. It is also important, however, that nurses help patients understand the goals of clinical research and to, therefore, have realistic expectations from their participation.

Palliative Care

Palliative care is often equated with a do-nothing, keep them comfortable philosophy. Today, however, the definition of *palliative care* has changed. Even when there is no expectation of response, treatment can be given to palliate symptoms. The treatment decisions can include not only pain medications and blood transfusions, but also radiation and chemotherapy. Some hospices and insurance companies are beginning to recognize the benefit of palliative care.

Physicians often wait to refer a patient for hospice services until the patient is very debilitated and close to death. Sometimes, the delay in referral is due to the possibility that the patient may believe a hospice referral is a sign that the physician has given up. The medical community has an obligation to educate patients and families about the benefits of hospice care not only for the patient, but also for the family. Although a life expectancy of less than 6 months is a criterion for hospice referral, there are no rules that preclude a renewal of hospice benefits once the 6-month mark is reached. Similarly, a patient may withdraw from hospice if a new treatment option becomes available.

Hospices offer many wonderful services to help patients and their families adjust to the diagnoses and changes in lifestyle. Hospice benefits typically provide equipment and services without waiting for insurance authorizations. It is important not to overlook hospice referrals as a treatment option.

Patient Decision-making Issues

Role Adjustment

With the diagnosis of CRC, a fully functioning adult immediately becomes a *patient*. The changing role often takes a person from a position of control and self-assurance to a world of new terminology, loss of control, and fear of what the future will bring. It is not uncommon for patients to feel anger, frustration, and isolation.[52] The most intelligent person can immediately feel ignorant and helpless. Some patients cannot accept the situation and simply refuse to deal in reality. Others struggle to maintain control by rejecting sound medical advice and turning away from treatment recommendations. Still others may turn toward alternative, sometimes harmful, or useless therapies in an effort to assert their will.

Family Adjustment

At the time of diagnosis, the families are often faced with several issues: Is my loved one going to die? What will the financial burdens be? What can I do to help? Will I be strong enough, both mentally and physically, to face the future?

Having a supportive family is a great asset to a patient. However, some patients simply surrender their decision-making privileges to a family member either because the patient is unable to cope or because the family member's preferences simply overpower the patient. Strong-willed family members may overtly force unwanted decisions on a patient; weak, dependent family members may covertly, even inadvertently, force decisions.

Information Gathering

As the news of the diagnosis travels, everyone begins to gather information to "help." Family, friends, and acquaintances offer stories of others with the "same diagnosis," suggestions about treatment options, and warnings about side effects. Quasimedical articles in every popular magazine are clipped and mailed to the patient. Internet chat rooms are used to gather anecdotal information. Clearly, this kind of "help" can be very detrimental and, moreover, add to the confusion that the patient is already experiencing. Although the Internet contains a wealth of valuable information, understanding what is applicable to a specific patient's situation can be difficult without prior medical knowledge.

As noted at the beginning of this chapter, patients are often moved swiftly from the primary physician with whom there has been a long-standing, trusting relationship, to a gastroenterologist, a surgeon, and then a medical and/

or radiation oncologist. Each step along the way, the patient may be given a volume of information and asked to make decisions, some with potentially devastating consequences.

The Nurse's Role in Decision Making

Although oncology nurses are typically not involved in the early diagnostic process, they often meet the patient and family shortly after the initial diagnosis is made. Nurses are invaluable resources as educators and patient advocates.

Adjustment to the Diagnosis

Information can return power to a patient who is feeling helpless. Nurses must assist patients in understanding and interpreting information about the diagnosis and stage of the illness. This is the first step in helping them accept the diagnosis and begin to deal with the decisions that lie ahead.

It is important to start by asking the patient to verbalize his or her understanding of the diagnosis. Some patients will not have heard anything that was already said. As much as time will allow, provide information in small doses, asking the patient to repeat the information in their own words. The use of pictures, especially when discussing surgery, is very helpful. Take care to use layperson's language, regardless of the educational level of the patient.

Sometimes, the greater challenge is assisting the patient's family to cope with the diagnosis. Often, the family's anxiety overrides the patient's concerns and interferes with the patient's ability to concentrate on decision making. When the patient has always been the emotional strength in a family, this burden will typically remain, sometimes leaving the patient with no one on whom to lean. Family members may also have agendas that are different from each other's or from the patient's.

Clarifying Misconceptions

As discussed earlier, patients often have misconceptions, either through their own misunderstanding of information or because of misinformation given by a well-meaning friend. As mentioned earlier, the Internet, a source of valuable information, can also be a source of misconceptions. Chat rooms prevail, and although some messages provide good resource material, patients must be cautioned about those who use this venue to vent their frustrations and fears.

Patients searching for better results than standard therapies provide often explore alternative therapies. Do not dismiss these patient queries as quackery or not worthy of discussion. Proponents of questionable therapies use testimonials from "cured" patients as proof that the treatment works.[53] Typically, this type of therapy has not been subjected to the rigors of clinical trials or peer review. It is important to discuss this emotionally charged area of information logically. To stay abreast of current information in the area of alternative therapies, contact the American Cancer Society at 1-800-227-2345 or visit the website, called "Questionable Cancer Therapies", at www.quackwatch.com/01QuackeryRelatedTopics/cancer.html.

Understanding Side Effects

During consultations with patients, physicians typically concentrate their discussions on the disease and treatment options. Side effects of the treatment are reviewed, but the discussion of their management is rarely discussed in detail. Often the patients' major concerns surround the effects of the therapy on their quality of life or on their appearance.

Nurses can provide patients with important information that helps them not only cope with the treatment, but also tolerate the therapy. Successful management of side effects, for example, diarrhea and vomiting, has a significant impact on the patient's ability to receive maximum doses. Suggestions about wigs, scarves, and makeup can help a female patient maintain her appearance and, often, fight depression. Helping patients differentiate between the symptoms of the cancer and the side effects of the therapy will also help them successfully manage the therapy. Understanding what to expect and how to cope with the symptoms or side effects helps patients make decisions that fit into their lifestyles.

Exploring Patient Preferences

Nurses should encourage patients to share their thoughts and concerns. Do not presume that you already know what the patient is thinking. Ask open-ended questions, allowing the patients to express their own thoughts. Developing an open relationship is imperative for patients to trust and confide in the nurse. Patients often perceive that the physicians are too busy to be bothered, but they are willing to talk with nurses if given the chance.

Providing References

Many good written resources are available to help patients and their families understand CRC. The American Cancer Society has many publications available, including a book, *Colorectal Cancer*, by Bernard Levin, MD. Pharmaceutical companies that market chemotherapy agents and devices used in CRC often provide patient education materials. These are valuable resources for helping patients achieve a better understanding of the situation and therefore make more informed decisions. (See Chapter 15 for additional resource suggestions.)

Some patients and families benefit from support groups. Others benefit from private discussions with social workers or spiritual counselors. Other patients, however, do not find comfort in talking about the situation. Knowing your patients and their preferences will help you to define the best way to support them through the decision-making process.

Conclusion

Compared with a decade ago, there are now many CRC treatment options, and more on the horizon. This is an exciting time for oncology nurses; however, the challenge of staying abreast of the new surgical approaches, chemotherapy agents, radiation, and novel treatment options can be overwhelming. Understanding the treatment options and the rationales that support them are crucial to the most important nursing role—patient advocate.

Acknowledgment

The author acknowledges Lee S. Rosen, MD, for his professional contribution.

References

1. Kemeny N. Colorectal cancer—An undertreated disease. Anticancer Drugs. 1996; 7(6):623–629.
2. Redmond K. Treatment choices in advanced cancer: Issues and perspectives. Eur J Cancer Care. 1998; 7(1):31–39.
3. Northover JMA. Staging and management of colorectal cancer. World J Surg. 1997; 21: 672–677.
4. Hoebler L. Colon and rectal cancer. In: Groenwald SL, Frogge MH, Goodman M, et al., eds. Cancer Nursing: Principles and Practice, 4th ed. Sudbury, MA: Jones and Bartlett Publishers, 1997: 1036–1054.

5. Lindmark G, Gerdin B. Prognostic predictors in colorectal cancer. Dis Colon Rectum. 1994; 37: 1219.

6. Girard P, Ducreux M, Bladeyrou P, et al. Surgery for lung metastases from colorectal cancer: Analysis of prognostic factors. J Clin Oncol. 1996; 14(7):2047–2053.

7. Bast RC, Bates S, Bredt A, et al. Clinical practice guidelines for the use of tumor markers in breast and colorectal cancer. Adopted on May 17, 1996 by the American Society of Clinical Oncology. J Clin Oncol. 1996; 14(10):2843–2877.

8. Bast RC, Desch CE, Hayes DF, et al. 1997 update of recommendations for the use of tumor markers in breast and colorectal cancer. Adopted on November 7, 1997 by the American Society of Clinical Oncology. J Clin Oncol. 1998; 16: 793–795.

9. Hoebler L, Irwin MM. Gastrointestinal tract cancer: Current knowledge, medical treatment, and nursing management. Oncol Nurs Forum. 1992; 19:1403–1415.

10. Nivatvongs S. Surgical management of early colorectal cancer. World J Surg. 2000. On-line publication, 3 July 2000. Available at http://link.springer-ny.com/search.htm Accessed August 6, 2000.

11. Cohen AM, Minsky BD, Schilsky RL. Cancer of the colon. In: DeVita VT Jr, Rosenberg SA, Hellman S, eds. Cancer Principles & Practice of Oncology, 5th ed. Philadelphia, PA: Lippincott-Raven, 1997: 1144–1197.

12. Adjuvant therapy for patients with colon and rectum cancer. NIH Consensus Statement Online. April 16–18, 1990; 8(4):1–25. Available at: http://isis.nlm.nih.gov/nih/cdc/www/79txt.html Accessed August 6, 2000.

13. Follow-up after primary therapy for colorectal cancer. Available at: http://intouch.cancernetwork.com/canmed/Ch121/121-17.htm Accessed August 6, 2000.

14. Benson AB, Engstrom PE, Gansler T, et al.

Colon and Rectal Cancer, Treatment Guidelines for Patients. Atlanta, GA: National Comprehensive Cancer Network & American Cancer Society, 2000.

15. Moertel CG, Fleming TR, MacDonald JS, et al. Intergroup study of fluorouracil plus levamisole as adjuvant therapy for Stage II/ Stage B_2 colon cancer. J Clin Oncol. 1999; 13(12):2936–2943.

16. Mamounas E, Wieand S, Wolmark N, et al. Comparative efficacy of adjuvant chemotherapy in patients with Stage B versus Stage C colon cancer: Results from four National Surgical Adjuvant Breast and Bowel Project Adjuvant Studies (C-01, C-02, C-03, and C-04). J Clin Oncol. 1999; 17(5):1349–1355.

17. Nathanson SD, Schultz L, Tilley B, et al. Carcinoma of the colon and rectum: A comparison of staging classifications. Am Surg. 1996; 52: 428–438.

18. Leichman CG, Fleming TR, Muggia FM, et al. Phase II study of fluorouracil and its modulation in advanced colorectal cancer: A Southwest Oncology Group study. J Clin Oncol. 1995; 13(6): 1303–1311.

19. Haller DG, Catalano PJ, MacDonald JS, et al. Fluorouracil, leucovorin, and levamisole adjuvant therapy for colon cancer: Five year final report of INT-0089. Proc Am Soc Clin Oncol. 1998; 982:256a (abstr).

20. O'Connell MJ, Laurie JA, Kahn M, et al. Prospectively randomized trial of postoperative adjuvant chemotherapy in patients with high-risk colon cancer. J Clin Oncol. 1998; 16(1): 295–300.

21. Groenwald SL, Frogge MH, Goodman M, et al. Colon and rectal cancer. In: Comprehensive Cancer Nursing Review, 4th ed. Sudbury, MA: Jones and Bartlett Publishers, 1998: 410–419.

22. Ellis Fischel Cancer Center. Cryotherapy for hepatic colorectal carcinoma metastases. Available at: www.muhealth.org/~ellisfischel/cryotherapy.shtml Accessed August 6, 2000.

23. Yoon SS, Tanabe KK. Surgical treatment and

other regional treatments for colorectal cancer liver metastases. Oncologist. 1999; 4(3):197–208.

24. Fong Y, Cohen AM, Forner JG, et al. Liver resection for colorectal metastases. J Clin Oncol. 1997; 15:938–946.

25. Nakamura S, Suzuki S, Baba S. Resection of liver metastases of colorectal carcinoma. World J Surg. 1997; 21:741–747.

26. Berry DP, Maddern GJ. Other in situ ablative techniques for unresectable liver tumors. Asian J Surg. 2000; 23(1):22–31.

27. Kokudo N, Ski M, Ohta H, et al. Effects of systemic and regional chemotherapy after hepatic resection for colorectal metastases. Ann Surg Oncol. 1998; 5(8):706–712.

28. Kemeny N, Juang Y, Cohen AM, et al. Hepatic arterial infusion of chemotherapy after resection of hepatic metastases from colorectal cancer. N Engl J Med. 1999; 341(27):2039–2048.

29. Kemeny N, Ron IG. Hepatic arterial chemotherapy in metastatic colorectal patients. Semin Oncol. 1999; 26(5):524–535.

30. McCormick PM, Martini N. A current view of surgical management of pulmonary metastases. In: Economou SG, Witt TR, Deziel DJ, et al. Adjuncts to Cancer Surgery. Philadelphia, PA: Lea & Febiger, 1991: 246–251.

31. Avis F. Surgical treatment of isolated metastases to the liver, lungs, and brain. In: Wittes RE, ed. Manual of Oncologic Therapeutics. Philadelphia, PA: Lippincott, 1991: 308–309.

32. Groen KA. Primary and metastatic liver cancer. Semin Oncol Nurs. 1999; 15(1):48–57.

33. Birnkrant A, Sampson J, Sugarbaker PH. Ovarian metastases from colorectal cancer. Dis Colon Rectum. 1986; 29:767.

34. Saltz LB, Cox JV, Blanke C, et al. Irinotecan plus fluorouracil and leucovorin for metastatic colorectal cancer. N Engl J Med. 2000; 343(13): 905–914.

35. Douillard JY, Cunningham D, Roth AD, et al. Irinotecan combined with fluorouracil com-

pared with fluorouracil alone as first-line treatment for metastatic colorectal cancer: A multicentre randomised trial. Lancet. 2000; 355(9209):1041–1047.

36. Willett CG, Kaufman DS, Efird J, et al. Postoperative radiation therapy for high-risk colon carcincoma. J Clin Oncol. 1993; 11(6):1112–1119.

37. Stubbs RS, Cannan R. Active treatment of colorectal hepatic metastases. Available at: www .rnzcgp.org.nz/nzfp/ISSUES/AUG99/orstubbs .htm Accessed August 6, 2000.

38. Who is at risk for recurrence after colon and rectal cancer resection? Available at: http:/// isis.nlm.nih.gov/nih/cdc/www/79txt.html Accessed August 6, 2000.

39. Follow-up after primary therapy for colorectal cancer. Available at: http://intouch .cancernetwork.com/myths/colon/CH121/121-17 .htm Accessed August 6, 2000.

40. Steele G Jr. Colorectal cancer. In: Murphy GP, Lawrence W, Lenhard RE, eds. American Cancer Society Textbook of Clinical Oncology, 2nd ed. Atlanta, GA: ACS, 1995: 247.

41. Sugarbaker P. Repeat hepatectomy for colorectal metastases. J Hepato-Biliary-Pancreatic Surg. 1999; 6(1):30–38.

42. Muto T, Watanabe T. Special report: Colorectal carcinoma: Recent advances in its biology and treatment. J Cancer Res Clin Oncol. 1999; 125(3/4):245–253.

43. Nakazawa S. Recent advances in endoscopic ultrasonography. J Gastroenterol. 2000; 35(4): 257–260.

44. Willet CG, Haller D, Steele G. Controversies in the management of localized rectal cancer. Proc Am Soc Clin Oncol. 1999; 18: 212–221.

45. Radiotherapy for rectal cancer. Available at: http://medweb.bham.ac.uk/cancerhelp/public/ specific/colorect/treat/radio/rectal.html Accessed July 5, 2000.

46. Meijer S, Rahusen FD, van der Plas LG. Palliative cryosurgery for rectal carcinoma. Int J Colorectal Dis. 1999; 14(3):177–180.

47. Berg DT, Lilienfeld C. Therapeutic options for treating advanced colorectal cancer. Clin J Oncol Nurs. 2000; 5(4):209–216.

48. Sargent D, Goldberg R, MacDonald J, et al. Adjuvant chemotherapy for colon cancer is beneficial without significantly increased toxicity in elderly patients: Results from a 3351 patient meta-analysis. Proc Am Soc Clin Oncol. 2000; 19:933 (abstr).

49. Grobovsky L, Kaplon M, Krozser-Hamati A, et al. Features of cancer in frail elderly patients. Proc Am Soc Clin Oncol. 2000; 19:2469 (abstr).

50. Knight RD, Miller LL, Pirotta N, et al. First-line irinotecan, fluorouracil, leucovorin especially improves survival in metastatic colorectal cancer patients with favorable prognostic indicators. Proc Am Soc Clin Oncol. 2000; 19:991 (abstr).

51. Murphy GP, Lawrence W Jr, Lenhard RE Jr. General approach to the patient. In: Murphy GP, Lawrence W, Lenhard RW, eds. American Cancer Society Textbook of Clinical Oncology, 2nd ed. Atlanta, GA. ASC, 1995: 71.

52. Coping with colorectal cancer. Available at: http://intouch.cancernetwork.com/myths/colon/Co107.htm Accessed August 6, 2000.

53. Barrett S, Herbert V. Questionable cancer therapies. Available at: http://www.quackwatch.com/01QuackeryRelatedTopics/cancer.html Accessed August 6, 2000.

CHAPTER 7 | Surgical Aspects of Colon Cancer

Anne Robin Waldman, MSN, RN, C, AOCN

Mary Ellen Crane, RN, BSN, CETN

Introduction

Surgery is the accepted standard of care for patients with colon and rectal cancers. Depending on location, lesions may be removed endoscopically, laparoscopically, or by open laparotomy with curative intent. It is essential that nurses caring for these patients understand their physical and emotional needs, as well as the special needs associated with each surgical procedure.

Management of Polyps

Polyps found during sigmoidoscopy and/or colonoscopy can safely be snared and removed during the procedure. If they are found during sigmoidoscopy, the patient should be evaluated by colonoscopy to ensure that there are no more lesions in the remaining large bowel. If the tumor has clear margins and is confined within the head of the polyp, the patient needs no more treatment and should undergo routine surveillance, with a repeat colonoscopy at 1 year and, if negative, again in 3 to 5 years.[1] Tumors within a polyp that have inadequate margins and sessile polyps with an invasive carcinoma require surgery to ensure that all disease has been safely removed[2] (Figure 7.1).

Laparoscopic Colon Resection

Traditionally, surgery for these polyps has been through an open laparotomy. Since the early 1990s, laparoscopic colectomy has become popular for the management of these early-stage

105

Colonoscopy + Polypectomy

Diminutive Polyp   Pedunculated Polyp   Sessile Polyp

Biopsy   Snare   Snare
                          (completely excised)

Hyperplastic   Adenoma   Adenoma   Adenoma with   Adenoma   Adenoma with
                                    invasive Ca   Invasive Ca

Future   Repeat
Colonoscopy?   Colonoscopy   ⊖ Vascular Invasion   ⊕ Vascular Invasion
               1 yr.   ⊖ Lymphatic Invasion   ⊕ Lymphatic Invasion
                              Favorable Histology   Unfavorable Histology
        ⊕   ⊖   Adeq. Margin   Close Margin

Colonoscopy   Colonoscopy   Colectomy
1 yr.   3–5 yrs.   (Lymph nodes ⊕ 10%)
                                                       Local Recurrence 5%

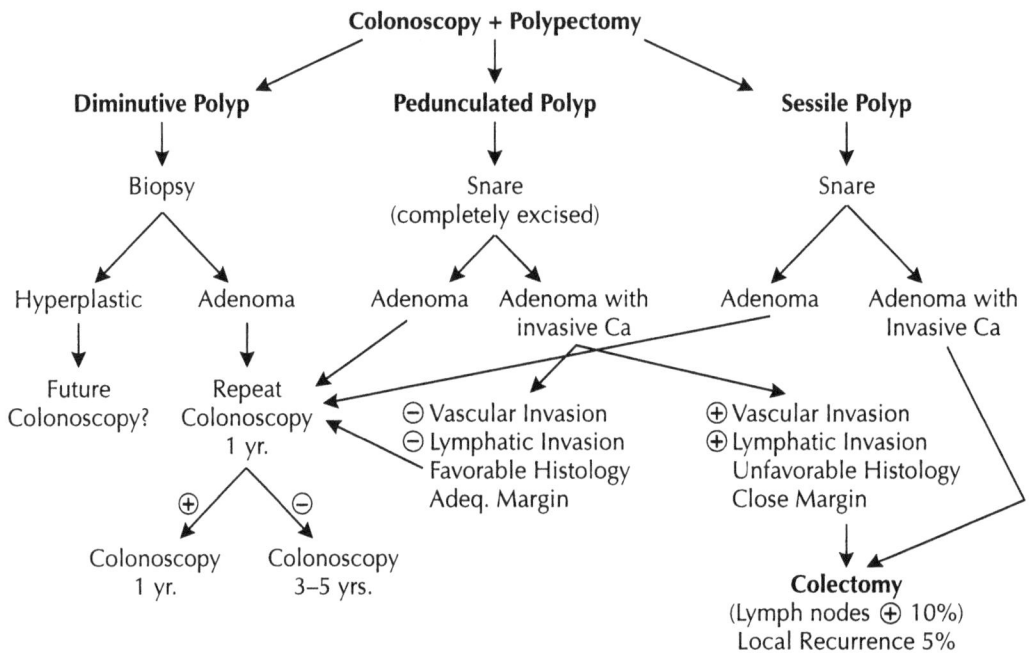

Figure 7.1   Management of polyps.

Source: Kodner IJ, Fry RD, Fieshman JW, Birnbaum EH, Read TE. Colon, rectum and anus. In Schwartz SI, Shires GT, Spencer FC, Daly JM, Fischer JE, Galloway AC (eds.), *Principles of Surgery,* 7th ed. Vol 2. New York: McGraw-Hill, 1999, p 1345. Used with permission from McGraw-Hill.

lesions and is thought by many to be safe and comparable, in the short term, to conventional open procedures.[3] Advocates for laparoscopic colonic resection cite the advantages as those provided in Table 7.1. Potential disadvantages

of the procedure are outlined in Table 7.2. A number of studies have positively favored the safety of laparoscopic colonic resection for early-stage disease.[4–7] However, at the present

Table 7.1   Advantages of Laparoscopic Colonic Resection

1. Limited abdominal wall trauma
2. Reduced postoperative pain
3. Possible more rapid return of bowel function
4. Possible reduced length of hospital stay
5. Possible hastened postoperative recovery
6. Similar staging opportunities compared with open procedures
7. Short-term outcome similar to that of traditional procedures
8. Possible protection of immune function

Source: From Green F. Laparoscopic management of colorectal cancer. CA Cancer J Clin. 1999; 49(4):222. With permission.

Table 7.2   Potential Disadvantages of Laparoscopic Colonic Resection

1. Reduced ability to explore the peritoneum
2. Reduced ability to palpate and localize the colonic lesion
3. Mechanical manipulation of the tumor, leading to cellular disbursement
4. Increased operating room time and cost
5. Possibility of port-site tumor seeding
6. Possible detrimental effects of conversion to open procedures
7. Questionable detrimental effect on recurrence rates and survival

Source: From Green F. Laparoscopic management of colorectal cancer. CA Cancer J Clin. 1999; 49(4):226. With permission.

time, the National Comprehensive Cancer Network (NCCN) guidelines do not recommend this procedure to perform lymph node harvest for disease staging unless the procedure is performed in the context of a well-designed clinical trial.[8]

The National Cancer Institute is currently conducting a high-priority, phase III, randomized study of laparoscopic-assisted colectomy versus open colectomy for colon cancer to (1) compare the disease-free and overall survival rates of patients with colon cancer randomized to laparoscopic-assisted colectomy versus open colectomy, (2) assess the frequency of treatment-related early and late morbidity and 30-day mortality of patients on both arms, and (3) compare the differences in costs and cost effectiveness between the two arms.[9]

Surgical Management

Surgery is the accepted standard of care for patients with colon cancer. The specific procedure and timing of the surgery depends on the tumor location. There are five basic principles governing colorectal cancer resection. It offers the opportunity to perform a full intraabdominal assessment; visceral metastases can be identified and confirmed; there is a safe creation of an anastomosis or stoma, where applicable; there are adequate longitudinal and radial margins of resection; and full mesenteric and nodal dissections are ensured.[3] The ideal surgical margin has a 5-cm margin of normal bowel on either side of the tumor; however, satisfactory margins can be achieved with 2 cm of disease-free tissue if adequate mesentery is resected.[1]

Cancers of the Ascending, Transverse, and Descending Colon

In an effort to improve the accuracy of staging at the time of initial diagnosis, the effectiveness of sentinel lymph node (SLN) mapping techniques are being studied in colon cancer patients. SLN mapping has been used successfully for identifying lymph node involvement in breast cancers[10–12] and melanoma.[13] Using these techniques, Saha et al.[14] successfully mapped SLNs in 85 of 86 patients. They found that in 53 of 56 patients in which the SLNs were negative, the non-SLNs were also negative. In the remaining 29 patients, the SLNs were positive for metastases, with 14 of 29 patients having other non-SLNs positive for metastasis and 15 of 29 patients having micrometastasis only in the SLN. They concluded that SLN mapping can be performed easily in colorectal cancer patients, with an accuracy of more than 95%, and that 18% of the 85 patients in their study were upstaged from stage I/II to stage III. Because there is a lack of data supporting the effectiveness of postoperative adjuvant therapy in patients with AJCC stage I/II disease, they usually do not receive therapy outside of a clinical trial. However, in this study, 15 patients were found to have micrometastasis only in the SLN, making them eligible for adjuvant therapy. Further work on this approach to staging needs to be done to evaluate long-term survival.

Uncomplicated carcinomas of the right colon, hepatic flexure, and transverse colon are generally treated with a right or extended right colectomy. The tissue removed during this procedure usually includes a 10-cm portion of the terminal ileum,[1] the cecum, proximal transverse colon, the accompanying mesocolon and lymphatic channels, and the ileum and left transverse colon are anastomosed (Figures 7.2, 7.3, and 7.4, pages 108 and 109). Because a portion of the terminal ileum is excised, caution is taken not to remove more than 50 cm, to minimize the affect on vitamin B_{12} and bile salt absorption.[15] Poor bile salt absorption may result in the malabsorption of nutrients and chronic diarrhea, while a lack of B_{12} may result in anemia.

Carcinomas of the mid transverse colon can be treated in two ways: transverse colectomy

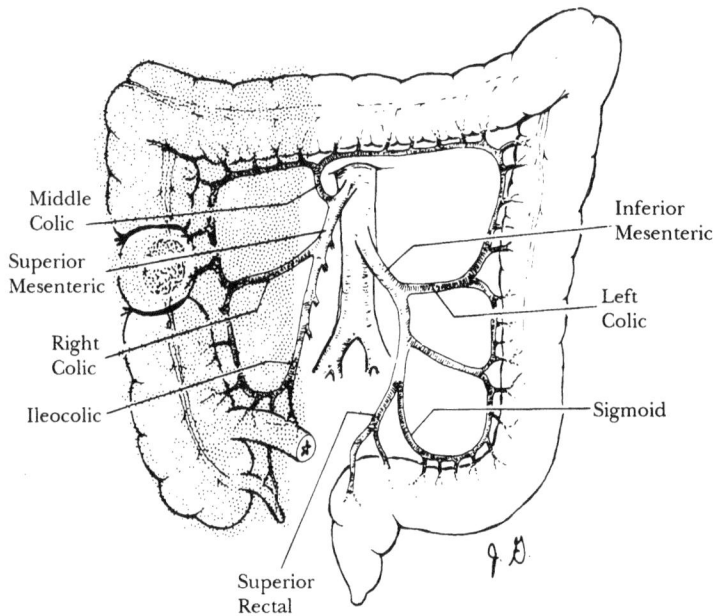

Figure 7.2   Right colectomy.
Source: Hoebler L. Colon and rectal cancer. In: Groenwald SL, Frogge MH, Goodman M, et al. Cancer Nursing Principles and Practice. 4th ed. Sudbury, MA: Jones & Bartlett, 1997: 1036–1054.

and extended right hemicolectomy. With a transverse colectomy, only the transverse colon is removed; the middle colic artery is ligated to interrupt lymphatic drainage to the area, and the ascending and descending colons are anastomosed (Figure 7.3). With an extended right hemicolectomy, the ileum and proximal descending colon are anastomosed (see Figure 7.4). This is the preferred procedure for elderly patients, in whom there is concern for having a well-vascularized anastomosis.[16]

Uncomplicated lesions in the splenic flexure and the descending colon are treated with a left colectomy. With a left colectomy for a splenic flexure lesion, the mid and distal transverse colon and the descending colon are removed, and the right transverse colon and the sigmoid colon are anastomosed. With a left colectomy for a descending colon lesion, the distal transverse colon, the descending colon, and a portion of the sigmoid colon are removed, and the right transverse colon and distal sigmoid colon are anastomosed (Figures 7.5 and 7.6, page 110).

Obstructing lesions may require one of three approaches. The first is either a two-stage or a traditional three-stage surgical approach. The two-stage approach utilizes the Hartmann procedure, by which, initially, the tumor is resected, the proximal colon is brought to the skin as an end-colostomy, and the distal colon is sutured or stapled closed. This is followed by a second operation several months later to reestablish intestinal continuity. The traditional three-stage resection, used primarily for left-sided lesions, involves, first, a diverting transverse colostomy or a cecostomy, followed by involved tumor resection 10 to 14 days later, and then reestablishment of intestinal continuity several months later.[17] A second approach is resection with a permanent stoma or, as a third approach, resection, intraoperative bowel lavage, and primary anastomosis. Uncomplicated lesions in the sigmoid, rectosigmoid, and upper rectum are managed with an anterior resection, with preservation of the sympathetic nerves (Figure 7.7, page 111).

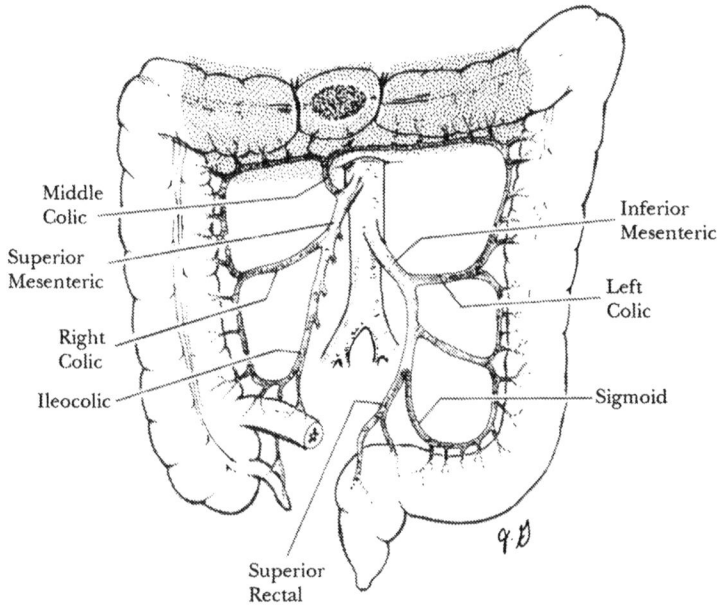

Figure 7.3 Transverse colectomy.

Source: Hoebler L. Colon and rectal cancer. In: Groenwald SL, Frogge MH, Goodman M, et al. Cancer Nursing Principles and Practice. 4th ed. Sudbury, MA: Jones & Bartlett, 1997: 1036–1054.

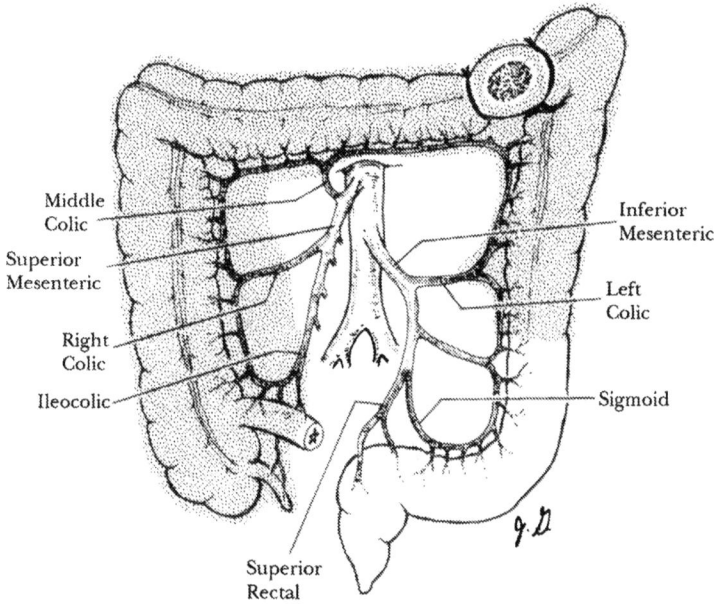

Figure 7.4 Extended resection for transverse colon carcinoma.

Source: Hoebler L. Colon and rectal cancer. In: Groenwald SL, Frogge MH, Goodman M, et al. Cancer Nursing Principles and Practice. 4th ed. Sudbury, MA: Jones & Bartlett, 1997: 1036–1054.

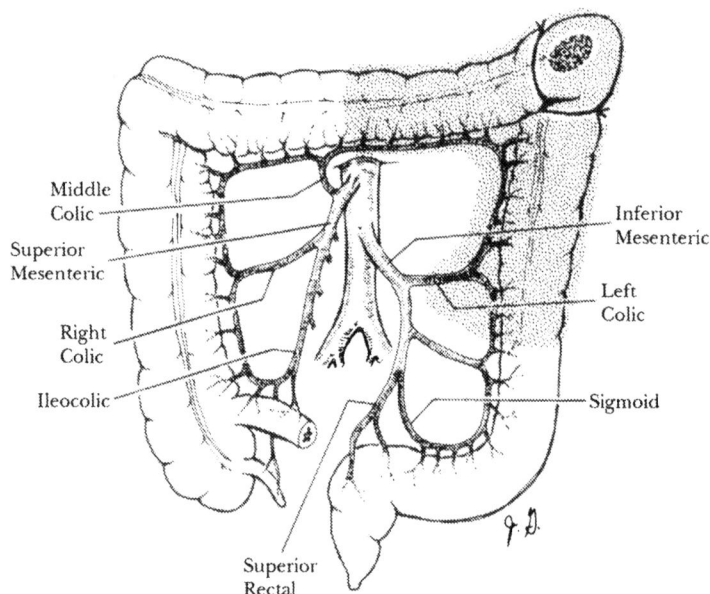

Figure 7.5   Colectomy for splenic flexure carcinoma.

Source: Hoebler L. Colon and rectal cancer. In: Groenwald SL, Frogge MH, Goodman M, et al. Cancer Nursing Principles and Practice. 4th ed. Sudbury, MA: Jones & Bartlett, 1997: 1036–1054.

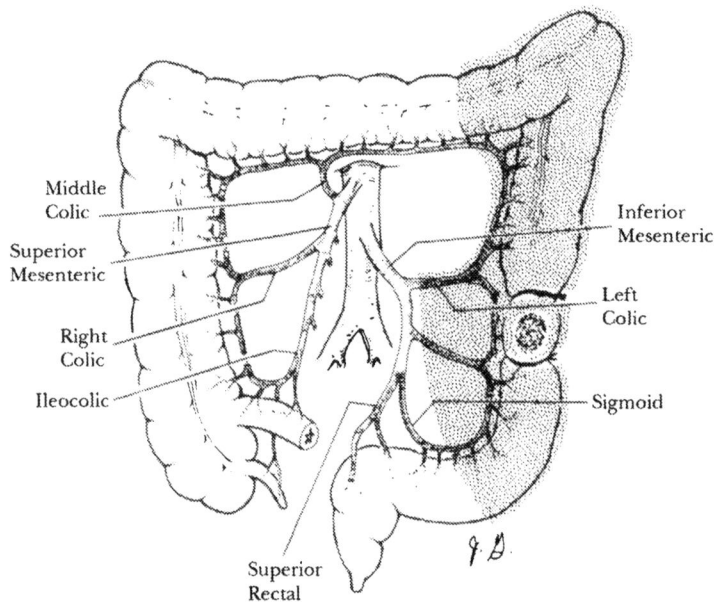

Figure 7.6   Left colectomy.

Source: Hoebler L. Colon and rectal cancer. In: Groenwald SL, Frogge MH, Goodman M, et al. Cancer Nursing Principles and Practice. 4th ed. Sudbury, MA: Jones & Bartlett, 1997: 1036–1054.

Cancer of the Rectum

The management of rectal lesions has become increasingly complex, as the curative treatment may be a local incision, sphincter-preserving abdominal surgery, or abdominoperineal resection. Clinical staging factors determining whether local therapy or radical resection will be the treatment modality are the depth of invasion into the rectal wall, the size and macro-

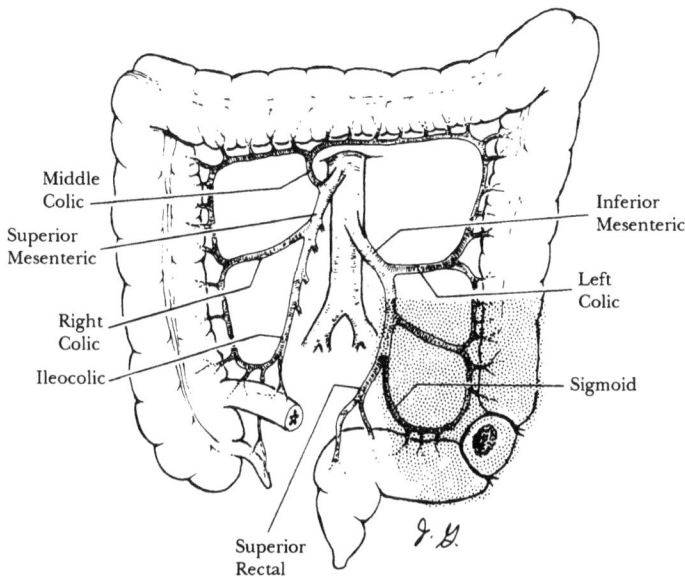

Figure 7.7 Sigmoid colectomy.

Source: Hoebler L. Colon and rectal cancer. In: Groenwald SL, Frogge MH, Goodman M, et al. Cancer Nursing Principles and Practice. 4th ed. Sudbury, MA: Jones & Bartlett, 1997: 1036–1054.

scopic appearance of the cancer, the presence or absence of regional lymph node metastasis, and the level above the anal verge.[16] (See Chapter 5 for details of the preoperative work-up and staging description.)

Transanal excision of rectal lesions is feasible for well-differentiated superficial lesions, limited to the submucosa, that are less than 3 to 4 cm in diameter; these can be completely excised with negative margins (T_1). Ideally, the clear surgical margin should be 1 cm, and perirectal fat should be included to try to detect nodal spread.[17]

Uncomplicated lesions of the mid and lower rectum can be managed with a low anterior resection (LAR) or coloanal anastomosis, with preservation of the sympathetic and parasympathetic nerves, only if the anastomosis provides for an excellent blood supply, no tension, and adequate sphincter muscle function[1] (Figure 7.8). Abdominoperineal resection (APR) may be necessary if the sphincter muscles are involved or if the tumor extends to within 2 cm of the dentate line (Figure 7.9).

Perforation

Sealed, perforated lesions may be resected with anastomosis, but open perforations are generally resected with a primary stoma.

Lesions Invading Adjacent Organs

Lesions invading adjacent organs are managed with an in-continuity resection, in which adherent or invaded viscera are removed with the primary tumor and then intestinal continuity is reestablished with a primary anastomosis.

Metastatic Tumor Resection

Colon tumors most frequently metastasize to the liver and lungs. When there are discrete lesions of less than 5 cm, surgical resection or ablative techniques such as cryoablation, radiofrequency ablation, ethanol injection, transarterial chemoembolization, hepatic artery transfusion, or systemic chemotherapy may be considered.

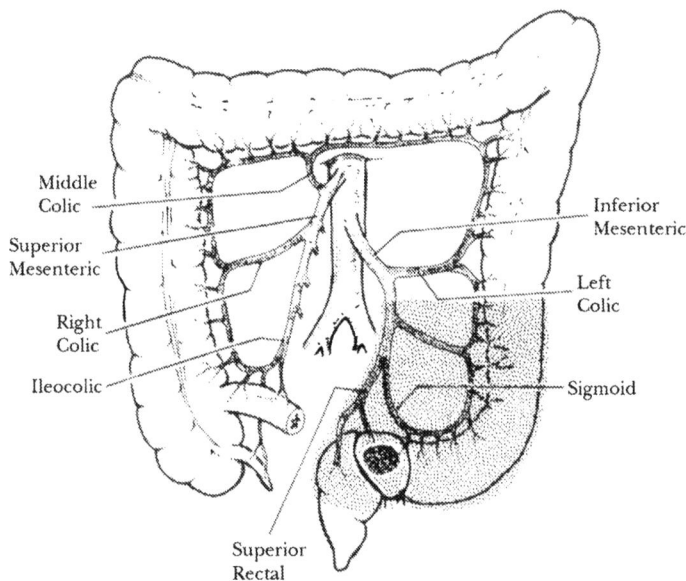

Figure 7.8   Anterior rectal resection.

Source: Hoebler L. Colon and rectal cancer. In: Groenwald SL, Frogge MH, Goodman M, et al. Cancer Nursing Principles and Practice. 4th ed. Sudbury, MA: Jones & Bartlett, 1997: 1036–1054.

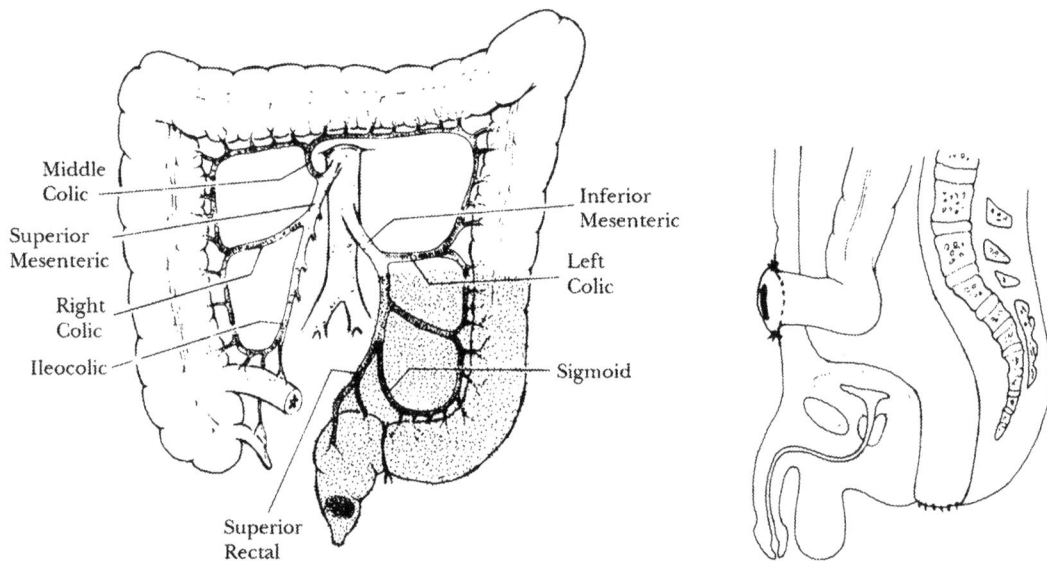

Figure 7.9   Abdominoperineal resection.

Source: Hoebler L. Colon and rectal cancer. In: Groenwald SL, Frogge MH, Goodman M, et al. Cancer Nursing Principles and Practice. 4th ed. Sudbury, MA: Jones & Bartlett, 1997: 1036–1054.

The goals of surgical resection of metastatic colon lesions are to achieve at least 1 cm of uninvolved margin and to minimize the loss of normal tissue.[18] The lesions are usually removed via standard resection; the primary tumor must show evidence of being eradicated; there can be no other unresectable lesions; and the patient must be in good physical condition.[19]

Liver tumors are the most common site of colorectal metastases. Systemic chemotherapy may prolong survival, but that survival is usually not longer than 2 years. The median survival rate for patients who undergo liver resection of colorectal metastases is 28 to 40 months,[20] and Sheele et al.,[21] Jamison et al.,[22] and Fong et al.[23] have reported a 10-year survival rate of approximately 20% for some patients undergoing liver resection. Therefore, hepatic resection has been accepted as standard treatment for resectable colorectal liver metastases.[20]

In an attempt to refine patient selection criteria for liver resection, long-term postresection outcomes have been studied,[21-25] and, based on this analysis, the only absolute contraindications to liver resection are the presence of extrahepatic disease and the inability to resect all hepatic disease.

The preoperative work-up focuses on evaluating the patient's medical fitness for general anesthesia and surgery and should include chest, abdominal, and pelvic computerized tomography (CT), with CT portography for the abdominal CT to evaluate the number of hepatic lesions. If the lesion is close to major vessels or biliary structures, magnetic resonance imaging (MRI) or ultrasound should be done to visualize vascular structures and to distinguish metastatic lesions from benign cysts, hemangiomas, and fibronodular hyperplasia.

During surgery, intraoperative ultrasound may be utilized to further define the tumor's location and characteristics. Up to 80% to 90% of the liver can be removed safely, and within 3 to 6 weeks, the liver regenerates to approxi-mately its normal size.[26] Based on hepatic anatomy, segmental resection is preferred over wedge resection.[27] Wedge resection may be used for small peripheral lesions, but, for other lesions, it has been associated with histologically positive margins in up to 35% of cases.[21] The types of liver resection for metastatic disease are shown in Figure 7.10.

Postoperative complications from liver resection range from 20% to 50% and have been reported most commonly as liver-related (hemorrhage, bile fistula, perihepatic abscess), as wound infections, and as general complications, primarily cardiac and pulmonary.[21,23,28] The mortality rate is 4% to 5%.[20]

When metastatic disease causes an intestinal obstruction, surgery is indicated for only those patients with a good performance status. Obstruction may be extrinsic from studding of the bowel or abdominal carcinomatosis or intrinsic from tumor extension within the lumen of the bowel itself. Typical signs and symptoms are nausea and vomiting, crampy abdominal pain, constipation, abdominal distention, and abnormal bowel sounds. Conservative management consists of nasogastric or nasointestinal decompression and administration of parenteral fluids to restore fluid and electrolyte balance for approximately 3 days. If this is unsuccessful in relieving the obstruction, surgery is indicated. In this circumstance, the morbidity rate can be as high as 50% and the mortality rate at least 10%.[29]

If the patient is treated conservatively and intubation is required for more than a few days, the nasogastric or nasointestinal tube is replaced with a gastrostomy tube. This helps reduce the chance of the obstruction recurring and improves patient comfort. Nursing measures that improve patient comfort include providing frequent mouth care, care of the nares while the nasogastric or nasointestinal tube is in place, good pain management, and monitoring fluid- and electrolyte-replacement therapy.

A

B

C

D

E

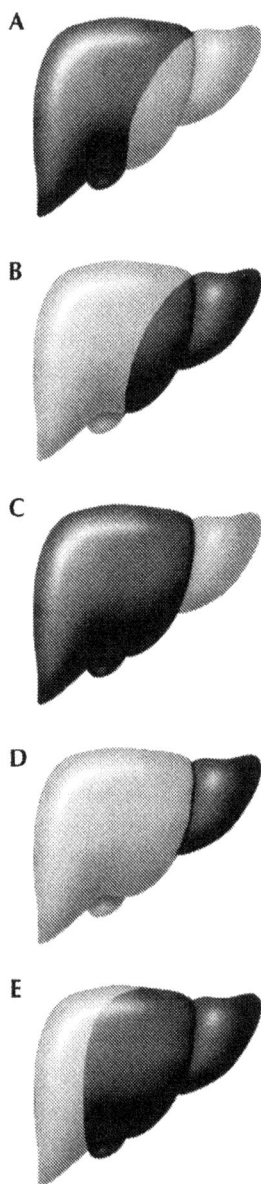

Figure 7.10   Common liver resections for metastatic colorectal cancer. **A:** Right lobectomy; **B:** Left lobectomy; **C:** Right trisegmentectomy; **D:** Left lateral segmentectomy; and **E:** Left trisegmentectomy.

Source: Fong Y. Surgical therapy of hepatic colorectal metastasis. CA Cancer J Clin. 1999; 49:231–255. With permission.

Ostomy Management

Introduction

Patients in whom the sphincter muscles are involved or where the tumor extends to within 2 cm of the dentate line will require an abdominal perineal resection with the creation of an ostomy, a fecal diversion,[30] where the intestines are brought through an opening on the surface of the abdominal wall. Healthcare professionals working with the patient need to keep in mind that the patient is being presented with information about a disease, which is frightening, and has to face a change in body image and body function. The enormity of the psychosocial impact of this treatment modality will bring a challenging experience for the patient and significant others. Because each person presents with a variety of coping skills in a new situation, significant others should be included in teaching and counseling sessions.[31–33]

Types of Interventions

A colostomy is the result of a diversion performed on the large intestine. Colostomies are most commonly performed in the cecum, transverse colon, left descending colon, and sigmoid colon. Intestinal ostomies are divided into two categories. The placement of the ostomy depends on the specific area identified above the cancerous lesions. The consistency of the output of a colostomy depends on the location of the ostomy.

An ileostomy is the result of ostomy surgery performed on the small intestine. Most ileostomies are performed on the distal small bowel, usually the terminal ileum. The common area for placement of an ileostomy and cecostomy, just distal to the ileocecal valve, is the right lower abdominal quadrant.[30] Drainage from an ileostomy is watery.

A cecostomy and ascending colostomy produces a mixture of mushy stool and water. Transverse colostomies can be placed on either the left or right upper abdominal quadrant. A transverse colostomy produces mushy to semi-formed stool. Descending colon and sigmoid colostomies are usually located in the left lower quadrant.[30] A descending and sigmoid colostomy produces semiformed to formed stool.

The opening to the skin surface of the abdomen is called a stoma. Presently, there are three common surgical constructions of a stoma: end, loop, and double barrel[30]:

An end stoma is formed by cutting the colon and bringing the proximal end to the abdominal surface and creating one stoma. This is usually a permanent stoma, with the distal portion of the colon being removed.[30]

A loop stoma is formed by pulling a loop of the colon to the surface and cutting an opening by creating a reverse fold in the intestine. Many times, this stoma may be reversed at a later date; therefore, it is referred to as a temporary ostomy.[30]

A double-barrel stoma is constructed by cutting the colon and bringing both ends to the abdominal wall, creating two stomas.[30] For the patient with a double-barrel colostomy, the proximal end of the stoma will drain the output from the bowel. The distal end will present with occasional discharge of mucus produced from the bowel wall in the lower portion of the colon. If the mucus is produced in larger quantities, causing leakage or mucus plug formation, the doctor may recommend periodic irrigation of the lower colon.

In preparation for an ostomy procedure, the patient should meet with an enterostomal therapy nurse (CWOCN) prior to surgery for teaching and siting of the stoma.[30,34] The CWOCN will perform a comprehensive assessment of the abdominal area and obtain a patient history to determine the best location for the position of the ostomy. The stomal site will be marked for the surgery, because placement of the stoma is crucial. A stoma in folds or creases of the abdomen that cannot be pouched complicates the containment of the drainage. The stoma site will be marked with a nontoxic marker and covered with a plastic transparent dressing, if available, to prevent the area from being scrubbed, which would remove the markings. Due to emergency situations such as perforation, obstruction, or total intestinal malfunction, immediate surgery may be necessary. If this occurs, siting for the stoma may not be possible.[30,35]

Although age is not a deciding factor in determining the ability of patients to care for their ostomy independently, mental status, hand dexterity, vision, and coordination are important and will need to be addressed when choosing a containment device. Acceptance of the ostomy will come with knowledge and easy adaptation. Having patients participate in the care as soon as possible postoperatively and encouraging them to ask questions will help in their adjustment.[34–37] In a study done by Pieper and Mikols[38] specific concerns were documented, reflecting predischarge and postdischarge concerns of ostomy patients (Tables 7.3 and 7.4).

Postoperative Care

Postoperatively, a pouching system is placed around the stoma. The drainage consists of mucus and bloody exudate for the first 3 to 5 days. As the diet increases from liquid to solid food, the effluent becomes thicker. The thickness depends on the location of the colon dissection. The bowel returns to normal function above the level of the stoma, and, within 3 to 5 days, flatulence begins to escape through the stoma. The bag needs to be opened periodically throughout the day to release the trapped air.

Table 7.3   Top-rated Predischarge Concerns of Ostomy Patients

1. Fear of stool leaking*
2. Odor*
3. Needing further treatment*
4. Wearing a pouch*
5. Changing a pouch*
6. Participating in sports*
7. Going out to eat
8. Interest in sex
9. Participation in sexual love play or intercourse*
10. Ability to have sex
11. Satisfaction after sexual intercourse
12. Caring for self in other people's homes
13. Change in body appearance*
14. Touching the stoma
15. Relationship with spouse or significant other

*Item appears on both the predischarge and postdischarge lists.

Source: Adapted with permission from Pieper B, Mikols C. Predischarge and postdischarge concerns of persons with an ostomy. JWOCN. 1996; 23:108.

Table 7.4   Top-rated Postdischarge Concerns of Ostomy Patients

1. Fear of stool leaking*
2. Odor*
3. Participating in sports*
4. Change in sleep habits
5. Needing further treatment*
6. Wearing a pouch*
7. Moods
8. Ability to work outside the home
9. Change in body appearance*
10. Changing a pouch*
11. Clothing
12. Energy level
13. Participation in sexual love play or intercourse*
14. Feeling embarrassed
15. Feeling like a whole person

*Item appears on both the predischarge and postdischarge lists.

Source: Adapted with permission from Pieper B, Mikols C. Predischarge and postdischarge concerns of persons with an ostomy. JWOCN. 1996; 23:108.

Choosing a Product

Choice of products depends on the location of the stoma site, drainage consistency, peristomal skin condition, and the convexity of the circumference of the stoma. After surgery, the nurse will assess the abdomen for proximity of the stoma and the incision. Correct fit of the appliance is crucial in preventing leakage of the fecal fluid. Most manufacturers recommend that the flange stay in place from 4 to 7 days[35] and only be changed if there is leakage. This helps to preserve the peristomal skin.[39]

There are many pouching systems from which to choose. All have a flange, which is a faceplate that makes contact with the skin surface. The consistency may be a skin barrier wafer, adhesive surface, or a synthetic surface. It can be flat, convex, a pre-cut system, a cut-to-fit system, a one-piece system (the bag and the flange are attached), a two-piece system (the bag and the flange are two separate pieces and must match), a stationary flange, or a floating flange. Each product has a different feel of flexibility.[35] Bag options include the length, the type of backing, and whether it contains a filter that automatically releases flatulence.

Allergies must be considered when choosing the product. Some products have plastic, latex, pectin, or tape backings to allow for contour and adherence to the area around the stoma. Allergic reactions may cause the appliance to come off prematurely, due to skin erosion, blistering, or seepage or peeling at the contact level, usually the epidermal level of the skin.[35]

Skin barriers come in many types. Their purpose is to put a protective barrier between the skin and the appliance. This also protects the skin from fecal leakage, which can erode the tissue. Caution is needed if the patient has any open areas, as some products have an alcohol base, which can sting the patient.[40]

Use of lotions and soaps on the peristomal skin area prevents the flange from adhering to the skin surface. The chemical composition of soap products may also cause allergic dermatitis.[41]

Care of the Ostomy

Maintenance of the stoma requires washing gently with warm water to remove any mucus and fecal matter. The flange should be cut approximately one-fourth-inch larger than the stoma, but care must be taken not to have the opening too large where the peristomal skin will be exposed to the fecal material. Postoperatively, a one-piece system is usually placed until the area heals and becomes less tender. There are now some two-piece systems with floating flanges that prevent pain and injury to the area until healing is completed. Two-piece systems may be easier for patients who are able to care for their ostomy independently. Each bag has hooks attached for extra security, and a belt can be inserted into the hooks and placed around the waist. This is especially useful while engaging in activities and sports.[35] Table 7.5 provides step-by-step directions for changing the ostomy bag and flange.

Table 7.5   Directions for Changing the Ostomy Bag and Flange

1. Remove the soiled bag and flange.
2. Wash the area around the stoma with mild soap and water. Do not use a soap with a lotion or cream base, as it will prevent the new product from adhering to the skin.
3. Allow the area to dry.
4. Apply skin protector or barrier film. This usually comes as an individually packaged 1-inch pad or in a lollipop form. This protects peristomal skin from erosion from the adhesive barrier and feces.
5. Allow the area to dry.
6. Cut the flange. This is the backing part of the bag that will adhere to the skin. It should be cut one-fourth of an inch larger than the stoma to prevent irritation to the stoma or leakage under the flange. Remove the paper backing from the flange.
7. Apply stoma adhesive paste, if needed. This product comes in a tube and should be applied to the flange adhesive side about one-fourth of an inch in from the edge. Apply like toothpaste and let dry.
8. When the stoma adhesive paste and the skin are totally dry, carefully apply the flange to the skin, making sure the opening is not covering any portion of the stoma.
9. If using the two-piece system, attach the bag and clamp the lower end of the bag.
10. If teaching patients, ask for a return demonstration of steps 1 through 9, as well as having them practice unclamping and clamping the bag as if they were emptying the bag. The bag should be emptied whenever it is half full, to prevent bag explosion. After emptying the bag, wipe the open end with toilet tissue and then reclamp the bag.

NOTE: The bag will periodically fill with flatus. Tell patients to open the clamp and release the air to prevent bag explosion. Patients are sometimes reluctant to perform this task due to the odor of the flatus, and should be encouraged to use a private area to prevent embarrassment. Room deodorizer sprays or deodorizers for inside the bag can be helpful.
Source: Courtesy of Mary Ellen Crane.

Sexuality

Sexual activity can resume as soon as the patient's abdominal discomfort dissipates. This may be very difficult for the patient and partner, due to the body-image change. There are products that can cover the pouch to make intimacy more comfortable. Both patient and partner need to be candid about their concerns. Sexuality is a combination of many emotions, beliefs, and past experiences, which both partners bring to the new situation.[33,34] As a result of the surgery, patients may experience impotency, vaginal dryness, or other problems. These issues should be discussed with the doctor.[31,32,42]

Irrigation

Ostomies on the lower part of the colon can be regulated to continent colostomies through irrigation. By irrigating with warm water, the ostomy can be evacuated at the same time each day.[13] Patients with a double-barrel or loop ostomy may have movement of mucus plugs from the sigmoid into the rectal area and complain of feeling that they are releasing a bowel movement through the rectum. Irrigating the lower bowel through the distal end of the stoma washes the excess mucus plug out through the rectal area, and this should relieve the pressure. For some patients, this needs to be a routine process, which will alleviate the leakage and concerns about leakage.[43]

Ordering Supplies

Ostomy supplies are purchased through any Durable Medical Company that carries ostomy products. To order, the company will need the numbers and manufacturer's name. Most products are partially or fully covered by medical insurance.[44]

Each company carries a varied number of

Table 7.6 Toll-free Telephone Numbers for Ostomy Suppliers

Bard	1-800-526-4455
Convatec	1-800-631-5244
Hollister	1-800-323-4060
Coloplast	1-800-533-0464
Marlen	1-216-292-7060
Incutec	1-800-699-4232
Nu Hope Laboratories Inc.	1-800-899-5017
Smith-Nephew	1-800-876-1261
Torbot-Group Inc.	1-800-545-4254
VIP (Cook)	1-800-843-4851

products, and patients are encouraged to call the manufacturing company for a product catalogue. Each also has a customer service representative available to assess the needs of the patient and provide sample products, if a change is required. A list of toll-free telephone numbers for the various suppliers can be found in Table 7.6.

Nursing Care of Patients with Bowel Surgery

Preoperative Preparation

Preoperative bowel preparation for colorectal surgery is important for preventing wound infection and intraabdominal abscess formation. Instituting a regime of mechanical cleansing and antibiotic administration cleans the bowel and reduces the number of bacteria exposed in the operative field.

Mechanical cleansing can be achieved using mono- and dibasic sodium phosphate purgatives or whole-gut lavage with polyethylene glycol (PEG).[1] Patients prepping with mono- and dibasic sodium phosphate usually drink a bottle of Fleet's phospha soda and 24 oz of clear liquid at 12 P.M. and 6 P.M. on the day prior to surgery. Caution should be taken with patients with renal failure or those on sodium-restricted diets, as they have the potential to develop hypocalcemia, hyperphosphatemia, hypernatremia, or acidosis. PEG (Go-Lytely or Co-Lyte), an isotonic lavage solution in a balanced salt solution, acts as an osmotic purgative. It reduces the absorptive power of the small bowel, clears feces from the colon, is not associated with the production of explosive colonic gas, and is not a culture medium for bacteria. However, for this method of bowel preparation to be effective, the patient must drink an average of 4 L over a period of 4 hours. The PEG solution has an unpleasant taste and should not be altered with flavorings, but refrigerating it does make it more palatable.

Either oral or intravenous antibiotics are given the day before surgery to reduce the bacterial concentration in the colon. A common regime calls for 1 g each of neomycin sulfate (Mycifradin) and erythromycin (E-Mycin) at 1 P.M., 2 P.M., and 11 P.M. on the day before surgery and an intravenous broad-spectrum antibiotic immediately before surgery.

As with all patients undergoing general anesthesia, those undergoing surgery for colorectal cancer will be NPO after midnight. Most patients will be admitted to the hospital the morning of the day of surgery. This means that, except for the preoperative intravenous antibiotic, the entire preparation will be done at home, leaving little time for in-depth patient instruction prior to the day of admission to the hospital.

Ideally, once admitted to the hospital, the patient should receive an explanation of what can be expected during the hospitalization. Issues needing to be addressed are the hospital routine, which includes the nursing history, the physician's history, and physical examination; operative identification procedures; skin prep; preoperative antibiotics and medications; and postoperative expectations, such as the stay in the postanesthesia care unit, indwelling tubes and catheters, pain management, coughing and deep breathing, ambulation, and dietary progression.

Postoperative Care

Postoperatively, the nurse's attention is focused on preventing complications and promoting convalescence. The potential complications from a colectomy include atelectasis or pneumonia, pain, fluid and electrolyte imbalances, leakage from the anastomotic site, poor wound healing, abdominal distention, paralytic ileus, inadequate dietary intake, and weight loss. In addition, patients with an abdominoperineal resection may have problems with urinary retention and impotence. See the nursing care plan in Table 7.7 for specific nursing diagnoses and interventions.

Most patients undergoing surgery for colon cancer will be hospitalized from 4 to 6 days. The current healthcare environment has been an impetus for institutions to develop clinical care pathways that are cost effective, that identify best practice, that assist in establishing a standard of care, that coordinate care across the continuum, and that streamline documentation. The Bowel Resection with Ostomy Pathway, presented in the Appendix, is from St. Joseph Mercy–Oakland in Pontiac, Michigan. Since implementing it, they have had an average cost reduction of $2,500 per case, improved patient education, and a 2-day decrease in length of stay. It has proved its value as a care plan, an education plan, and an education record.[45]

Summary

Surgical treatments for colorectal cancer are performed with the intent to cure the disease while maintaining normal bowel function. Alterations in normal bowel function are associated with surgeries on lesions of the rectum. All surgical options should be discussed at length with patients and their significant others.

Nurses need to provide appropriate nursing care and know the community resources available for supportive care of these patients.

Table 7.7   Plan of Care for Patients Undergoing Surgery for Treatment of Colon Cancer (Colectomy/Anterior–Posterior Resection)

Nursing Diagnosis: Knowledge deficit regarding surgery
Expected Outcome: The patient will verbalize an understanding of the disease, the planned treatment, the preoperative preparation, and postoperative care.
Nursing Interventions:
1. Assess the patient's knowledge of colon cancer and the planned procedure.
2. Educate the patient regarding the following: need for and elements of bowel preparation; NPO after midnight; pain management; coughing and deep breathing and incentive spirometry; antiembolism stockings, leg exercises, and early ambulation; purpose of catheters, drains, or ostomy; incision, dressing checks and changes; vital sign monitoring; postoperative nutrition; potential alteration in sexual function.

Nursing Diagnosis: Risk for fluid and electrolyte imbalance
Expected Outcome: Electrolytes will be within normal parameters. Patient will maintain a urinary output of at least 30 mL/h.
Nursing Interventions:
1. Monitor electrolytes and report abnormal values to the physician.
2. Maintain IV therapy as prescribed.
3. Monitor intake and output q8h.
4. Report a decrease in urinary output to the physician.
5. Report any changes in mental status to the physician.

Nursing Diagnosis: Risk for bleeding related to surgery
Expected Outcome: The patient will have stable vital signs and no overt signs of bleeding.
Nursing Interventions:
1. Assess dressings, catheter, drains, and nasogastric tube for signs of bleeding.
2. Monitor vital signs for hypotension and tachycardia.
3. Monitor hemoglobin and hematocrit. Notify the physician of a decrease in hemoglobin of 1 g or greater.
4. Assess for signs of hypoxia with pulse oximetry if the patient displays the following symptoms: lethargy, anxiety, restlessness, change in mental status.

Nursing Diagnosis: Risk for thrombophlebitis and pulmonary embolism
Expected Outcome: The patient will not develop thrombophlebitis or a pulmonary embolism.
Nursing Interventions:
1. Assess the patient for shortness of breath.
2. Assess the patient's calf for signs of thrombophlebitis: warmth, pain, redness, edema.
3. The patient wears antiembolism stockings when in bed and performs leg exercises.
4. The patient is out of bed and walking on postop day 1.
5. Administer anticoagulant therapy as prescribed.

Table 7.7 *Continued*

Nursing Diagnosis: Alteration in comfort related to pain
Expected Outcome: The patient will verbalize an acceptable level of comfort throughout the postoperative phase.
Nursing Interventions:
1. Assess for quantity, quality, location, and duration of pain.
2. Ensure that the patient uses patient-controlled anesthesia correctly and/or administer narcotics for pain as prescribed.
3. Reinforce preoperative teaching regarding splinting the incision when getting in and out of bed, and coughing and deep breathing.
4. Implement comfort measures: changing position, straightening bed linen, back rub, comfortable lighting, muted sounds.

Nursing Diagnosis: Impaired skin integrity related to surgical wounds, breaks in the integument, drains, and tubes
Expected Outcome: Incision and breaks in the integument will heal without postoperative wound complications.
Nursing Interventions:
1. Assess the incision, IVs, and catheters for signs of infection: warmth, redness, tenderness, drainage.
2. Maintain a strict aseptic technique when changing dressings and caring for IVs, drains, and tubes.
3. Assess the skin surrounding the stoma for itching, burning, or stinging.
4. Protect fragile skin from breakdown.

Nursing Diagnosis: Risk for anastomotic leak
Expected Outcome: The patient will have stable vital signs and no overt signs of anastomotic leak.
Nursing Interventions:
1. Assess for mild temperature elevation on postop days 4 to 7.
2. Assess the wound for signs of a fecal fistula.
3. Assess for an increase in abdominal pain.

Nursing Diagnosis: Body image disturbance related to the presence of an ostomy
Expected Outcome: The patient and significant others will adapt to the altered body image.
Nursing Interventions:
1. Assess the ability of the patient and significant others to use their usual coping mechanisms to adjust to the patient's altered body image.
2. Encourage the patient and significant others to discuss feelings related to the presence of the ostomy.
3. Encourage the patient and significant others to participate in ostomy care.
4. Offer an opportunity for the patient to talk with someone who has adapted successfully to an ostomy.
5. Refer the patient and family to the United Ostomy Association.

Nursing Diagnosis: Altered sexuality patterns related to abdominal/perineal resection
Expected Outcome: The patient and significant other will verbalize that they have achieved satisfactory sexual relations.
Nursing Interventions:
1. Review with the patient and significant other the potential alterations in sexual function that may occur as a result of surgery: positions, impotency, vaginal dryness.

(continues)

Table 7.7 *Continued*

2. Review with the patient and significant other behavioral interventions to relieve sexual dysfunction: creating a sensual environment, exploring alternative forms of sexual expression, use of mechanical devices, use of pouch covers, use of vaginal lubricants.
3. Encourage the patient and significant other to express their sexual concerns.
4. Refer the patient to appropriate resources for management of impotency or vaginal dryness.

Nursing Diagnosis: Altered nutrition (less than body requirements)
Expected Outcome: The patient will consume sufficient calories to meet daily nutrition requirements.
Nursing Interventions:
When the patient is no longer NPO:
1. Assess for nausea prior to mealtime. If nausea is present, administer antiemetics before food is served.
2. Encourage the patient to gradually increase the amount and consistency of food intake.
3. Offer liquid food supplements if the patient is not tolerating solid foods.

Nursing Diagnosis: Risk for constipation
Expected Outcome: The patient will have a bowel movement without straining.
Nursing Interventions:
1. Assess for bowel sounds.
2. Assess for abdominal distention.
3. Encourage early ambulation.
4. Encourage adequate fluid intake.
5. Administer anticonstipation therapy as ordered.

Source: Data from refs. 46 through 50.

APPENDIX—Bowel Resection with Ostomy Pathway

Source: Reprinted with permission from St. Joseph Mercy-Oakland, Pontiac, Michigan.

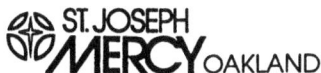

ST. JOSEPH MERCY OAKLAND

CODE: <u>362.2</u>
LOS: 5 <u>Days</u>

Post-Op Day 1 and 2	Date:					
KEY PATIENT OUTCOMES: (Y = Yes, N = No, C = Carry over to the next day. If N or C, document in Narrative Notes.)						Met/Initial
1. Patient/family verbalizes feelings/concerns regarding hospitalization/illness.						
2. Patient/family concurs with plan of care (Document every day).						
3. Verbalizes tolerance of ADL and up in room without respiratory distress						
4. Patient verbalizes pain controlled (<4 or less on pain scale of 0-10)						
5. Absence of respiratory complications AEB lung expansion – patient verbalizes lack of distress						
6. Adequate urinary output 60 cc/2 hrs.						
INTERVENTIONS: **TIME** (√ = Assessment Normal, * = Assessment Abnormal, → Abnormal Unchanged)						
ADL assistance (FA = Family assisted, S = Staff, I = Independent) whenever performed/ADL tolerance. (√ = Assessment Normal, * = Assessment Abnormal, → Abnormal Unchanged)						
Respiratory assessment q shift & prn						
GI assessment q shift & prn						
GU assessment q shift & prn						
DB & C Incentive Spirometer 10 x 1 hr. w.a. (Document average # cc reached)						
Assess stoma q shift & prn						
Refer to other forms: ☐ Episodic Flow Record ☐ Unit Specific Flow Record						
INITIALS						
ACTIVITY/EXERCISE **TIME**						
Activity (A = Ambulation, B = Bedrest, BSC = Bedside Commode, BRP = Bathroom Privileges, C = Chair, D = Dangle, U = Up ad lib, W = Wheel Chair)						
Distance/Duration (Distance in feet or duration in minutes if appropriate)						
# Assist (Number of people assisting with activity if appropriate, S = Staff, FA = with family member, I = Independent)						
Assistive devices (B – Brace, C = Cane, W = Walker, CR = Crutches if Appropriate)						
Activity/ Exercise Tolerance (√ = Assessment Normal, * = Assessment Abnormal, → Abnormal Unchanged)						
INITIALS						

BOWEL RESECTION WITH OSTOMY CLINICAL PATHWAY   ©

ADDITIONAL INTERVENTIONS:
Incorporate patient's belief system/spiritual and/or cultural beliefs into plan of care, if appropriate.
Assess existence of Advanced Directive and Code Status (Document in TDS)
Triflo 10 x q hr   JP drain   Ostomy care
Foley catheter – I/O   N/G irrig q 4 hrs & prn

EDUCATIONAL OUTCOMES: (Y = Yes, N = No, C = Carry over to the next day) Patient/Family will:

	Met/Initial
1. Demonstrate correct technique for DB & C	
2. Demonstrate use of Incentive Spirometer	

EDUCATIONAL INTERVENTIONS: Initial in appropriate shift to indicate intervention complete. Place "NR" or "needs reinforcement" when intervention needs to be reinforced.

	7p – 7a	7a – 7p
1. Assess readiness to learn - Place the appropriate letter from key below in the box corresponding to your shift, followed by your initials and make Narrative Notes as needed. A = Anxious, B = Language Barrier, E = Eager to learn, D = Denies need for education, I = Uninterested, C = Cognitive Concern, M = Memory Problems, N = Not assessed, U = Uncooperative		
2. Reinforce DB & C		
3. Reinforce use of Incentive Spirometer (10 x q hr)		
4. Give patient/family copy of Patient Pathway		

DIET: - NPO

DIAGNOSTIC TESTS
Labs   **Radiology**   **Other**
CBC, Lytes

MEDICATIONS:
PCA, IV Therapy (antibiotics)   * Antipyretics should not generally be given for temperature elevation, check with physician
Heparin SQ   * No suppositories or enemas post-op unless ordered by attending surgeon

CONSULTS – check and initial in space
☐ Social Worker _____   ☐ Pharmacy _____
☐ Pastoral Care _____   ☐ Dietitian _____
☐ Respiratory Therapy _____

DISCHARGE PLANNING - check and initial in space
☐ CRC _____   *See Notes

SIGNATURES Each person initialing this pathway must sign full signature, title and initials once.

SIGNATURE AND TITLE	INITIALS	SIGNATURE AND TITLE	INITIALS	SIGNATURE AND TITLE	INITIALS

"This guideline was designed to assist clinicians by providing an analytic framework for the evaluation and treatment of patients, and is not intended either to replace a clinician's judgement or to establish a protocol for all patients with a particular condition. A guideline will rarely establish the only approach to patient care."

FORM #: 90681
9/00

BOWEL RESECTION WITH OSTOMY CLINICAL PATHWAY

ST. JOSEPH
MERCY OAKLAND

CODE: <u>362.2</u>
LOS: 5 <u>Days</u>

Post-Op Day 3	Date:					
KEY PATIENT OUTCOMES: (Y = Yes, N = No, C = Carry over to the next day. If N or C, document in Narrative Notes.)						Met/Initial
1. Patient/family verbalizes feelings/concerns regarding hospitalization/illness.						
2. Patient verbalizes pain controlled (<4 or less on pain scale 0-10)						
3. Absence of respiratory complications AEB lung expansion – patient verbalizes lack of distress						
4. Return of GI function – passing flatus tolerating diet, functioning ostomy						
5. Patient verbalizes feelings related to loss/disfigurement						
6. Adequate urinary output AEB: no urinary retention						
INTERVENTIONS: **TIME** (√ = Assessment Normal, * = Assessment Abnormal, → Abnormal Unchanged)						
ADL assistance (FA = Family assisted, S = Staff, I = Independent) whenever performed/ADL tolerance. (√ = Assessment Normal, * = Assessment Abnormal, → Abnormal Unchanged)						
Respiratory assessment q shift & prn						
GI assessment q shift & prn						
GU assessment q shift & prn						
Assess incision/drsg/ q shift & prn						
DB & C Incentive Spirometer 10x q 1 hr w.a. (Document average # cc reached)						
Response to participation in ostomy care q shift & prn						
Assess stoma q shift & prn						
Refer to other forms: ☐ Episodic Flow Record ☐ Unit Specific Flow Record **INITIALS**						
ACTIVITY/EXERCISE **TIME**						
Activity (A = Ambulation, B = Bedrest, BSC = Bedside Commode, BRP = Bathroom Privileges, C = Chair, D = Dangle, U = Up ad lib, W = Wheel Chair)						
Distance/Duration (Distance in feet or duration in minutes if appropriate)						
# Assist (Number of people assisting with activity if appropriate, S = Staff, FA = with family member, I = Independent						
Assistive devices (B – Brace, C = Cane, W = Walker, CR = Crutches if Appropriate)						
Activity/ Exercise Tolerance (√ = Assessment Normal, * = Assessment Abnormal, → Abnormal Unchanged)						
INITIALS						

BOWEL RESECTION WITH OSTOMY CLINICAL PATHWAY   ©

ADDITIONAL INTERVENTIONS:
Incorporate patient's belief system/spiritual and/or cultural beliefs into plan of care, if appropriate.
Assess existence of Advanced Directive and Code Status (Document in TDS)
Foley D/C
I/O   TEDS off 1 hr/shift   Ostomy care
JP drain   N/G Tube D/C   Ostomy appliance: 1 piece # _____   2 piece # _____

EDUCATIONAL OUTCOMES: (Y = Yes, N = No, C = Carry over to the next day) Patient/Family will:	Met/Initial	
1. Demonstrate Incentive Spirometer (level 1500 cc)		
2. Verbalize and demonstrates ostomy care before discharge		
3. Verbalize understanding of Discharge Care Pathway		
4. Verbalize understanding ostomy care		

EDUCATIONAL INTERVENTIONS: Initial in appropriate shift to indicate intervention complete. Place "NR" or "needs reinforcement" when intervention needs to be reinforced.	7p – 7a	7a – 7p
1. Assess readiness to learn - Place the appropriate letter from key below in the box corresponding to your shift, followed by your initials and make Narrative Notes as needed. A = Anxious, B = Language Barrier, E = Eager to learn, D = Denies need for education, I = Uninterested, C = Cognitive Concern, M = Memory Problems, N = Not assessed, U = Uncooperative		
2. Reinforce Incentive Spirometer (10 x q hr)		
3. Give patient/family Discharge Care Pathway		
4. Teach patient self care re: Incision, ostomy care		
5. Patient/S.O. view ostomy film		

DIET: - Liquid
DIAGNOSTIC TESTS
Labs   Radiology   Other

MEDICATIONS:
Oral analgesics   * Antipyretics should not generally be given for temperature elevation, check with physician
                       * No suppositories or enemas post-op unless ordered by attending surgeon
CONSULTS – check and initial in space
☐ Social Worker _____   ☐ Pharmacy _____
☐ Pastoral Care _____   ☐ Dietitian _____
☐ Respiratory Therapy _____

DISCHARGE PLANNING - check and initial in space
☐ CRC _____   *See Notes

SIGNATURES Each person initialing this pathway must sign full signature, title and initials once.

SIGNATURE AND TITLE	INITIALS	SIGNATURE AND TITLE	INITIALS	SIGNATURE AND TITLE	INITIALS

"This guideline was designed to assist clinicians by providing an analytic framework for the evaluation and treatment of patients, and is not intended either to replace a clinician's judgement or to establish a protocol for all patients with a particular condition. A guideline will rarely establish the only approach to patient care."

FORM #: 90618   **BOWEL RESECTION WITH OSTOMY CLINICAL PATHWAY**
9/00

ST. JOSEPH MERCY OAKLAND

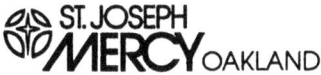

CODE: <u>362.2</u>
LOS: 5 <u>Days</u>

Post-Op Day 4	Date:				
KEY PATIENT OUTCOMES: (Y = Yes, N = No, C = Carry over to the next day. If N or C, document in Narrative Notes.)					Met/Initial
1. Patient/family concurs with plan of care (Document every day)					
2. Absence of respiratory complications AEB lung expansion – patient verbalizes lack of distress					
3. Return of GI function AEB passing flatus, functional ostomy, tolerating diet					
4. Patient states pain controlled (<4 on pain scale 0-10)					
5. Patient verbalizes feelings of disfigurement					
INTERVENTIONS: **TIME** (√ = Assessment Normal, * = Assessment Abnormal, → Abnormal Unchanged)					
ADL assistance (FA = Family assisted, S = Staff, I = Independent) whenever performed/ADL tolerance. (√ = Assessment Normal, * = Assessment Abnormal, → Abnormal Unchanged)					
Respiratory assessment q shift & prn					
GI assessment q shift & prn					
GU assessment q shift & prn					
Assess incision/drsg q shift & prn					
Response to participation in ostomy care q shift & prn (Document in narrative notes)					
DB & C Incentive Spirometer 10x q 1 hr. w.a. (Document average # cc reached)					
Assess stoma q shift & prn					
Refer to other forms: ☐ Episodic Flow Record ☐ Unit Specific Flow Record **INITIALS**					
ACTIVITY/EXERCISE **TIME**					
Activity (A = Ambulation, B = Bedrest, BSC = Bedside Commode, BRP = Bathroom Privileges, C = Chair, D = Dangle, U = Up ad lib, W = Wheel Chair)					
Distance/Duration (Distance in feet or duration in minutes if appropriate)					
# Assist (Number of people assisting with activity if appropriate, S = Staff, FA = with family member, I = Independent					
Assistive devices (B – Brace, C = Cane, W = Walker, CR = Crutches if Appropriate)					
Activity/ Exercise Tolerance (√ = Assessment Normal, * = Assessment Abnormal, → Abnormal Unchanged)					
INITIALS					

FORM #: 90618
9/00

BOWEL RESECTION WITH OSTOMY CLINICAL PATHWAY ©

ADDITIONAL INTERVENTIONS:
Incorporate patient's belief system/spiritual and/or cultural beliefs into plan of care, if appropriate.
Assess existence of Advanced Directive and Code Status (Document in TDS)
TEDS – off 1 hr q shift   Ostomy care
I/O   Ostomy appliance: 1 piece # _____   2 piece # _____

EDUCATIONAL OUTCOMES: (Y = Yes, N = No, C = Carry over to the next day) Patient/Family will:	Met/Initial	
1. Verbalize home care before discharge		
2. Verbalize and demonstrates ability to change ostomy appliance		

EDUCATIONAL INTERVENTIONS: Initial in appropriate shift to indicate intervention complete. Place "NR" or "needs reinforcement" when intervention needs to be reinforced.	7p – 7a	7a – 7p

1. Assess readiness to learn - Place the appropriate letter from key below in the box corresponding to your shift, followed by your initials and make Narrative Notes as needed.
     A = Anxious, B = Language Barrier, E = Eager to learn, D = Denies need for education,
     I = Uninterested, C = Cognitive Concern, M = Memory Problems, N = Not assessed,
     U = Uncooperative		

2. Reinforce information from Discharge Care Pathway		
3. Reinforce skills as indicated		
4. Reassess need to see ostomy film again before discharge		

DIET: - As tolerated

DIAGNOSTIC TESTS
Labs   Radiology   Other

MEDICATIONS:
Oral analgesics   * Antipyretics should not generally be given for temperature elevation, check with physician
                         * No suppositories or enemas post-op unless ordered by attending surgeon

CONSULTS – check and initial in space
☐ Social Worker _____   ☐ Pharmacy _____
☐ Pastoral Care _____   ☐ Dietitian _____
☐ Respiratory Therapy _____

DISCHARGE PLANNING - check and initial in space
☐ CRC _____   *See Notes

SIGNATURES Each person initialing this pathway must sign full signature, title and initials once.

SIGNATURE AND TITLE	INITIALS	SIGNATURE AND TITLE	INITIALS	SIGNATURE AND TITLE	INITIALS

"This guideline was designed to assist clinicians by providing an analytic framework for the evaluation and treatment of patients, and is not intended either to replace a clinician's judgement or to establish a protocol for all patients with a particular condition. A guideline will rarely establish the only approach to patient care."

FORM #: 90618
9/0

BOWEL RESECTION WITH OSTOMY CLINCIAL PATHWAY

ST. JOSEPH MERCYOAKLAND

CODE: <u>362.2</u>
LOS: 5 <u>Days</u>

Post-Op Day 5	Date:				
KEY PATIENT OUTCOMES: (Y = Yes, N = No, C = Carry over to the next day. If N or C, document in Narrative Notes.)					Met/Initial
1. Patient/family concurs with plan of care (Document every day).					
2. Absence of respiratory complications AEB lung expansion – patient verbalizes lack of distress					
3. Return of GI functions AEB passing flatus, functional ostomy tolerating diet					
INTERVENTIONS: **TIME** (√ = Assessment Normal, * = Assessment Abnormal, → Abnormal Unchanged)					
ADL assistance (FA = Family assisted, S = Staff, I = Independent) whenever performed/ADL tolerance. (√ = Assessment Normal, * = Assessment Abnormal, → Abnormal Unchanged)					
Respiratory assessment q shift & prn					
GI assessment q shift & prn					
GU assessment q shift & prn					
Assess incision/drsg q shift & prn					
Response to participation in ostomy care prn (Document in narrative notes)					
Assess stoma q shift & prn					
Refer to other forms: ☐ Episodic Flow Record ☐ Unit Specific Flow Record **INITIALS**					
ACTIVITY/EXERCISE **TIME**					
Activity (A = Ambulation, B = Bedrest, BSC = Bedside Commode, BRP = Bathroom Privileges, C = Chair, D = Dangle, U = Up ad lib, W = Wheel Chair)					
Distance/Duration (Distance in feet or duration in minutes if appropriate)					
# Assist (Number of people assisting with activity if appropriate, S = Staff, FA = with family member, I = Independent					
Assistive devices (B – Brace, C = Cane, W = Walker, CR = Crutches if Appropriate)					
Activity/ Exercise Tolerance (√ = Assessment Normal, * = Assessment Abnormal, → Abnormal Unchanged)					
INITIALS					

FORM #: 90618
9/00

BOWEL RESECTION WITH OSTOMY CLINICAL PATHWAY ©

ADDITIONAL INTERVENTIONS:
Incorporate patient's belief system/spiritual and/or cultural beliefs into plan of care, if appropriate.
Assess existence of Advanced Directive and Code Status (Document in TDS)

EDUCATIONAL OUTCOMES: (Y = Yes, N = No, C = Carry over to the next day) Patient/Family will:	Met/Initial	
1. Verbalize knowledge of ostomy care		

EDUCATIONAL INTERVENTIONS: Initial in appropriate shift to indicate intervention complete. Place "NR" or "needs reinforcement" when intervention needs to be reinforced.	7p – 7a	7a – 7p
1. Assess readiness to learn - Place the appropriate letter from key below in the box corresponding to your shift, followed by your initials and make Narrative Notes as needed. A = Anxious, B = Language Barrier, E = Eager to learn, D = Denies need for education, I = Uninterested, C = Cognitive Concern, M = Memory Problems, N = Not assessed, U = Uncooperative		
2. Reinforce information from, "How To Care For Your Ostomy"		

DIET: - General

DIAGNOSTIC TESTS
Labs   Radiology   Other

MEDICATIONS:
Oral analgesics

CONSULTS – check and initial in space
☐ Social Worker _____   ☐ Pharmacy _____
☐ Pastoral Care _____   ☐ Dietitian _____
☐ Respiratory Therapy _____

DISCHARGE PLANNING - check and initial in space
☐ CRC _____   *See Notes

SIGNATURES   Each person initialing this pathway must sign full signature, title and initials once.

SIGNATURE AND TITLE	INITIALS	SIGNATURE AND TITLE	INITIALS	SIGNATURE AND TITLE	INITIALS

"This guideline was designed to assist clinicians by providing an analytic framework for the evaluation and treatment of patients, and is not intended either to replace a clinician's judgement or to establish a protocol for all patients with a particular condition. A guideline will rarely establish the only approach to patient care."

BOWEL RESECTION WITH OSTOMY CLINICAL PATHWAY

ST. JOSEPH MERCY OAKLAND

Pain Med_____   Date: _____

Med Change to_____.

(Reassess pain score and relief within one hour of intervention)

TIME																
10	•	•	•	•	•	•	•	•	•	•	•	•	•	•	•	•
9	•	•	•	•	•	•	•	•	•	•	•	•	•	•	•	•
8	•	•	•	•	•	•	•	•	•	•	•	•	•	•	•	•
7	•	•	•	•	•	•	•	•	•	•	•	•	•	•	•	•
Pain 6	•	•	•	•	•	•	•	•	•	•	•	•	•	•	•	•
Score 5	•	•	•	•	•	•	•	•	•	•	•	•	•	•	•	•
4	•	•	•	•	•	•	•	•	•	•	•	•	•	•	•	•
3	•	•	•	•	•	•	•	•	•	•	•	•	•	•	•	•
2	•	•	•	•	•	•	•	•	•	•	•	•	•	•	•	•
1	•	•	•	•	•	•	•	•	•	•	•	•	•	•	•	•
0	•	•	•	•	•	•	•	•	•	•	•	•	•	•	•	•
Pain relief acceptable ✓, Rx, or ✽																

Pain Management Education

Comfort Goal:_____   Informed that pain relief is important ☐ Yes ☐ No ☐ N/A

Instructed patient to notify RN if in pain ☐ Yes ☐ No ☐ N/A   Patient notified of changes made to pain medication ☐ Yes ☐ No ☐ N/A

Patient Assessment (for IV pain meds)				INFUSION INFORMATION Medication_____						SHIFT TOTALS				Epidural and Intrathecal patients only			
Time	Resp Rate	Level of Sedation	Side Effects	System Check	Bolus Dose	Basal Rate	PCA Dose	Delay Time	Hourly Lockout	Total Mg. Infused	Injections			*Motor		*Sensory	
											Attempts	Injection		RL	LL	RL	LL

CODES FOR ASSESSMENT

SYSTEM CHECK GUIDELINES	LEVEL OF SEDATION	SIDE EFFECTS	MOTOR FUNCTION(BROMAGE) EPIDURAL OR INTRATHECAL	SENSORY EPIDURAL OR INTRATHECAL
Infusion system securely taped, tubing's are patent, and pump has volume and is infusing as ordered. PCA-Patient button within reach and functioning properly. Place (✓) in box if assessment meets normal. Place (✽) in box if abnormal and document	S- Sleeping: easy to arouse 1 – Awake and alert 2 – Occasionally drowsy: easy to arouse 3 – Frequently drowsy: arousable, drifts off to sleep during conversation 4 – Somnolent; difficult to arouse; minimal or no response to stimuli (Notify Anesthesia)	0 – None N – Nausea V – Vomiting I – Itching CM- change of mentation UR – Urinary Retention C – Constipation H – Hypotension (Notify Anesthesia) R – Respiratory Depression (RR< 10) (Notify Anesthesia)	0 – No motor block 1 - Inability to raise leg (Notify Anesthesia) 2 - Inability to flex knee (Notify Anesthesia) 3 - Inability to flex ankle (Notify Anesthesia) X - Immobilized, can wiggle toes	1- WNL 2- Numbness 3- Tingling If patient has 2 or 3 and did not receive local anesthetic, NOTIFY ANESTHESIA ASAP

Multidisciplinary Care Planning

☐ Patient/Family   ☐ Physician   ☐ RNCM   ☐ CRC   ☐ Social Worker

☐ Pastoral Care   ☐ Dietary   ☐ Pharmacy   ☐ PT   ☐ OT

☐ Speech   ☐ Other

Prioritized Plan of Care:

_____

_____

_____

_____

_____

_____

_____

_____

_____

_____

Signature: _____

FORM # 90799   **PAIN MANAGEMENT/PLAN OF CARE RECORD**

References

1. Kodner IJ, Fry RD, Fleshman JW, et al. Colon, rectum, and anus. In: Schwartz SI, et al., eds. Principles of Surgery, 7th ed. New York, NY: McGraw-Hill, 1999: 1265–1382.
2. Eckhauser FE, Knol JA. Surgery for primary and metastatic colorectal cancer. Gastroenterol Clin North Am. 1997; 26:103–128.
3. Greene F. Laparoscopic management of colorectal cancer. CA Cancer J Clin. 1999; 49:221–228.
4. Franklin ME, Rosenthal D, Abrego-Medina D, et al. Prospective comparison of open vs laparoscopic colon surgery for carcinoma: Five-year results. Dis Colon Rectum. 1996; 39:S35–S46 (suppl 10).
5. Franklin ME, Rosenthal D, Norem RF. Prospective evaluation of laparoscopic colon resection versus open colon resection for adenocarcinoma. A multicenter study. Surg Endosc. 1995; 9:811–816.
6. Milsom JW, Bohm B, Hammerhofer KA, et al. A prospective, randomized trial comparing laparoscopic versus conventional techniques in colorectal cancer surgery: A preliminary report. J Am Coll Surg. 1998; 187:46–54.
7. Kakisako K, Koichi S, Yosuke A, et al. Laparoscopic colectomy for Dukes A colon cancer. Surg Laparosc Endosc Percutan Tech. 2000; 10: 66–70.
8. Colon and Rectal Cancer Treatment Guidelines for Patients. Version 1, March 2000. American Cancer Society and the NCCN. Atlanta, GA: ACS.
9. NCI high-priority clinical trial. Available at: http://cancernet.nci.nih.gov/cgibin/srch... col&ZUI=199_10431&SFMT=prot_summary/ 1/0/0 Accessed October 28, 2000.
10. Krag DN, Weaver DI, Alex JC, et al. Surgical resection and radiolocalization of the sentinel lymph node in breast cancer using a gamma probe. Surg Oncol. 1993; 2:335–339.
11. Guiliano A, Jones R, Brennan M, et al. Sentinel lymphadenectomy in breast cancer. J Clin Oncol. 1997; 15:2345–2350.
12. Albertini J, Lyman G, Cox C, et al. Lymphatic mapping and sentinel node biopsy in patient with breast cancer. JAMA. 1996; 276:1818–1822.
13. Morton D, Wen D, Wong J, et al. Technical details of intraoperative lymphatic mapping for early stage melanoma. Arch Surg. 1992; 127: 392–399.
14. Saha S, Wiese D, Badin J, et al. Technical details of sentinel lymph node mapping in colorectal cancer and its impact on staging. Ann Surg Oncol. 2000; 7:120–124.
15. Kettlewell MG. Colorectal cancer and benign tumours of the colon. In: Morris PJ, Malt RA, eds. Oxford Textbook of Surgery. New York, NY: Oxford University Press, 1994: 1060–1087.
16. Bleday R, Steele G. Colorectal cancer surgery. In: Rustgi AK, ed. Gastrointestinal Cancers: Biology, Diagnosis, and Therapy. Philadelphia, PA: Lippincott-Raven Publishers, 1995: 455–475.
17. Guillem JG, Cohen AM. Current issues in colorectal cancer surgery. Semin Oncol. 1999; 26: 505–513.
18. Asbun HJ, Hughes KS. Management of recurrent and metastatic colorectal carcinoma. Surg Clin North Am. 1993; 73:145–165.
19. Rosato E. Hepatobiliary malignancy. Presented at Thomas Jefferson University Oncology Grand Rounds. Philadelphia, PA, October 11, 2000.
20. Fong Y. Surgical therapy of hepatic colorectal metastasis. CA Cancer J Clin. 1999; 49:231–253.
21. Sheele K, Stang R, Altendorf-Hoffman A, et al. Resection of colorectal liver metastases. World J Surg. 1995; 19:59–71.
22. Jamison RI, Donohue JH, Nagorney DM, et al. Hepatic resection for metastatic colorectal cancer results in cure for some patients. Arch Surg. 1997; 132:505–511.

23. Fong Y, Fortner J, Sun R, et al. Clinical score for predicting recurrence after hepatic resection for metastatic colorectal cancer: Analysis of 1001 consecutive cases. Ann Surg. 1999; 230: 309–318.

24. Fong Y, Cohen AM, Fortner JG, et al. Liver resection for colorectal metastases. J Clin Oncol. 1997; 15:938–946.

25. Jenkins LT, Milikan KW, Bines SD, et al. Hepatic resection for metastatic colorectal cancer. Am Surg. 1997; 63:605–610.

26. Fong Y, Blumgart LH. Surgical therapy of liver cancer. In: Zakim D, Boyer TD, eds. Hepatology: A Textbook of Liver Disease, 3rd ed. Philadelphia, PA: WB Saunders Company, 1996: 1548–1564.

27. Jarnagin WR. Hepatic colorectal metastases: Surgical management. In: Perry MC, ed. ASCO Clinical Practice Forum Book. Alexandria, VA: American Society of Clinical Oncology, 2000: 69–72.

28. Dosi R, Gennari L, Gignami P, et al. Morbidity and mortality after hepatic resection of metastases from colorectal cancer. Br J Surg. 1995; 82: 337–381.

29. Fischer JE, Nussbaum MS, Chance WT, et al. Manifestation of gastrointestinal disease. In: Schwartz SI, Shires GT, Spencer FC, et al., eds. Principles of Surgery, 7th ed. New York, NY: McGraw-Hill, 1999: 1033–1079.

30. Hampton BG, Bryant R. Ostomies and continent diversions. St. Louis, MO: Mosby–Year Book, 1992: 1–128.

31. Turnell E. Mindfulness and people with stomas. JWOCN. 1996; 23:38–45.

32. Klula A, Kristjanson LJ. Development and testing of the Ostomy Concerns Scale: Measuring ostomy-related concerns of cancer patients and their partners. JWOCN. 1996; 23:166–170.

33. Northouse L, Schafer J, Tipton J, et al. The concerns of patients and spouses after the diagnosis of colon cancer: A qualitative analysis. JWOCN. 1999; 26:8–17.

34. Piwonka MA, Merino J. A multidimensional modeling of predictors influencing the adjustment to a colostomy. JWOCN. 1999; 26: 298–305.

35. Rolstad BS, Boarini J. Principles and techniques in the use of convexity. Ostomy/Wound Manage. 1996; 42(1):325–346.

36. Erwin-Toth P. The effect of ostomy surgery between the ages of 6 and 12 years on psychosocial development during childhood, adolescence, and young adulthood. JWOCN. 1999; 26:77–85.

37. Manworren R. Developmental effects on the adolescent of temporary ileostomy. JWOCN. 1996; 23:210–217.

38. Pieper B, Mikols C. Predischarge and postdischarge concerns of persons with an ostomy. JWOCN. 1996; 23:105–109.

39. Erwin-Toth P. Prevention and management of peristomal skin complications. Adv Skin Wound Care. 2000; 13(4):175–178.

40. Campbell K, Woodbury G, Whittle H, et al. A clinical evaluation of 3M no-sting barrier film. Ostomy/Wound Manage. 2000; 46:24–30.

41. Kirsner R, Froelich C. Soaps and detergents: Understanding their composition and effect. Ostomy/Wound Manage. 1998; 44:62S–70S.

42. Golis A. Sexual issues for the person with an ostomy. JWOCN. 1996; 23:33–37.

43. Roberts D. The pursuit of colostomy continence. JWOCN. 1997; 24:92–97.

44. Halvorson M, Kertz J. Changes in Medicare reimbursement for ostomy supplies: An overview. JWOCN. 1996; 23:26–32.

45. Jones K, Denomme V. Bowel resection pathway saves $2,500 per case, cuts LOS. Hosp Case Manage. 2000; 7:103–106.

46. Black JM, Matassarin-Jacobs E. Medical-Surgical Nursing: Clinical Management for Continuity of Care, 5th ed. Philadelphia, PA: WB Saunders Company, 1997: 484–492, 1811–1816.

47. Mischler MA. Interventions for intraoperative clients. In: Ignatavicius DD, Workman ML,

Mishler MA, eds. Medical-Surgical Nursing: A Nursing Process Approach, 2nd ed. Philadelphia, PA: WB Saunders Company, 1994: 360–377, 409–430.

48. Carpenito LJ. Nursing Care Plans and Documentation, 2nd ed. Philadelphia, PA: JB Lippincott Co., 1995: 484–498, 780–798.

49. Ellis C, Saddler DS. Colorectal cancer. In: Yarbro CH, Frogge MH, Goodman M, et al., eds. Cancer Nursing: Principles and Practice, 5th ed. Sudbury, MA: Jones and Bartlett, 2000: 1117–1137.

50. Brunner DW, Iwamoto RR. Altered sexual health. In: Groenwald SL, ed. Cancer Symptom Management. Sudbury, MA: Jones and Bartlett, 2000: 523–551.

CHAPTER 8 | Radiation Therapy

Tracy K. Gosselin, RN, MSN, AOCN

Introduction

Patients diagnosed with colorectal cancer face myriad treatment options and a disease trajectory that is often unpredictable. Radiation therapy is one type of treatment modality for patients diagnosed with colorectal cancer, and the decision to use radiation therapy is based on individual patient characteristics. The focus of this chapter is on the role of external beam radiation therapy in the management of colorectal cancer, as well as the role of intraoperative radiation therapy, combined-modality treatment, and the nursing management that is essential to the quality of life for patients undergoing treatment.

Radiation oncology is a term used to describe the clinical as well as scientific discipline dedicated to the treatment of a person with cancer, using ionizing radiation.[1] The radiation therapy treatment team consists of the radiation oncologist, radiation therapist, physicist, dosimetrist, and nurse. Treatment facilities may also have social workers, dietitians, and cancer patient support programs, to which patients can be referred, depending on their individual needs. If clinical trials are being conducted, research staff will be involved with the coordination of patient care.

Radiation therapy in the colorectal patient can be classified as neoadjuvant or adjuvant, depending on the patient's staging and prognostic factors. In the neoadjuvant setting, the goal is to reduce the tumor burden, making the tumor more resectable, thus sparing healthy tissue at the time of surgical resection, and to downstage the tumor so that the chance of the patient requiring a permanent colostomy is decreased. In the adjuvant setting, the goal is to eradicate any remaining tumor cells and to reduce the risk of local recurrence. Patients may also receive chemotherapy in addition to radiation therapy. The goal of radiation therapy is to deliver a therapeutic dose of ionizing radiation to the tumor while minimizing injury to surrounding healthy tissues.[1] Doing this requires the integration and application of therapeutic principles across all disciplines.

The linear accelerator is the most common treatment-delivery machine in use today (Figure 8.1, see page P-3 of insert). The *linac*, as it is sometimes called, produces both electrons (superficial penetrating radiation) and photons (deep penetrating radiation); this is what is referred to as *external beam radiation therapy*. The radiation is then considered to be either electromagnetic or particulate. Electromagnetic radiation has high energy and consists of gamma rays and x-rays. This type of radiation has no mass and can penetrate tissues deeply, thus sparing the skin. Particulate radiation includes electrons, neutrons, protons, and a variety of other high-energy particles that have a mass, which limits their ability to penetrate into deep tissues. Patients with colorectal cancer are generally treated with high-energy photons.

Radiation therapy is typically fractionated; this means that the total treatment dose is divided over a set number of days or weeks. Patients typically receive one fraction per day, whereas in hyperfractionation, the patient receives more than one treatment per day. For cell death to occur, the DNA needs to be damaged by the ionizing radiation. In understanding fractionation, it is important to understand the four Rs of radiobiology:

1. *Repair* is the ability of the cells to recover from sublethal radiation injury between radiation treatments. Normal cells have the ability to repair between treatments, whereas the

ability of the tumor cells to repair diminishes over time with continued radiation.

2. *Reproduction* (repopulation) is the ability of the normal irradiated cells to successfully undergo mitosis between radiation doses. Tumor cells are less successful in undergoing mitosis, due to injury from the radiation.

3. *Redistribution* is when the remaining tumor cells move into mitosis, which is considered to be the most sensitive phase of the cell cycle with each consecutive radiation treatment.

4. *Reoxygenation* of cells occurs between successive doses of radiation, which is also known as *fractionation*. Well-oxygenated cells are more sensitive to the effects of radiation.

Pretreatment Evaluation and Studies

Before patients are scheduled to start radiation therapy, they are seen in consultation by the radiation oncologist. At this initial visit, they undergo a thorough history and physical examination. In addition, laboratory and radiographic studies are discussed, and treatment recommendations, including acute and late side effects, are reviewed. The radiation nurse provides the patients and their families with symptom management and patient education materials that are pertinent to the treatment plan and consistent with their educational and cultural backgrounds.

Typical studies that are performed prior to consultation with the radiation oncologist may include a computed tomography (CT) scan or magnetic resonance imaging (MRI) of the abdomen and pelvis, colonoscopy or barium enema, chest x-ray, and a transrectal ultrasound. Patients also may undergo carcinoembryonic antigen (CEA), complete blood count, serum chemistry, and liver function tests. Additionally, pathology will be reviewed to confirm diagnosis.

Treatment Planning

The goal of treatment planning is to define the target volume to be treated with external beam radiation and to minimize the dose of radiation to healthy tissue/organs in the surrounding area. Factors that are taken into consideration during the planning process include the patients' age and performance status, prognosis and stage of disease, tumor histology, tumor size and location, the known patterns of disease spread, acute and late side effects, and available treatment equipment. The radiation oncologist, who develops and oversees the therapy, uses this information to develop an appropriate treatment plan.

Simulation

Simulation is done prior to the initiation of radiation therapy and typically takes an hour in patients with colorectal cancer. The simulator mimics the actual treatment machine, in how it moves, but does not deliver radiation (Figure 8.2, see page P-3 of insert). Patients are asked to drink oral barium contrast 30 to 60 minutes prior to the simulation to provide better visualization of the small bowel, and they may also receive intravenous contrast, if indicated. A Foley catheter, rectal tube, and/or a contrast enhanced vaginal cylinder also may be placed to assist with identification of anatomic structures (vagina, bladder, and anus). Approximately 60 mL of barium may be placed in the rectal tube to assist in visualizing the anus. In postoperative patients, the rectal contrast should not be inserted until after anterior and lateral radiographs have been obtained to ascertain the position of surgical clips, which are sometimes left to mark the tumor bed.[2] To outline the incision, postoperative patients will have a small wire wrapped in tape placed on the scar to ensure that adequate treatment is provided to the area. Immobilization devices such as an alpha cradle are typically used in patients with colorectal cancer (Figure 8.3, see page P-4 of insert).

The use of contrast may cause patients to feel "a fullness" in the rectal area, and it is important that patients be made aware of this sensation. If patients receive oral contrast, they should be instructed to take a dose of Milk of Magnesia or another laxative, to wash the small bowel contrast out of the intestine, as it can cause constipation in some patients.

During simulation, patients are asked to lie still on the treatment table, which is often referred to as the "treatment couch." The preferred patient position is prone, to allow better visualization of the sacrum on the lateral radiograph and to promote a gravitational shift of small bowel out of the pelvis.[2] This is done to reduce the risk of future small-bowel obstruction. Various techniques can be used to decrease the amount of radiation to the small bowel, such as the use of a belly board or having patients have a full bladder (Table 8.1). Patients who have had prior abdominal surgery or are to receive radiation postoperatively are also at risk for small-bowel obstruction. In women who have had a hysterectomy, the absence of the uterus allows additional loops of bowel to drop into the pelvic radiation field, and, in addition, postsurgical adhesions may cause trappings of loops of small bowel within the radiation field.[3] Patients who are going to receive postoperative radiation may have a mesh sling or pedicle flap placed at the time of surgery to decrease the amount of bowel in the treatment field.

Fluoroscopy is used to assist with identifying the treatment field during simulation. Radiographs are taken at this time to assist with determining treatment volume (Figure 8.4, see page P-4 of insert). The radiographs are also used to assist with reproduction of the treatment

Table 8.1   Techniques to Decrease Radiation Toxicity in Small Bowel

1. High-energy (≥ 6 MV) linear accelerators.
2. Treatment 5 days per week and all fields each day.
3. Port films once per week or more often if clinically indicated.
4. Pelvic field: Multiple-field technique (posterior-anterior plus laterals or posterior-anterior–anterior-posterior plus laterals) is recommended. If the patient is male (the genitalia are commonly in the treatment field), there is a large volume of small bowel in the pelvis, or if a colostomy is present, a three-field technique (posterior-anterior plus laterals) is recommended.
5. Boost field: Opposed laterals.
6. Computerized dosimetry optimizing between minimizing the lateral hot spots and small bowel dose and increasing the homogeneity within the target volume. In thin patients, a combination of 6 MV for the posterior fields and 10 to 15 MV for the lateral fields may result in more homogeneous dosimetry.
7. Shaped blocks and, if needed, wedges on the lateral fields.
8. Small bowel contrast. Shield as much small bowel as possible in the lateral parts.
9. Rectal contrast. Barium sulfate is injected with a 16-French Foley catheter. A wire is placed on the catheter to identify the anal verge.
10. Prone position.
11. Full bladder, only if it does not make the patient so uncomfortable as to cause movement.
12. The only portion of the perineum at risk for recurrence after an abdominoperineal resection is the scar. The remaining perineum can be blocked. The entire perineum can be blocked after a low anterior resection. Use wire to outline the portion of the perineum that is not at risk for recurrence and block it on the lateral fields.
13. Immobilization molds (belly boards) and abdominal wall compression may be helpful.
14. Dose considerations
    A. Limit whole pelvis dose to 4500 to 4680 cGy.
    B. Limit boost to 5000 to 5040 cGy if the small bowel is in the boost field.
    C. Total dose: Preoperative, 5040 cGy; postoperative; 5040 cGy or if the small bowel is excluded from the high-dose field, the boost dose can be increased to 5400 cGy. If there is microscopic or gross residual disease, then higher doses (5500–6000 cGy) are needed; however, this may be associated with increased toxicity.
    D. Standard fractionation in patients receiving combined-modality therapy is 180 cGy per day and in patients receiving radiation therapy alone is 180–200 cGy per day.

Source: With permission, from Minsky B. Rectal cancer. In: Leibel SA, Phillips TL, eds. Textbook of Radiation Oncology, 3rd ed. Philadelphia, PA: WB Saunders Company, 1998: 686–702.

field; these are often referred to as *portal images*. Portal images are x-rays that show the actual treatment field, and are taken at regular intervals (determined by physician/institution) during the patients' treatment. The physician then compares these x-rays with the simulation films to verify the treatment field and to make any changes. The number of portal images taken depends on the number of treatment fields; patients with colorectal cancer typically have a three-field or four-field treatment plan. This means that the radiation beam is directed at the patient from three to four different directions, which can be from the front, back, left, or right side. Patients may often ask what the x-rays that were taken while they were on the

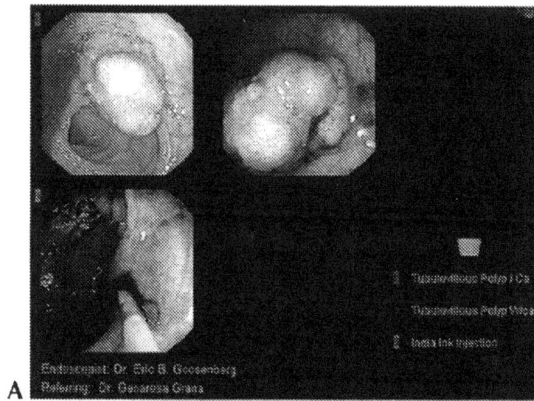
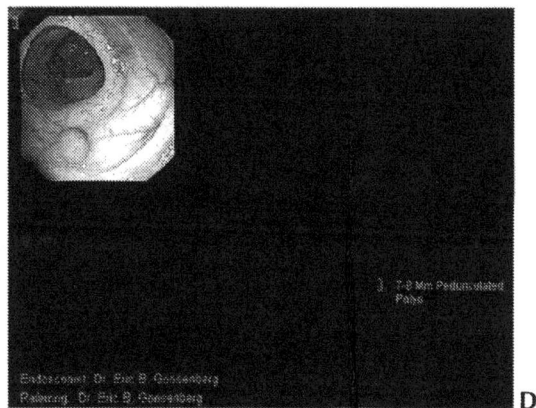
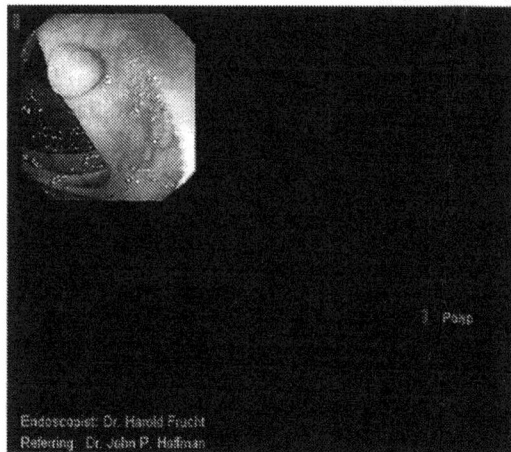
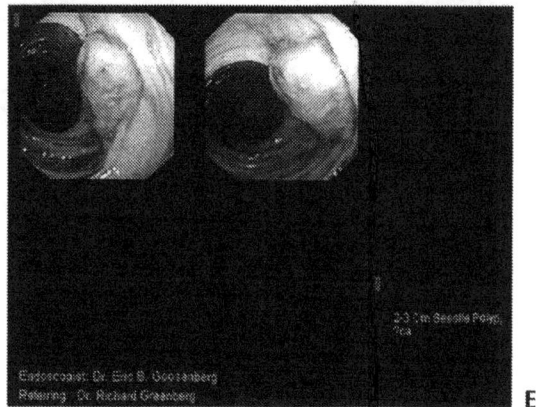
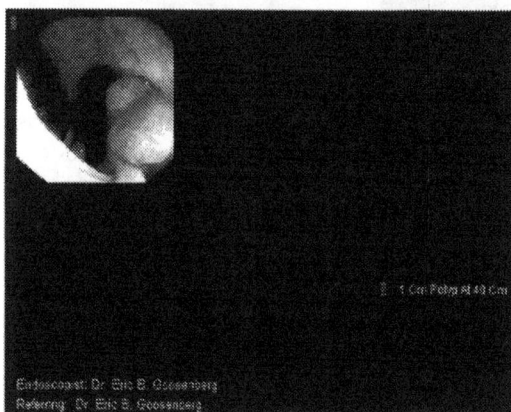
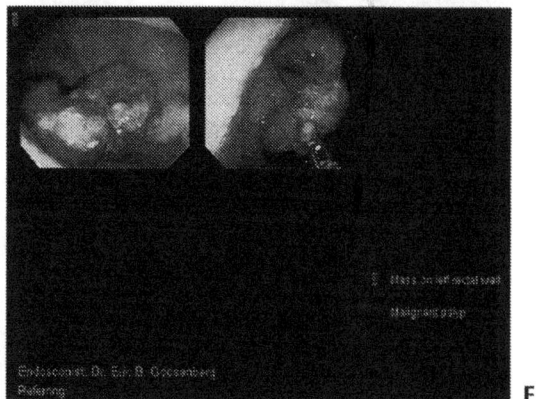

Figure 5.4 Views of polyps, utilizing the Optical Biopsy System. **A:** Tubulovillous polyp. **B:** Polyp on a short stalk. **C:** Snare around a polyp. **D:** Pedunculated polyp. **E:** Sessile polyp. **F:** Malignant polyp in rectum.

Source: Photos courtesy of Dr. Eric B. Goosenberg.

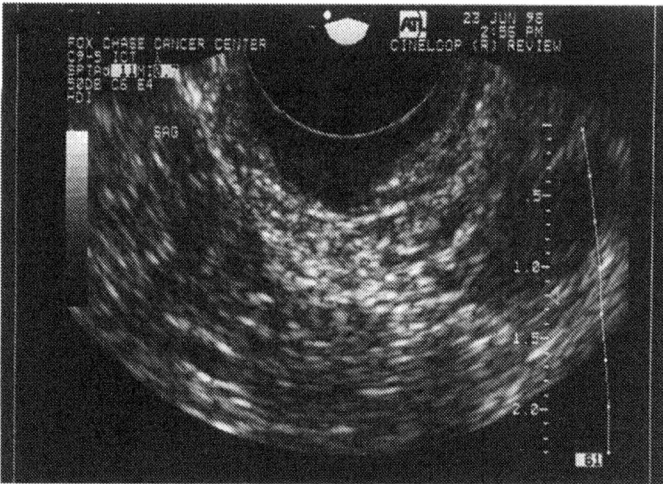

Figure 5.5 Endorectal ultrasound showing well-defined anterior rectal mass. Thickness varies from 0.4 to 0.6 cm. No invasion through the rectal wall.

Source: Photo courtesy of the Fox Chase Cancer Center, Department of Radiology.

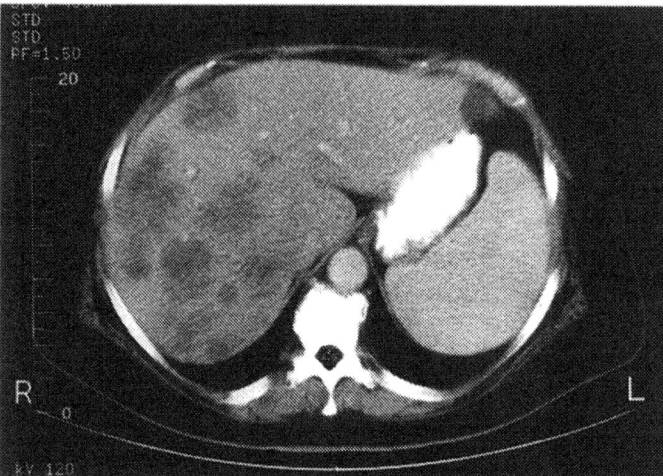

Figure 5.6 CT scan showing widespread metastatic liver disease.

Source: Photo courtesy of the Fox Chase Cancer Center, Department of Radiology.

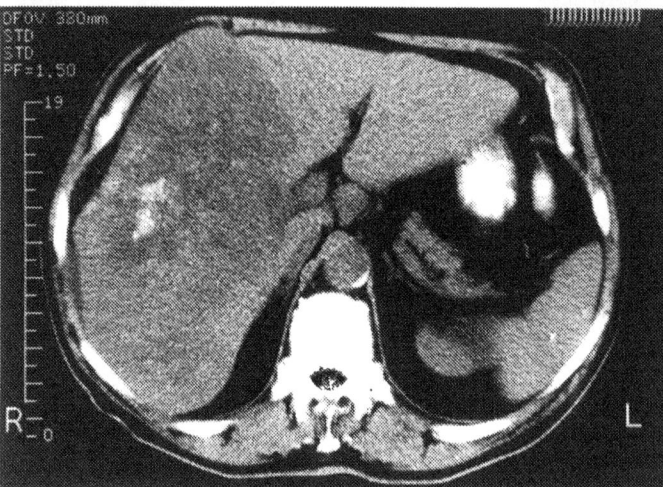

Figure 5.7 CT scan showing extensive metastatic liver disease.

Source: Photo courtesy of the Fox Chase Cancer Center, Department of Radiology.

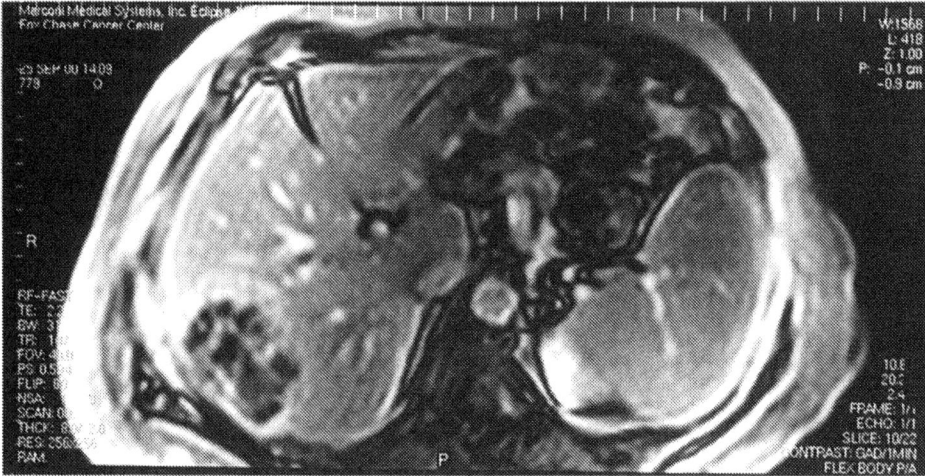

Figure 5.8 MRI demonstrating two masses in the liver consistent with metastatic colon cancer.
Source: Photo courtesy of the Fox Chase Cancer Center, Department of Radiology.

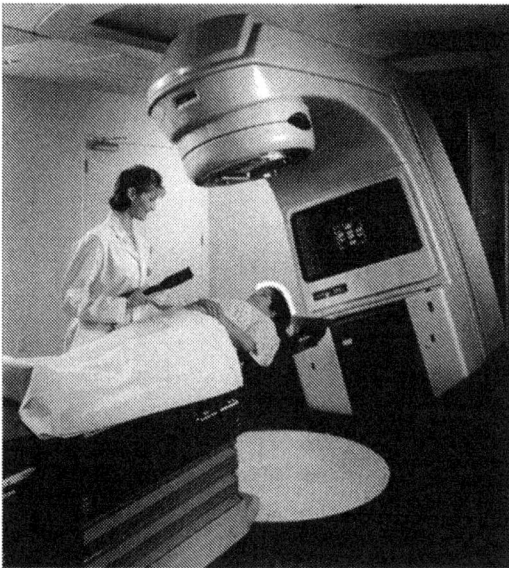

Figure 8.1 Linear accelerator.
Source: Courtesy of Duke University Medical Center, Department of Radiation Oncology, Durham, North Carolina.

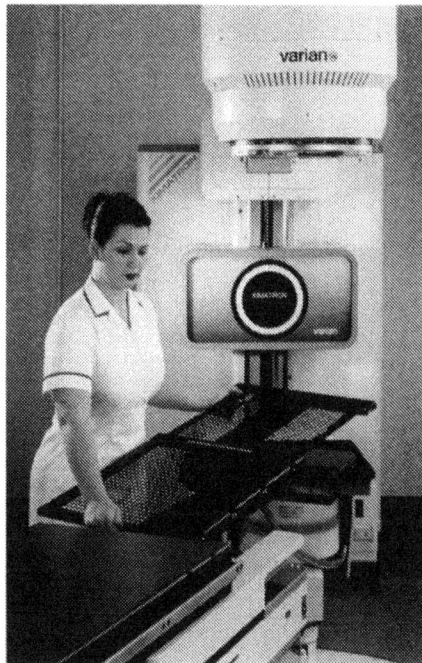

Figure 8.2 Simulator.
Source: Courtesy of Duke University Medical Center, Department of Radiation Oncology, Durham, North Carolina.

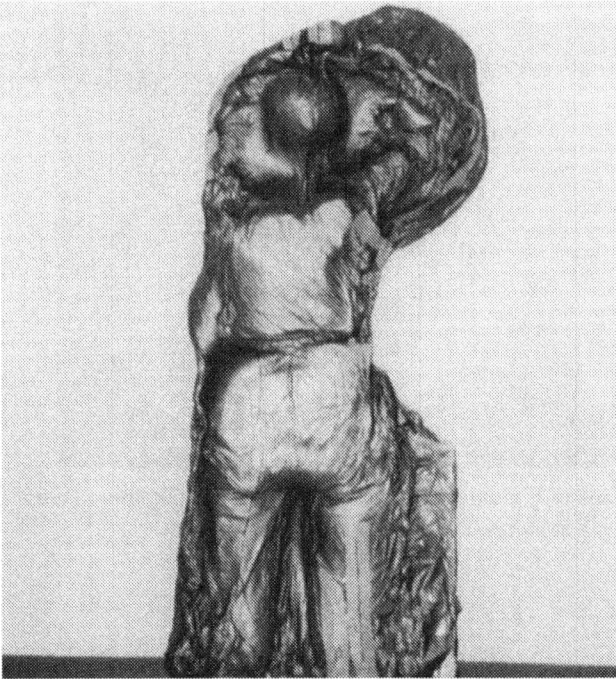

Figure 8.3 Alpha cradle.

Source: Courtesy of Duke University Medical Center, Department of Radiation Oncology, Durham, North Carolina.

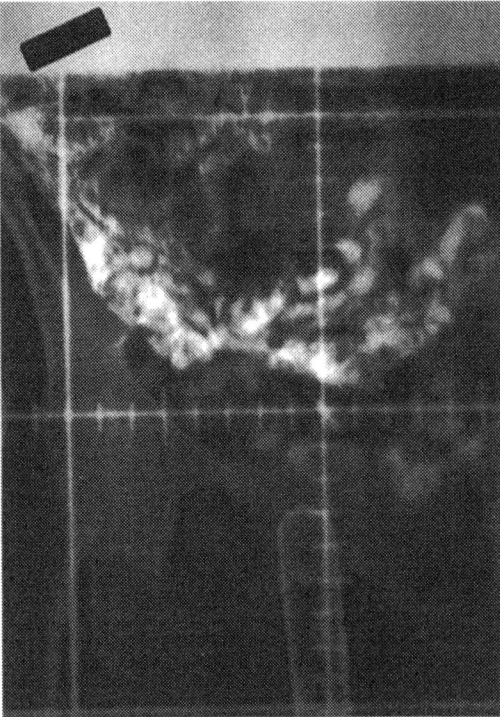

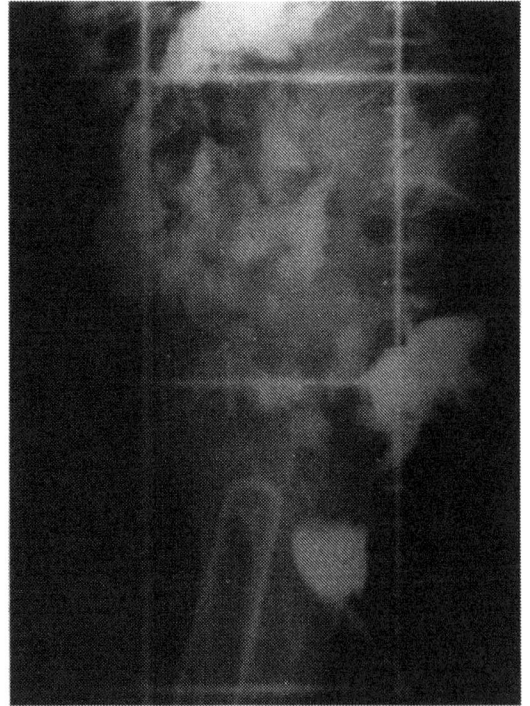

Figure 8.4 Simulation radiograph AP/PA.

Source: Courtesy of Duke University Medical Center, Department of Radiation Oncology, Durham, North Carolina.

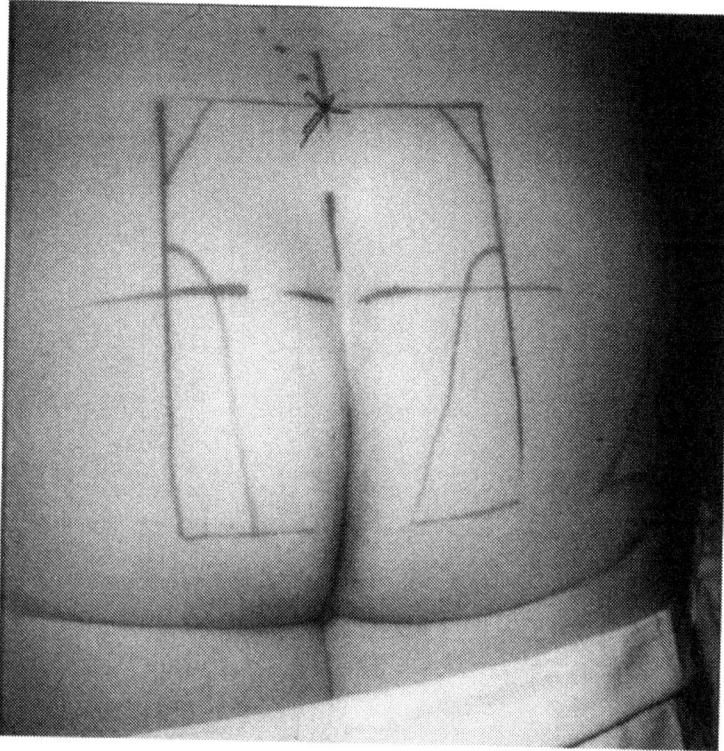

Figure 8.5 Skin markings at time of simulation.

Source: Courtesy of Duke University Medical Center, Department of Radiation Oncology, Durham, North Carolina.

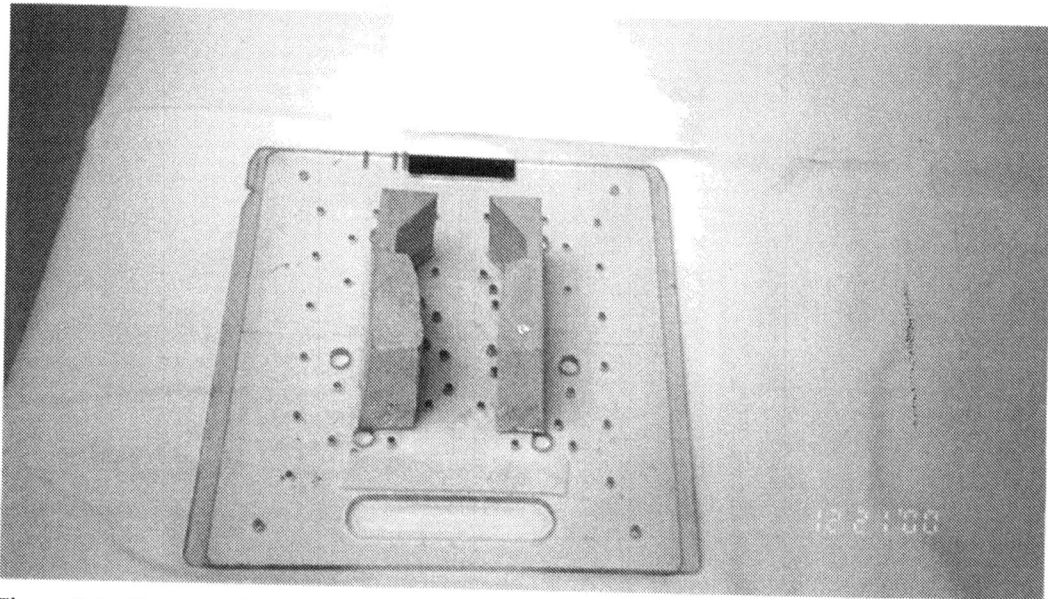

Figure 8.6 Treatment block.

Source: Courtesy of Duke University Medical Center, Department of Radiation Oncology, Durham, North Carolina.

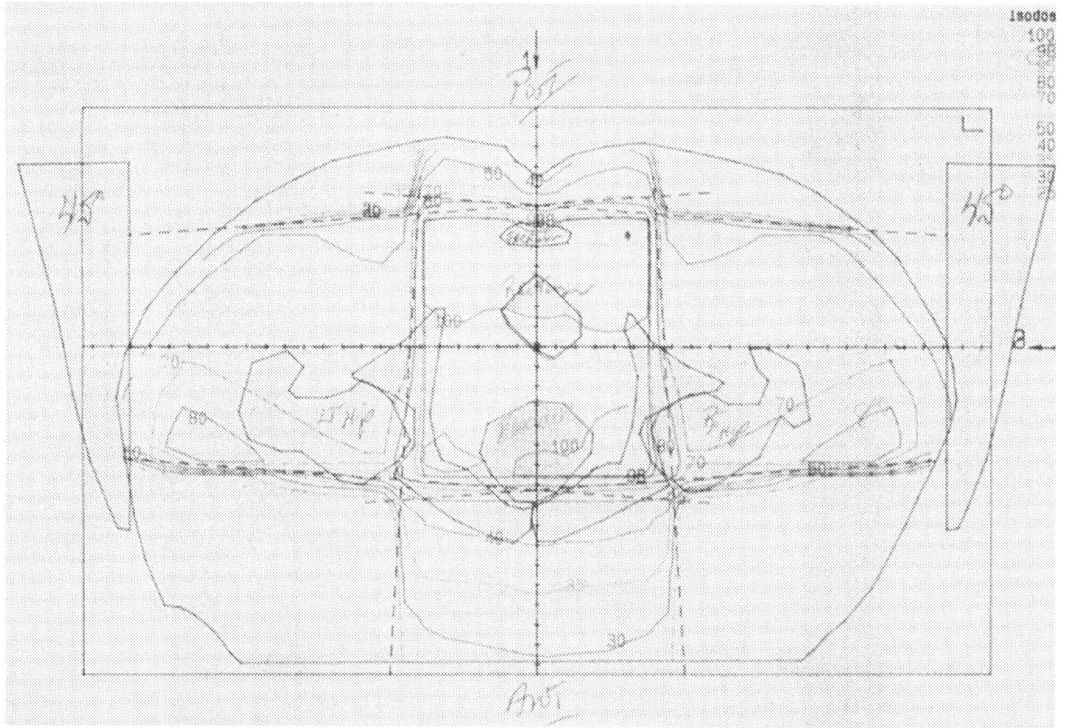

Figure 8.7 Isodose treatment plan.
Source: Courtesy of Duke University Medical Center, Department of Radiation Oncology, Durham, North Carolina.

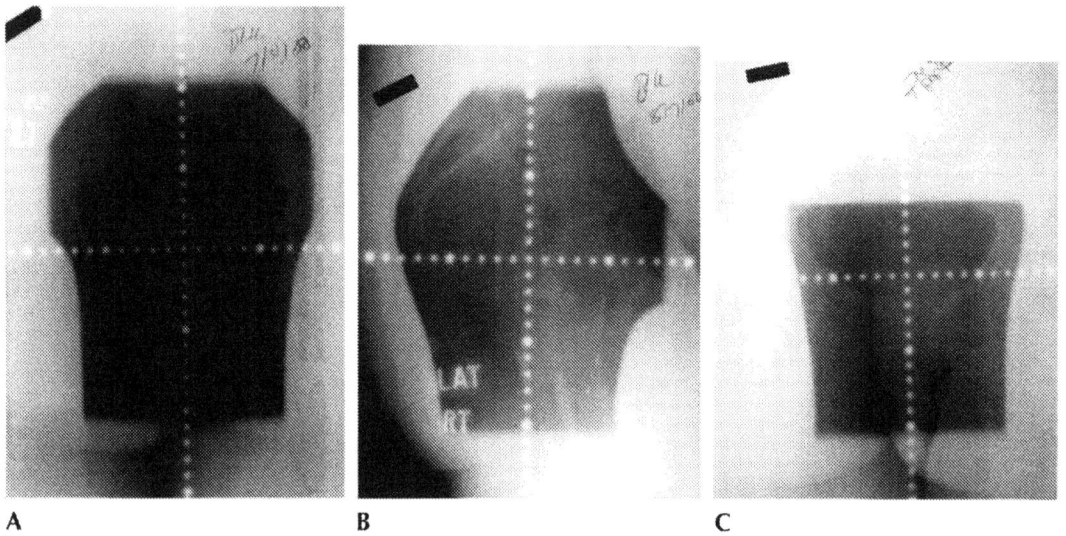

A   B   C

Figure 8.8 AP/PA and lateral film. **A:** AP/PA. **B:** Lateral. **C:** Boost.
Source: Courtesy of Duke University Medical Center, Department of Radiation Oncology, Durham, North Carolina.

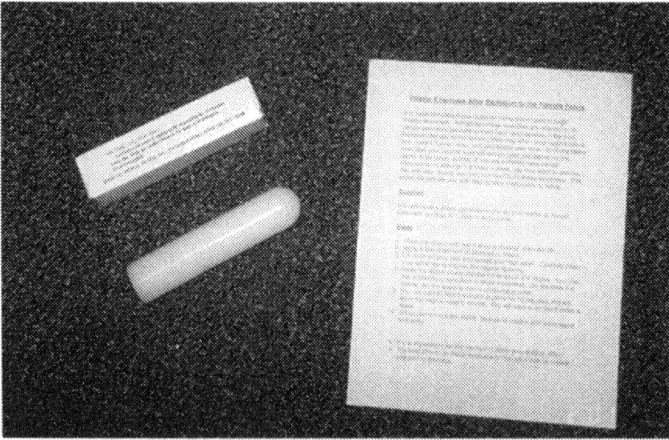

Figure 8.11 Female dilator and instruction sheet.

Source: Courtesy of Duke University Medical Center, Department of Radiation Oncology, Durham, North Carolina.

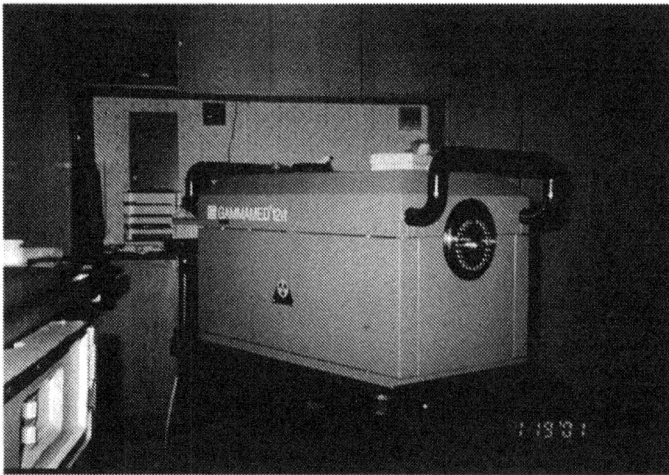

Figure 8.12 High-dose rate brachytherapy machine.

Source: Courtesy of Duke University Medical Center, Department of Radiation Oncology, Durham, North Carolina.

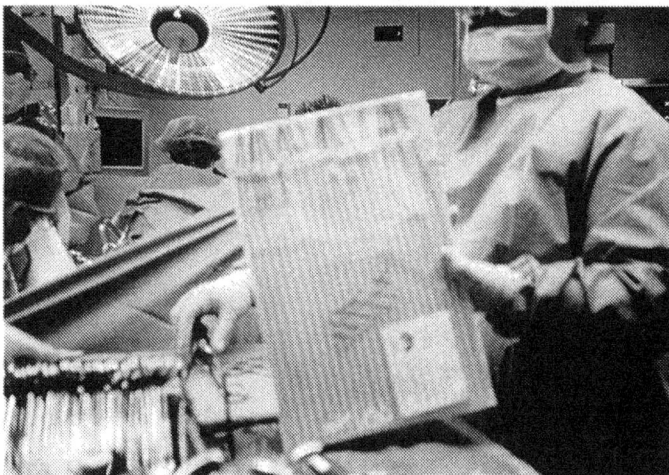

Figure 8.13 The Harrison-Anderson-Mick (HAM) applicator (developed at Memorial Sloan-Kettering Cancer Center).

Source: Courtesy of Duke University Medical Center, Department of Radiation Oncology, Durham, North Carolina.

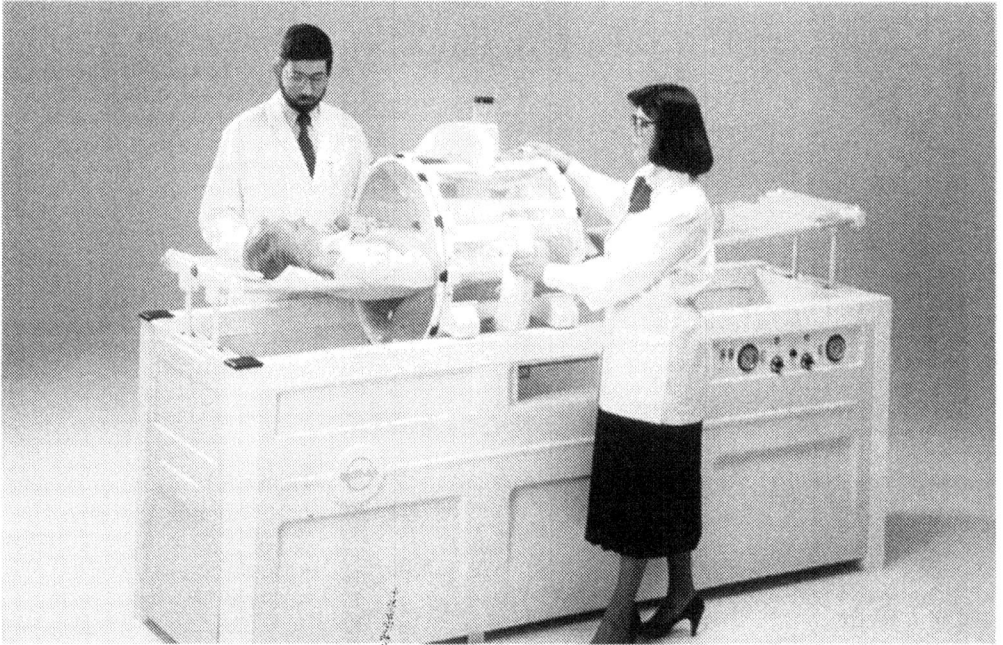

Figure 8.14 Deep hyperthermia machine.
Source: Courtesy of Duke University Medical Center, Department of Radiation Oncology, Durham, North Carolina.

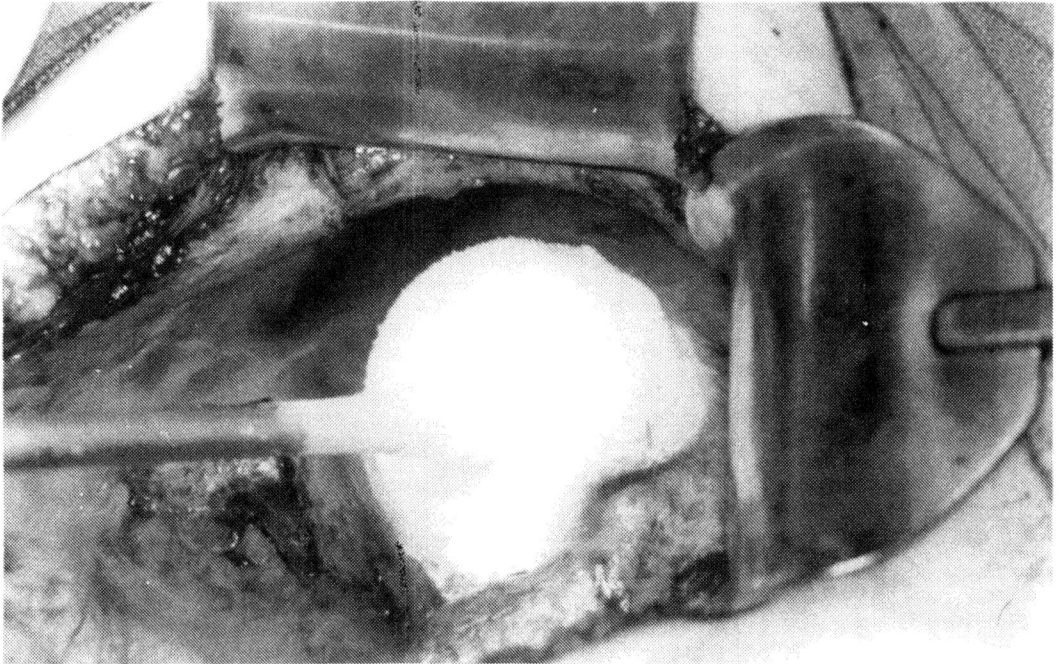

Figure 11.8 Cryosurgery utilizes extreme temperature of liquid nitrogen through a probe to freeze the tumor. A ball of ice is formed during cryo-assisted surgical resection of liver cancer.
Source: Photo courtesy of The Johns Hopkins Hospital.

treatment table showed, and it is important for them to know that these are not diagnostic x-rays, but a way to verify treatment planning.

Reproducibility of the treatment field is accomplished through the use of three laser lights that intersect at a consistent point on the patient. The laser lights are mounted into walls of the simulator room and also in the treatment rooms. These lights are used to assist in reproducing the treatment field each time. Other methods that are used to reproduce the treatment field include the use of skin marks, photographs, and tattoos. Skin markings are done on the day of simulation and define the treatment field on the patient (Figure 8.5, see page P-5 of insert). These markings are not to be washed off by patients until they begin treatment. India ink may be used to make the tiny tattoos once the patient has started treatment. These tattoos are small permanent dots that are used if the skin marks get washed off during treatment to recreate the treatment field or if the treatment field needs to be identified months to years after treatment.

Lead blocks are made to shape the radiation beam as it comes out of the linear accelerator and are used to minimize the dose of radiation to normal tissue (Figure 8.6, see page P-6 of insert). The beam is either square or rectangular, and the collimater of the treatment machine can adjust the size of the beam. Lead blocks are made after the radiation oncologist has drawn on the simulation films which body structures are to be excluded from the treatment field. This film is then used as a template for the development of the blocks. Multileaf collimators (MLCs) also have been increasingly used to shape the radiation beam as a replacement for conventional blocks. An MLC is a computer-programmed device that allows direct beam collimation (shaping) during the treatment without the use of any blocks.

Computerized treatment planning is the next step and integrates information from the simu-

lation and CT done of the patient to identify vital structures. The physicist and dosimetrist use this information, which is in a computer software program, to then formulate the isodose plan, which shows the dose distribution of radiation (Figure 8.7, see page P-6 of insert). The treatment should be designed with the use of computerized radiation dosimetry and be delivered by high-energy linear accelerators ($\geq$ 6MV), which, by nature of their depth-dose characteristics, deliver a higher dose to the tumor volume while sparing the surrounding normal tissues.[4] Patients with colorectal cancer may initially have two isodose plans done; one for a three-field plan and the other for a four-field plan. The radiation oncologist then selects the appropriate plan for the patient. Patients may also have Intensity Modulated Radiation Therapy (IMRT), which is a computer software program that generates the most conformal treatment plan by using highly sophisticated MLCs to adjust dose intensity during actual treatment, minimizing the radiation dose to surrounding tissue without compromising the tumoricidal therapeutic dose.

External Beam Therapy

External beam radiation or teletherapy is the most common method of delivering radiation therapy. Treatment is typically delivered once a day, Monday through Friday, unless patients are in a clinical trial. The treatment itself is only 3 to 5 minutes, but the actual time patients are in a treatment room is 10 to 15 minutes, and this accounts for patient and linear accelerator set-up time.

In most settings, patients will see their radiation oncologist and nurse once a week during treatment. During this appointment the patients' weight and vital signs may be checked, in addition to an assessment of how they are responding to treatment. The radiation oncologist will review the patients' treatment plan, assess the skin in the treatment field, and review any laboratory work or other studies that have been done. This is an opportune time for the nurse to reinforce patient education regarding fatigue, pain management, nutritional management, or any other issues that need to be addressed.

Treatment Field and Technique

The radiation treatment field runs along an X (width) and Y (length) axis that meets in iso-center; this is measured in centimeters. The typical treatment field for a patient with colo-rectal cancer is a multifield approach that is either three-field or four-field, although a two-field approach may be used. Multifield tech-niques are useful with primary lesions of the sigmoid colon, but for lesions in other parts of the colon, parallel, opposed, anterior–posterior (AP):posterior–anterior (PA) fields are used for the major portion of treatment, unless CT stud-ies or clip placement suggests that multifield techniques can spare normal tissues.[5] The three-field method uses a PA and laterally opposed field approach (one treatment from each side). The four-field method utilizes the AP:PA and laterally opposed field approach (Figure 8.8, see page P-6 of insert). A three- or four-field approach is often preferred because it decreases the amount of bowel in the treatment field.

The typical daily dose of radiation for a pre-operative rectal patient is 180 cGy (25 fractions) to a total dose of 4,500 cGy. This is delivered to the area of greatest risk of tumor recurrence or to the actual tumor site and includes the regional lymph nodes and tissues (Figure 8.9). The patient may then receive what is called a "cone down" or "boost" (smaller treatment field) to the primary area of disease with a 2- to 3-cm margin around the tumor site. This is typically delivered at a daily dose of 180 cGy (3 fractions) to a dose of 540 cGy; the patient's total dose of radiation would then be 5,040 cGy.

Patients who receive treatment postoperatively may receive a higher total dose, depending on the institution.

Patients with colon cancer are most com-monly treated with radiation therapy if they have locally advanced disease at the time of surgery or if metastatic disease is present; then it is used for palliation. The daily postoperative dose is 180 cGy. The patient may then receive a boost to the postoperative site, as described, resulting in a total dose of 5,040 cGy (Figure 8.10). Again, the total dose may vary, based on the institution. For patients with metastatic disease receiving palliative treatment, the dose and treatment field vary, based on the site of disease.

Field size varies, based on the inclusion or exclusion of lymph nodes. For the AP set-up, the superior border of the treatment field typi-cally lies at the bottom of the L5 vertebra and at the top of the S1; the distal portion of the field is typically 3 cm below the primary tumor site. In the lateral set-up, the anterior border varies, depending on whether the external iliac lymph nodes are included; typically the internal iliac lymph nodes are always included. The posterior border is often 1.0 to 1.5 cm behind the anterior bony sacral border. Anteriorly, the lower third of the rectum abuts the posterior vaginal wall or prostate, and these structures should be included in patients with distal le-sions.[8] Blocks are then used to decrease the dose to the small intestine, bladder, and femur heads, pelvic bones, or the large bones of the hips.

Treatment of Colon Cancer

Radiation therapy is used on an adjuvant basis in some patients with colon cancer, though it is not indicated in patients with carcinoma in situ or in those with a T1-2 N0 M0. Patients may receive local or regional radiation therapy

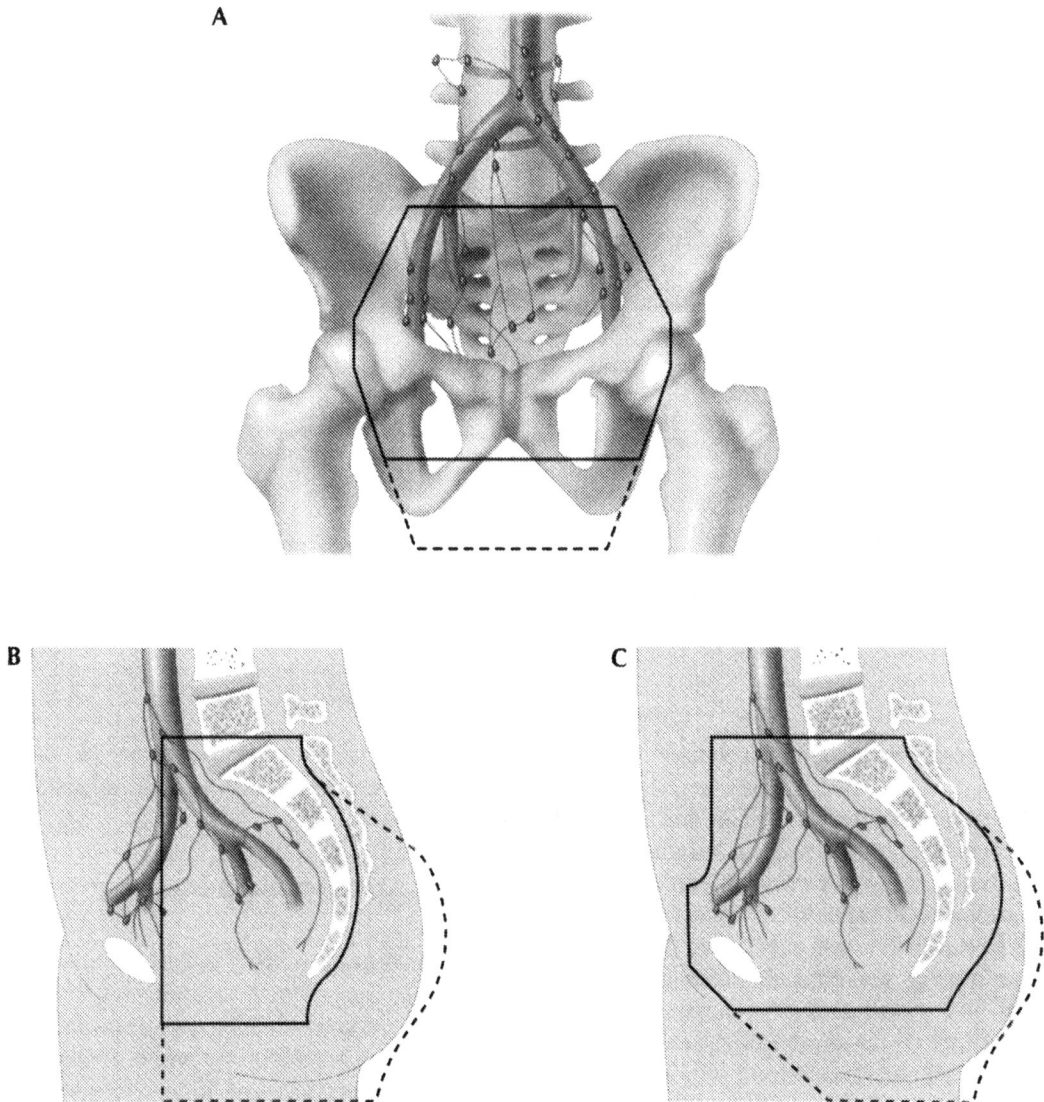

Figure 8.9   Rectal treatment field. Idealized irradiation fields for rectal cancer either preceding or following anterior resection or following abdominoperineal resection (APR): interrupted lines indicate alterations of fields after APR. **A:** AP:PA field. **B:** Lateral field when only internal iliac and presacral nodes are at risk. **C:** Lateral field when external iliac nodes are also at risk.

Source: From Gunderson LL, Martenson JA, Smalley SR, et al. Lower gastrointestinal cancers: Rationale, results and techniques of treatment. Front Radiat Ther Oncol. 1994; 28:140–154. With permission.

A

B

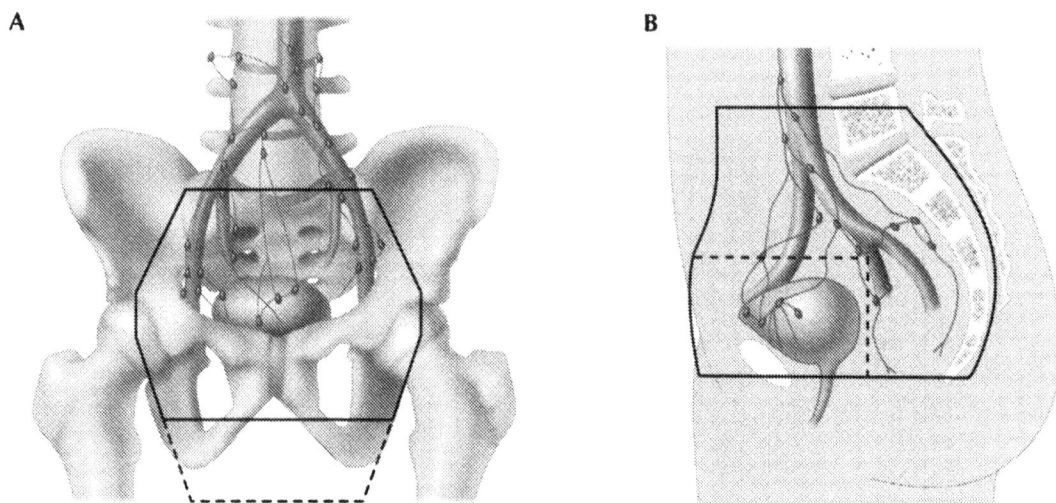

Figure 8.10   Colon treatment field. Idealized multiple field irradiation technique following resection of a sigmoid colon cancer that was adherent to the bladder (large field—solid lines: boost field—interrupted lines). **A:** AP:PA. **B:** Paired laterals.

Source: From Gunderson LL, Martenson JA, Smalley SR, et al. Lower gastrointestinal cancers: Rationale, results and techniques of treatment. Front Radiat Ther Oncol. 1994; 28:140–154. With permission.

or whole-abdomen radiation therapy. Local radiation is most commonly used in the postoperative setting in patients with bulky, locally advanced T3 or T4 disease. Whole-abdomen radiation therapy is used, although not as frequently as local radiation, in patients who are at risk of recurrence in the abdomen. The primary dose-limiting structures in patients receiving local or regional radiation therapy for colon cancer include the small bowel, stomach, liver, kidney, and the spinal cord.[6]

Guidelines from the National Comprehensive Cancer Network (NCCN) have been established to guide practitioners in treating patients with colon cancer. Their current recommendation for T1-3 N1-2 M0 is that the patient receive 5-fluorouracil (5-FU) and leucovorin, or 5-FU and leucovorin and radiation, if perforation is present.[7] For patients with T4 N1-2 M0, they recommend 5-FU and leucovorin, or 5-FU and leucovorin and radiation.[7] Adjuvant radiation

therapy for colon cancer should not be given except in the context of a formal, prospective clinical trial.[8]

Treatment of Rectal Cancer

Radiation therapy is used to treat rectal cancer in both the neoadjuvant and adjuvant settings. Both of these treatments have their own advantages and disadvantages. Radiation is also used for palliation of symptoms if the disease should recur. The U.S. Patterns of Care Study reported that 75% of patients received postoperative therapy, while only 22% received preoperative therapy.[10]

Preoperative Radiotherapy

The potential advantages of a preoperative approach over postoperative therapy are decreased tumor seeding, less acute toxicity, increased radiosensitivity, and enhanced sphincter preservation.[9] The major theoretical disadvantage of preoperative radiation therapy is possibly overtreating 10% to 15% of the patients (i.e., those patients with stages T1-2 N0 M0 disease who do not require adjuvant therapy).[4]

Preoperative radiation therapy may also be combined with chemotherapy to assist in downstaging of the tumor. One important goal of this strategy is to preserve sphincter function. Historically, preoperative, randomized clinical trials have shown an improvement in local control but not improved survival, until recently. Many of these clinical trials did not incorporate standard radiation doses (at least 45 Gy), the interval between completion of radiation and surgery was too short (4–6 weeks is recommended to allow maximal tumor downstaging and recovery of normal tissues within the radiation field), and the radiation techniques employed were suboptimal and known to be associated with an increased incidence of complications.[11] Two recent studies done by the Stockholm Rectal Cancer Study Group and the Swedish Rectal Cancer Study Group randomized patients to surgery alone or preoperative radiation therapy prior to surgery. Both of these trials demonstrated a decrease in local recurrence and also an improved overall survival rate.[9]

Postoperative Radiotherapy

The advantages of the postoperative approach include the following: (1) The stage is already known (thereby sparing the 10% to 15% of patients with T1-2 N0 M0 disease treatment) and (2) a more accurate definition of the tumor bed for radiation planning is obtained by the placement of clips at the time of surgery.[11] The aims of adjuvant therapy after resection for rectal cancer are to improve local tumor control, decrease distant metastasis, and improve survival.[9] Clinical trials looking at the role of post-operative radiation therapy have also been done. One randomized trial, by the National Surgical Breast and Bowel Project (NSABP) RO-1, confirmed an advantage in local control (with borderline significance) in patients who received radiation therapy versus surgery alone.[11] A principal finding in another study, which looked at sphincter control, showed that anorectal function, as measured both in the laboratory and clinically, was markedly inferior in patients with rectal cancer who had received radiotherapy after anterior resection than in patients who had been treated by surgery alone.[12]

The NCCN also has guidelines for the treatment of rectal cancer and recommends the following for unresectable tumors. For T1-2 N1-2 M0 or T3 N0-2 M0, the NCCN recommends 5-FU and radiation therapy before surgery, then 5-FU and leucovorin after surgery, or, if the patient does not receive neoadjuvant therapy, 5-FU and leucovorin are given after surgery, followed by 5-FU and radiation, then more 5-FU and leucovorin.[7] For any T4 cancer, the NCCN recommends, as primary therapy, 5-FU (given continuously or intermittently) and radiation therapy, followed by resection, if possible.

Side Effects of External Beam Radiotherapy

Radiation therapy side effects can be classified as acute or chronic, and patients receiving radiation therapy need to understand the implications and impact that these side effects may have on their quality of life (Table 8.2). Acute side effects are those that arise during treatment and typically resolve within a few weeks to months after treatment is completed. Late side effects may be the continuation of an acute side effect or may arise months to years after treatment has been completed. A variety of medications can be used to treat the side effects that may arise during therapy (Table 8.3).

Table 8.2   Acute and Late Side Effects of Radiation Therapy for Colorectal Cancer

Site	Acute	Late
Colon	Abdominal cramps	Fibrosis
	Diarrhea	Diarrhea
Rectum	Tenesmus	Fibrosis
	Rectal pain	Fistula
	Perianal pruritus	Proctitis
	Frequent stools	Frequent stools
	Urgency, incontinence	Adhesions
	Mucus or bloody discharge	Stenosis
Bladder	Frequency	Atrophy*
	Urgency, incontinence	Ulceration, bleeding*
	Dysuria	Fibrosis*
	Hematuria	Fistula
	Suprapubic pain	
Vagina	Vaginal irritation, dryness,	Thinning, atrophy
	pruritus	Fibrosis
	Mucus or bloody drainage	Narrowing, shortening
	Dyspareunia	Dryness
Ovary	Hot flashes	Vaginal dryness and dyspareunia
	Vaginal dryness and dyspareunia	
Bone marrow	Anemia	Chronic hypoplasia*
	Leukopenia	
	Thrombocytopenia	
Skin	Erythema	Fibrosis
	Dry desquamation	Telangiectasias
	Moist desquamation	

*Rare.

Source: Data from Frankel KJ. Gastrointestinal cancers. In: Dow KH, Bucholtz JD, et al., eds. Nursing Care in Radiation Oncology. Philadelphia, PA: WB Saunders Company, 1997: 152–183; and Coia LR, Robert RJ, Tepper JE. Later effects of radiation therapy on the gastrointestinal tract. Int J Radiat Oncol Biol Phys. 1995; 31:1213–1236.

Side effects for the patient with colorectal cancer undergoing radiation therapy are often predictable, based on the treatment site, daily dose of radiation, other therapies, the volume of area irradiated, and other individual differences. Side effects are also site-specific, in that they are localized to the area of the body receiving treatment. Patient education and symptom management among the patient, radiation oncologist, and radiation nurse is an ongoing process from the day of consultation into the follow-up phase.

Skin Reaction

Skin reactions are an expected side effect of radiation therapy and occur approximately 2 to 3 weeks into treatment. Skin reactions can be classified as either acute or late. An acute reaction is characterized by the following: ery-

Table 8.3   Commonly Used Symptom-Management Medications

Symptom	Medication	Dosing
Diarrhea	Loperamide hydrochloride	OTC 4 mg after 1st loose bowel movement, followed by 2 mg with each subsequent bowel movement, not to exceed 8 mg/day for more than 2 days
	Diphenoxylate hydrochloride with atropine sulfate	Initial, 2.5–5.0 mg tid-qid; maintenance, 2.5 mg bid-tid
	Paregoric (camphorated opium tincture)	5–10 mL 1–4 times/day (5 mL contains 2 mg of morphine)
	Cholestyramine resin	1 g 1–2 times/day
Dysuria	Phenazopyridine hydrochloride	200 mg tid; do not take longer than 2 days if taking antibiotic
Nausea	Prochlorperazine maleate	5–10 mg tid-qid (up to 40 mg daily)
	Promethazine hydrochloride	25 mg (usual); 12.5–25.0 mg every 4–6 hours as needed
	Ondansetron hydrochloride	8 mg 1–2 hours before radiotherapy, with subsequent doses 8 hours after the 1st dose for each day xrt is given
	Granisetron hydrochloride	2 mg once daily, taken within 1 hour of xrt
Bladder spasms	Oxybutynin chloride	5 mg bid-tid; maximum dose, 5 mg qid
Proctitis	Hydrocortisone (Proctocort)	1 applicator (90 mg) 1–2 times/day for 2–3 weeks; then every 2nd day

xrt, radiation therapy.

Source: Data from PDR Nurse's Drug Handbook. Montvale, NJ: Delmar Publishers and Medical Economics Company, Inc., 2001.

thema, dry desquamation, hyperpigmentation, and moist desquamation. Typically these side effects are progressive in nature. The perineal area of the body is warm and moist, has poor aeration, traps moisture, and is in constant contact with other skin or clothing, causing friction. Patients may complain of itching, burning, discomfort, and pain. Late effects include telangiectasias, fibrosis, and hyper- or hypopigmentation. Repair of tissue after early reactions involves progressive fibrosis, which is a major factor in late expression of radiation injury.[13] Men also may complain of scrotal tenderness or irritation.

Patients who are receiving treatment for colorectal cancer are at risk for skin reactions in the gluteal folds and perineum, and should be positioned prone to minimize skin reactions. Skin sparing is further reduced when the patient is in the supine position, because the gluteal folds are squeezed together, and when the beam is parallel with the skin surface, the skin-sparing effect of high-energy beams is decreased.[2] Special considerations need to be given to the patient receiving pelvic irradiation after low anterior or AP resection for rectal cancer.[14] Patients who are postoperative are at risk for infection if the site is not properly healed. Patients with an ostomy may need to remove the ostomy appliance and adhesive so as not to create a bolus effect on the skin, and the ostomy should be checked daily for problems. Patients who experience a severe skin reaction may need a treatment break to let the skin heal.

A variety of skin care products can be recommended to patients, and each treatment facility typically has its own skin-care protocol (Table 8.4). Patients may be instructed to use Aquaphor for erythema or dry desquamation, and for moist desquamation, Domeboro Astrin-

Table 8.4 Perineal-Rectal Skin Care Protocol

Routine Care

During morning care and after each episode of urination or defecation, the patient will receive the following care.
- Gently cleanse skin with tepid water or a mild cleansing agent followed by gently patting areas dry **or** cleanse with tepid to cool sitz baths.
- If open lesions are present, cleanse with a wound cleanser or normal saline solution and treat.
- Apply a moisturizing cream.
- Recommend cotton undergarments; avoid restrictive clothing.
- Perform a full assessment of the perineal-rectal skin.
- Perform a nutrition assessment followed by nutrition consult, if needed.
- Consult an enterostomal therapy or wound-care nurse as needed.

Assessment	Recommendations for Care

Erythema signs and symptoms
  Pink
  Tenderness
	Gently cleanse using a mild cleansing agent (perineal skin cleansers).
	Apply a moisturizing, protective cream.
	If cleanser is not accessible and soap must be used, use a soap without perfumes and thoroughly rinse all soap residues from the skin.
	Avoid lotions or creams containing perfume and talc (if receiving radiation therapy to area, avoid products containing metals or ointments or cleanse area prior to receiving radiation therapy).
	Frequency of skin care: Daily and after toileting

Dry desquamation signs and symptoms
  Scaling
  Flaking
  Pruritus
  Pain
	Cleanse with tepid water or a wound cleanser.
	Apply a protective cream.
	Assess for pruritus, if present.
	• Apply topical antihistamine creams.
	• Take a cool shower or bath.
	• Consider analgesics or antihistamines.
	Assess for fungal infection, if present.
	• Treat with topical antifungal or systemic antifungal agent.
	Frequency of skin care: Twice a day/as needed after toileting

gent Solution. For patients who complain of itchiness, Benadryl may be recommended for use at bedtime. A variety of occlusive dressings and/or hydrocolloid dressings also can be recommended. If the patient has moist desquama-tion, it is important to expose the area to as much air as possible to assist with healing. Topical Lidocaine Jelly may also be recommended for rectal discomfort. Two products typically not recommended to patients are cornstarch powder

Table 8.4 *Continued*

Assessment	Recommendations for Care
Moist desquamation signs and symptoms	
Pain	Recommend sitz bath, shower, whirlpool as needed.
Weeping	Cleanse with a wound cleanser as needed.
Sloughing	Apply a protective cream that will adhere to open skin.
Abscess	Apply an adhesive peripad or a pantyliner without deodorant to the undergarments.
	Assess need for analgesics, pain medications.
	If desquamation worsens, apply a wound hydrogel.
	Frequency of skin care: Twice a day/as needed after toileting
Possible complications of moist desquamation	
Vesicles	Consult with physician or advanced practice nurse for treatment and systematic antibiotics.
Furuncle	
Carbuncles	If vesicles are present, rule out herpes and treat
Abscess formation	appropriately.

Report to Physician	Documentation
Worsening of skin alteration	Anatomical area involved
Increase in inflammation	Size of involvement
Appearance of furuncle, carbuncles, abscess	• Area may be difficult to measure because of the perineal-rectal anatomy.
Appearance of vesicles	• Attempt to record in centimeters.
Pain or increase in pain, change in character of pain	• Measure from where the normal skin stops to where it begins again (use a disposable ruler). If open areas develop, measure width, length, and depth.
	• Record daily in acute care or weekly in home or long-term care.
	Changes in skin or wound conditions
	Colors of skin
	Drainage (i.e., amount, odor, color, consistency)
	Presence of sloughing or necrosis
	Presence and intensity of pain or pruritus
	Patient outcomes

Source: With permission, from Haisfield-Wolfe ME, Rund C. Nursing protocol for the management of perineal-rectal skin alterations. Clin J Oncol Nurs. 2000; 4:1. Copyright 2000 by Oncology Nursing Press, Inc.

and steroid cream. Cornstarch is to be avoided because of the potential for fungal growth, and steroid creams usually are not recommended because they can cause thinning and delayed healing of the skin, as well as mask a possible infection. If a foul odor or discharge is noted, the area should be cultured.

Patients need to receive education early on about caring for their skin. Both men and women will want to avoid tight-fitting pants and underwear, which will cause friction and irritation. Women also should avoid wearing pantyhose and girdles, which may be tight and not allow air to the skin. The use of loose, cotton clothing and underwear is recommended. Long-term, the patient will want to avoid chemical, mechanical, thermal, or other irritants to the skin (Table 8.5).

Fatigue

Fatigue is seen in approximately 95% of patients undergoing radiation therapy.[15] There are a variety of different theories as to why fatigue occurs in patients undergoing cancer therapy that can be related to a decrease in red blood cells, circulating cellular waste, and toxic metabolites inhibiting normal cell function. Treatment-related fatigue is initially noticed during the second or third week of treatment, peaks near the completion of therapy, and gradually resolves over the following weeks to months posttreatment. It is important that the healthcare provider be able to distinguish between acute and chronic fatigue in this population, especially if patients are undergoing combined-modality treatment with chemotherapy or are recovering from surgery. For some patients, just coming for treatment everyday may make them fatigued.

Initial and ongoing education throughout the course of treatment, to assess and address the multiple issues related to fatigue, is critical. The radiation oncology nurse plays a pivotal

Table 8.5   Long-Term Skin Care Following Radiation Therapy

Mechanical
Wash with hands; do not use a washcloth.
Pat dry with a soft, clean towel or use a hair dryer on a cool setting.
Use an electric shaver.
Avoid friction (e.g., wear loose-fitting clothing).
Avoid scratching the affected area.
Avoid using tape on the affected area.

Thermal
Use warm, not hot, water.
Avoid exposure to temperature extremes.
Do not apply ice packs or heat (e.g., heating pad, hot water bottle, sun lamp).

Chemical
Use mild soap and rinse thoroughly.
Apply only recommended substances.
Do not use deodorants in the affected area.
Wash clothing with mild detergent.

Other
Keep skin folds dry.
Wear absorbent cotton clothing.
Prevent skin infection.
Protect skin from direct sun exposure (cover or shade area).
Use dressings as needed for moist desquamation.

Source: Sitton E. Early and late radiation-induced skin alterations, part I: Mechanisms of skin changes. *Oncol Nurs Forum.* 1992; 19:801–807. With permission.

role in educating patients about cancer-related fatigue, as well as interventions to assist not only with activities of daily living, but also with memory and emotional stability. It is important for patients to be able to prioritize activities, take naps as needed, and follow a well-balanced diet.

Myelosuppression

Patients undergoing radiation therapy for colorectal cancer typically have their blood counts checked at regular intervals. In the adult, 15% to 25% of the marrow is located in the pelvis.[16]

Radiation therapy depletes stem cells, which then form erythrocytes, leukocytes, and platelets, which places patients at risk for infection, fatigue, and bleeding. The degree of myelosuppression is dependent on the size of the treatment field, dose of therapy prescribed, and whether patients are receiving combined-modality therapy.

Anorexia/Nausea

The nutritional needs of patients during radiation therapy should be assessed prior to the initiation of therapy and throughout the course of therapy. Patients may suffer from anorexia and nausea as a result of the treatment. Nausea is a common side effect in patients receiving radiation to the pelvic area. Patients typically experience nausea 1 to 2 hours posttreatment and should be encouraged not to eat a heavy meal prior to radiation therapy. Patients who experience persistent nausea may need to take an antiemetic prior to therapy or on a regular basis, as prescribed.

Appropriate dietary strategies to minimize nausea should be taught to patients and their families. A copy of "Eating Hints," produced by the National Cancer Institute, should be provided to patients, and specific side effects and interventions should be reviewed. A dietitian should also be consulted if weight loss becomes an issue. Patients should be encouraged to eat six small meals a day, to avoid foods that are odorous, and to bring crackers and other light snacks with them to eat after treatment.

Diarrhea

Diarrhea occurs from changes in the bowel due to radiation and the inability of the bowel to absorb nutrients. Although patients vary, 85% of those receiving radiation to the bowel experience diarrhea.[17] Patients are at risk for developing radiation-induced diarrhea if they have a large amount of bowel in the treatment field, are receiving concomitant chemotherapy, and/ or have had prior colorectal surgery. Acute radiation-induced enteritis is characterized by reduced mitotic activity of intestinal epithelial cells and shortening of the villi, both of which are histologic abnormalities caused by direct mucosal injury by ionizing radiation.[18] Once radiation therapy ends, the mucosal cells start to regenerate within several days; however, symptoms may persist for up to 6 months.[19] Late radiation-induced bowel changes may take years to develop and are typically characterized by small-bowel obstruction, fibrosis, adhesions, and fistulas. Clinically, it is often difficult to determine whether a patient with symptoms of mild to moderate diarrhea is demonstrating small-bowel injury or impaired rectal compliance.[20]

Patients may complain of increased frequency of liquid stool or formed stool, abdominal cramping, and tenesmus. Patients also may experience increased bloating and gas related to the treatment. Bloating and flatus can occur secondary to the radiation therapy, especially in patients receiving concomitant therapy. Light activity such as walking and stretching may help move gas along.

It is important that the patient understand that this is an expected side effect of treatment and that by following a low-residue diet (Table 8.6) and taking the recommended medications as ordered, the frequency of the diarrhea will be decreased. Patients should be encouraged to drink six to eight glasses of nonalcoholic, non-caffeinated fluids a day. A high-protein diet is often encouraged, and supplements should be used, as tolerated, by patients (Table 8.7). If patients are lactose intolerant, supplements may need to be diluted with water. Weight should continue to be monitored two to three times a week to determine whether they are stable, are

Table 8.6   Recommended Low-Residue Food List

Food Group	Foods Recommended	Foods to Avoid
Soup	Broth, bouillon, cream soups made from milk allowance, vegetable soup made with vegetable allowance	All others
Meat, fish, cheese, eggs or substitute	Tender baked, broiled, roasted, or stewed beef, chicken, fish, lamb, ham, liver, pork, turkey, shellfish, veal; cottage cheese, cream cheese, American cheese, farmers cheese, mild cheddar cheese, Swiss cheese; eggs; creamy peanut butter	Tough fibrous meats with gristle; chunk-style peanut butter; dried beans or peas; sardines, fried meats, barbecued meats
Potato or substitute	White potatoes without skin; whipped sweet potatoes or yams; macaroni, noodles, white rice	Brown and wild rice; barley, hominy, whole sweet potatoes, whole yams, potato skins
Vegetables and legumes	Vegetable juices; only tender cooked asparagus tips, beets, carrots, eggplant, green or wax beans, mushrooms, strained pumpkin, spinach, whipped winter squash, cooked spinach	All others, especially raw vegetables
Fruit	Any juice except prune; ripe banana; cooked or canned apple sauce, mandarin oranges, baked apple without skin	All others, especially berries and dried fruits, melon, other fresh fruits
Breads, cereals, and flour	Enriched white or light rye without seeds; Saltine or soda crackers; plain rolls, muffins, or biscuits; melba toast; zwieback; cooked, refined wheat, corn, or rice cereals; quick-cooking oatmeal; prepared cereals made from corn, rice, or oats; white enriched flour	Breads and crackers containing whole grains, bran, or seeds; whole grain cereals, bran shredded wheat; whole grain flours, cornbread
Fats and nuts	Butter, margarine, cooking fats; vegetable oils, crisp bacon; cream or half and half is limited to $\frac{1}{4}$ cups per day. Clear milk salad dressing	All nuts
Desserts	Plain cakes and cookies; fruit whips; gelatin; plain puddings, ice cream, and sherbert made from milk allowances	Desserts containing coconut, berries, nuts, seeds, skins,, or restricted fruits
Beverages and milk	Coffee, teas, decaffeinated coffee, carbonated beverages; any milk and plain milk products are limited to two (2) cups per day, flavored yogurt, yogurt with allowed ingredients	Yogurt containing berries and peelings
Sweets	Plain hard candy, honey, jelly, sugar, syrup, molasses	Jam, marmalade, coconut

Table 8.6 *Continued*

Food Group	Foods Recommended	Foods to Avoid
Miscellaneous	White sauce, mild catsup, gravy, vinegar, salt, pepper if tolerated, mild spices and herbs in moderation	Chili sauce, horseradish, olives, pickles, relish, popcorn, potato chips, mustard, garlic. Whole spices; poppy seed, caraway
Commercial supplements	Ensure, Ensure Plus, Sustacal, Sustacal Plus, Equate, Equate Plus, Boost, Boost Plus, Scandishake	

Source: Used with permission from Duke University Medical Center, Department of Radiation Oncology, Durham, North Carolina.

Table 8.7 **Nutritional Supplements**

Product	Serving Size	Calories	Grams Protein
Boost	8 oz	240	10
Boost High Protein	8 oz	240	15
Boost Energy Bar	1 bar	190	4
Carnation Instant Breakfast (plus milk)	8 oz	280	12
Enlive by Ensure	8.1 oz	300	10
Ensure	8 oz	254	9
Ensure High Calcium	8 oz	225	12
Ensure Plus	8 oz	360	13
Equate (WalMart)	8 oz	250	9
Equate Plus (WalMart)	8 oz	250	13
Resource	8 oz	180	9
ScandiShake (plus milk)	8 oz	600	16

Source: With permission, from Gosselin T, Pitz S. Anorexia. In: Nevidjon BM, Sowers KW, eds. A Nurse's Guide to Cancer Care. Philadelphia, PA: Lippincott Williams & Wilkins, 2000; 319–333.

continuing to decrease, or are increasing with the changes in eating.[21] Patients who have a history of Crohn's disease or irritable bowel syndrome should also be followed closely for exacerbation of symptoms related to therapy.

Radiation therapy and diarrhea can frequently cause a patient's hemorrhoids to become inflamed and irritated. Careful cleansing after each bowel movement is important to help reduce the irritation. Sitz baths and unscented baby wipes may be incorporated to assist with cleansing of the perineum. Medication may be prescribed to assist in the management of this side effect.

Cystitis

The bladder is in close proximity to the rectum and often becomes irritated during radiation therapy, although not as easily as the small bowel. Patients may verbalize concerns regarding increased frequency, dysuria, and urgency, and urinary tract infection needs to be ruled out. Rarely does the prostate in male patients become inflamed and obstruct urinary outflow. If this happens, a Foley catheter is placed and medications may be given. It is important that the patient drink 2 to 3 L of fluid a day to decrease bladder irritation. If the problem continues, the radiation oncologist may prescribe medication that will reduce the dysuria and frequency associated with urination.

Late cystitis is a rare late effect and can lead to stricture of the bladder, decreasing its capacity and irritation of the bladder wall lining, which can lead to bleeding and/or recurrent infections. Although this is quite rare after radiation for colon or rectal cancer, it may be helped with DMSO instillations and/or hyperbaric oxygen therapy.

Reproduction/Sexuality

Although colorectal cancer is often thought to be a disease of the middle aged or elderly, it does occur in patients who are young adults, and the impact that it has on sexuality should not be understated. Patients who are of childbearing age need to use contraception to prevent pregnancy during treatment. Women may experience changes in the normal vaginal flora from radiation therapy and complain of vaginal discharge, itching, and/or pain. This is often the result of irritation by the radiation to the vaginal vault. Impotence may occur in men receiving radiation therapy, although it is not well documented in the literature. The pathophysiology of radiation-associated impotence has been linked to possible radiation injury to the nerves, blood vessels, and testes.[17]

Premature menopause may also occur in women who still have ovarian function. The ovaries do not tolerate high doses of radiation and sterility may therefore occur. Generally, hormone replacement therapy (HRT) may be initiated to ease the symptoms of menopause and to continue to provide estrogen to the body. HRT may be prescribed by either the patients' radiation oncologist or gynecologist.

Vaginal stenosis is a late side effect that occurs in women who received pelvic radiation, and is often characterized by painful intercourse, narrowing of the vagina, and decreased vaginal lubrication. Patients may take hor-

mones to assist with vaginal lubrication, in the form of either a patch, a pill, or vaginal cream. The radiation oncologist and/or radiation nurse will also provide patients with a vaginal dilator (Syracuse Medical Devices, Inc.) and specific exercises that will need to be done to keep the vagina open, not only for intercourse, but also for future examinations (Figure 8.11, see page P-7 of insert). If patients are sexually active, they may not need to do the exercises, but should discuss this with their physician or nurse first. The exercises are typically done three times a week for 10 minutes. Patients may find that incorporating a lubricant such as KY Jelly or Astroglide during intercourse or while performing the exercises decreases the discomfort that may arise. Patients may also use Replens as a moisturizing agent on a regular basis.

The radiation nurse needs to be able to intervene effectively in the short-term and long-term for these patients. It is important to listen to patients and ascertain their fears and concerns regarding the impact radiation therapy has on their sexuality. Referrals to counselors may sometimes be needed and patients should be provided a copy of the American Cancer Society booklet, "Sexuality and Cancer," based on their specific gender. Alternative ways of expressing emotion should be reviewed with patients.

Endocavitary Radiation Therapy

Endocavitary radiation therapy is a treatment option that can be used in curative early-stage rectal cancer instead of surgery. It is typically performed on an outpatient basis with local anesthetic in the radiation therapy department. Endocavitary radiation therapy produces high rates of local control and long-term survival in appropriately selected patients with rectal cancer.[8] Patients typically receive four 30-Gy treatments separated by intervals of approximately 2 weeks.[8] Factors that need to be included in the treatment decision include (1) the accessibility of the lesion by treatment procto-scope, $\leq$ 10 cm above the anal verge, (2) no evidence of disease extension beyond the bowel wall on digital rectal examination, (3) a maximum tumor size of 3 cm $\times$ 5 cm, (4) no significant extension to the anal canal, (5) well- or moderately well-differentiated histological (6) exophytic morphology.[8] Endocavitary irradiation is typically well tolerated.[22] Approximately 35% of patients have minor rectal bleeding; rectal urgency occurs in about 20%.[22] Late effects include telangiectasia and mild fibrosis of the underlying tissue.[16]

Intraoperative Radiation Therapy

Intraoperative radiation therapy (IORT) can be delivered in one of two ways. The first method is through the use of a linear accelerator and the second is with high dose rate (HDR) brachytherapy. The major indications for use of IORT are to treat an exposed tumor bed or areas of unresectable gross tumors, and as a boost in combination with large-field external beam radiation therapy and surgical resection.[23] In either case, patients would have their planned surgery and resection in a specially designed room that is fully shielded for the delivery of the radiation therapy. All other necessary operating room equipment and supplies are modified so that when the radiation is being delivered, patients are alone in the room and the treatment team can still monitor them.

In the first approach, patients have surgery and then receive the intraoperative treatment with electrons to the operative bed. This treatment is delivered by a linear accelerator that is built into an operating room or patients are transported to the radiation therapy department. It is critical to define the area at highest risk for subsequent local relapse in order to determine the optimal position for the IORT field.[24] Challenges that are commonly associated with

this method include the costs associated with having a designated linear accelerator in an operating room, difficulty with targeting the surface with electron cones, and the possible overlapment of multiple treatment fields.

The second approach that is used is HDR IORT. The HDR machine (Figure 8.12, see page P-7 of insert) is not stationary, so it can be moved between the operating room and the radiation oncology clinic. This type of remote afterloader is most commonly used in the outpatient setting to deliver HDR brachytherapy. One type of applicator that is commonly used with the HDR unit for IORT is the HAM (Harrison-Anderson-Mick) applicator (Figure 8.13, see page P-7 of insert), which was developed at Memorial Sloan-Kettering Cancer Center. The applicator is made of a flexible 1-cm translucent pad that is often referred to as "super flab." Source guide tubes are placed into the center of the pad and the pad comes in various sizes. In particular, it is ideal for curved or complex surfaces, such as the pelvic side wall, presacral area, pubic region, or other abdominal or thoracic surfaces.[25] The applicator is placed into the surgical bed and secured with packing or sutures, and intraoperative shields are placed to protect surrounding tissues and/or structures. The source guide tubes are then connected to the HDR unit and the radioactive sources (iridium-192) leave the vault in the HDR unit, travel through the source guide tube to the designated area in the applicator, and deliver the appropriate amount of radiation. The time for treatment delivery depends on the electron energy used, number of fields, dose per field, and total dose.[26] After IORT is completed, the surgical team finishes the surgery and the patient is taken to the postanesthesia care unit.

It is important that nurses in the operating room and nurses on the inpatient unit providing care to these patients understand both the process and the procedure that patients go through, so they can provide quality nursing care. Side effects may include, but are not limited to, peripheral nerve damage; infection/abscess; damage to the ureter and/or blood vessels; delayed or impaired wound healing; fibrosis of the surgical anastomosis and/or fibrosis of the muscle, bone, or cartilage; and small-bowel obstruction.

Combined-Modality Therapy

The role of combined-modality treatment in the management of colorectal cancer continues to be an area of ongoing clinical research. Both preoperative and postoperative combined-modality therapy with standard radiation and 5-FU–based chemotherapy has been shown to improve clinical outcome in patients with resectable rectal cancer.[27] Most combined-modality therapy regimens include six cycles of 5-FU–based chemotherapy plus concurrent pelvic radiation.[9] Chemotherapy assists in the downstaging of the cancer prior to surgery and is also used to minimize systemic disease either before or after surgery in patients with colorectal cancer. Combined radiation therapy plus chemotherapy has less acute toxicity when it is delivered preoperatively than when delivered postoperatively.[28] Two studies, conducted by the Gastrointestinal Tumor Study Group (GITSG) and the North Central Cancer Treatment Group (NCCTG), found a significant survival benefit with combined-modality therapy, and the latter trial showed a significant reduction in both local recurrences (14% vs. 25%) and distant metastases (29% vs. 46%) with combined-modality treatment compared with postoperative radiation alone.[9] A recent study also concluded that a combination of high-dose preoperative radiochemotherapy followed by extended surgery can achieve clear resection margins in more than 80% of patients with locally advanced T4 rectal cancer.[29] The National Surgical Breast and Bowel Project is currently conducting another study, NSABP-03, looking at the benefits and complications of preoperative versus postoperative combined-modality therapy.

Patients undergoing combined-modality therapy may receive their chemotherapy as a bolus dose prescribed over several weeks or as a continuous infusion. The use of 5-FU is often incorporated in colorectal cancer treatment regimens with radiotherapy because it is thought to act as a radiosensitizer, thereby making the tumor more sensitive to the effects of radiation. 5-FU also may be used in conjunction with leucovorin and levamisole. In the U.S. Patterns of Care Process Survey on rectosigmoid and rectal cancer, it was noted that the majority of patients received combined-modality treatment.[10]

The acute and late side effects that were discussed earlier in this chapter also apply to patients receiving combined-modality treatment. One study found that the addition of 5-FU to pelvic radiation therapy results in higher rates of severe and life-threatening diarrhea, both during radiation therapy and during chemotherapy following radiation therapy, and that rates of toxicity are higher during adjuvant therapy after low anterior resection than after abdominoperineal resection.[30]

Lastly, patients may also undergo what is known as a "sandwich" approach in their treatment. Patients receive chemotherapy and radiotherapy preoperatively and again postoperatively. The goal of therapy is to improve resectability, local control, and survival in tethered and fixed rectal cancer.[31] The specifics of chemotherapy are deferred to Chapter 9, which discusses chemotherapeutic agents, their dosing regimens, routes of delivery, and side effects.

Hyperthermia

Hyperthermia is the use of heat to treat cancer. It is used in clinical trials to treat patients with rectal cancer as well as other types of cancers.

In patients with rectal cancer, hyperthermia is typically combined with external beam radiation therapy and/or chemotherapy and may be followed by surgery. The goal of treatment is for the area that is receiving treatment to heat to 42°C verify heat. Patients who are to receive this treatment should be carefully screened and shown the hyperthermia equipment prior to treatment (Figure 8.14, see page P-8 of insert). Catheters are placed in the rectum using CT guidance, and, if in female patients, in the vagina, to track the temperatures during the hyperthermia treatment. Patients are continuously monitored, and the treatment typically lasts 60 to 90 minutes. Side effects of the treatment may be exacerbated if a patient is receiving combined-modality treatment. Side effects may include skin erythema or blistering, diarrhea, and localized discomfort. Ongoing clinical research continues to explore the role of hyperthermia in conjunction with chemotherapy and external beam therapy in the treatment of rectal cancer, and further evaluation of this treatment appears warranted.[32]

Conclusion

The role of radiation therapy in the management of colorectal cancer spans the disease trajectory from cure to palliation. The role of the multidisciplinary team in providing care to this patient population is essential. Knowledgeable practitioners, who demonstrate technical expertise as well as clinical expertise, are needed to provide patients with an organized, coordinated plan of care. Symptom management strategies are essential to patient compliance and quality care.

References

1. Hilderly L. Principles of teletherapy. In: Dow KH, Bucholtz JD, Iwamoto RR, eds. Nursing Care in Radiation Oncology. Philadelphia, PA: WB Saunders Company, 1997: 6–20.
2. Bentel GC. Radiation Therapy Planning. New York, NY: McGraw-Hill, 1996: 439–489.
3. Rosen EM, Fan S, Goldberg ID, et al. Biological basis of radiation sensitivity. Part 1: Factors governing radiation tolerance. Oncology. 2000; 14: 543–550.
4. Minsky B. Rectal cancer. In: Leibel SA, Phillips TL, eds. Textbook of Radiation Oncology, 3rd ed. Philadelphia, PA: WB Saunders Company, 1998: 686–702.
5. Gunderson LL, Martenson JA, Smalley SR, et al. Lower gastrointestinal cancers: Rationale, results and techniques of treatment. Front Radiat Ther Oncol. 1994; 28:140–154.
6. Minsky B. Colon cancer. In: Leibel SA, Phillips TL, eds. Textbook of Radiation Oncology, 3rd ed. Philadelphia, PA: WB Saunders Company, 1998: 677–685.
7. National Comprehensive Cancer Network. Colon and rectal cancer treatment guidelines for patients. American Cancer Society, Inc. Version 1, March 2000. Atlanta, GA: ACS.
8. Martenson JA, Gunderson LL. Colon and rectum. In: Perez CA, Brady LW, eds. Principles and Practice of Radiation Oncology. Philadelphia, PA: Lippincott-Raven, 1997: 1489–1510.
9. Peeters M, Haller DG. Therapy for early-stage colorectal cancer. Oncology. 1999; 13:307–315.
10. Minsky BD, Coia L, Haller DG, et al. Radiation therapy for rectosigmoid and rectal cancer: Results of the 1992–1994 patterns of care process survey. J Clin Oncol. 1998; 16:2542–2547.
11. Minsky BD. The role of adjuvant radiation therapy in the treatment of colorectal cancer. Hematol Oncol Clin North Am. 1997; 11:679–697.
12. Lewis WG, Williamson ME, Kuzu A, et al. Potential disadvantages of post-operative adjuvant radiotherapy after anterior resection for rectal cancer: A pilot study of sphincter function, rectal capacity and clinical outcome. Int J Colorectal Dis. 1995; 10:133–137.
13. Sitton E. Early and late radiation-induced skin

alterations. Part 1: Mechanisms of skin changes. Oncol Nurs Forum. 1992; 19:801–807.

14. Iwamoto R. Radiation therapy. In: Otto SE, ed. Oncology Nursing. Philadelphia, PA: Mosby, 1997: 503–526.

15. Nail LM, Jones LS. Fatigue as a side effect of cancer treatment: Impact on quality of life. *Qual Life-A Nursing Challenge.* Meniscus Educational Institute. 1995; 4:8–13.

16. Hassey KM. Radiation therapy for rectal cancer and the implications for nursing. Cancer Nurs. 1987; 10:311–318.

17. Witt ME, McDonald-Lynch A, Grimmer D. Adjuvant radiotherapy to the colorectum: Nursing implications. Oncol Nurs Forum. 1987; 14: 17–21.

18. Darbinian JA, Coulston AM. Impact of radiation therapy on the nutrition status of the cancer patient: Acute and chronic complications. In: Bloch AS, ed. Nutrition Management of the Cancer Patient. Rockville, MD: Aspen, 1990: 181–191.

19. Chamberlin RS, Jacobs TS, Orkin BA. Radiation enteritis: A primer on bowel injury due to radiation treatment for cancer. Ostomy Q. 1999; 36:36–39.

20. Coia LR, Myerson RJ, Tepper JE. Late effects of radiation therapy on the gastrointestinal tract. Int J Radiat Oncol Biol Phys. 1995; 31: 1213–1236.

21. Gosselin T, Pitz S. Anorexia. In: Nevidjon BM, Sowers KW, eds. A Nurse's Guide to Cancer Care. Philadelphia, PA: Lippincott Williams & Wilkins, 2000: 319–333.

22. Chao KSC, Perez CA, Brady LW. Radiation Oncology: Management Decisions. Philadelphia, PA: Lippincott-Raven, 1999: 399–408.

23. Maher KE. Principles of radiation therapy. In: Nevidjon BM, Sowers KW, eds. A Nurse's Guide to Cancer Care. Philadelphia, PA: Lippincott Williams & Wilkins, 2000: 215–240.

24. Willett CG, Shellito PC, Gunderson LL. Primary colorectal EBRT and IOERT. In: Gunderon LL, ed. Intraoperative Irradiation. Totowa, NJ: Humana Press, 1999: 249–272.

25. Harrison LB, Enker WE, Anderson LL. High-dose-rate intraoperative radiation therapy for colorectal cancer. Oncology. 1995; 9:737–741.

26. Wojtas F, Smith R. Hyperthermia and intraoperative radiation therapy. In: Dow KH, ed. Nursing Care in Radiation Oncology. Philadelphia, PA: WB Saunders Company, 1997: 36–46.

27. Minsky BD. The role of radiation therapy in rectal cancer. Semin Oncol. 1997; 24:S18-25–S18-29 (suppl 18).

28. Minsky BD, Cohen AM, Kemeny N, et al. Combined modality therapy of rectal cancer: Decreased acute toxicity with the preoperative approach. J Clin Oncol. 1992; 10:1218–1224.

29. Rodel C, Grabenbauer GG, Schick C, et al. Preoperative radiation with concurrent 5-fluorouracil for locally advanced T4-primary rectal cancer. Strahlenther Onkol. 2000; 176:161–167.

30. Miller RC, Martenson JA, Sargent DJ, et al. Acute treatment-related diarrhea during postoperative adjuvant therapy for high-risk rectal carcinoma. Int J Radiat Oncol Biol Phys. 1998; 4: 593–598.

31. Chan AKP, Wong AO, Langevin JM, et al. "Sandwich" preoperative and postoperative combined chemotherapy and radiation in tethered and fixed rectal cancer: Impact of treatment intensity on local control and survival. Int J Radiat Oncol Biol Phys. 1997; 37:629–637.

32. Anscher MS, Lee C, Hurwitz H, et al. A pilot study of preoperative continuous infusion 5-fluorouracil, external microwave hyperthermia, and external beam radiotherapy for treatment of locally advanced, unresectable, or recurrent rectal cancer. Int J Radiat Oncol Biol Phys. 2000; 47:719–724.

CHAPTER 9 | Systemic Chemotherapy for Colorectal Cancer

Deborah T. Berg, RN, BSN

Introduction

Colorectal cancer (CRC) represents a significant health problem in the United States. Considering the U.S. population as a whole, it is the second leading cause of cancer and cancer-related death.[1] Five-year survival for CRC has improved over the past two decades, in part because of improvements in therapy.[2] For most stages of disease, the curative treatment option is surgical removal of the primary tumor and any regional lymph nodes. Depending on the stage of disease at the time of diagnosis, adjuvant chemotherapy and/or radiation therapy may be given. Unfortunately, due to residual tumor cells too small to detect at the time of curative surgery, many patients develop recurrent cancer in regional or distant sites, such as lymph nodes, liver, and lungs. Metastatic CRC affects the vast majority of individuals diagnosed with this disease, with approximately 25% of CRC patients initially presenting with metastatic disease; despite adjuvant therapy, another 50% ultimately progress with cancer in distant organs.[3] This chapter reviews the systemic chemotherapeutic treatment options available to patients with CRC.

Adjuvant Therapy

Overview

Because of the likelihood of residual cancer at the time of curative surgery, adjuvant chemotherapy with or without radiation therapy is now

157

considered standard care for specific stages of disease. However, even as recently as 10 years ago it was not common practice. The goal of adjuvant therapy, given along with potentially curative surgery, is to eradicate any residual malignant cells before they develop into new tumors. Specific treatment recommendations regarding the use of adjuvant therapy depend on the surgical pathologic stage of the primary tumor, which, despite research into other areas, continues to be the most important prognostic tool.

Stage I colon cancer is treated with curative surgery only, because additive therapy has not been shown to improve overall survival. Stage III colon cancer, disease that has spread outside the bowel wall to regional lymph nodes, is treated with curative surgery plus chemotherapy, which has been shown to decrease the risk of tumor recurrence by 50% and to prolong survival.[4] Adjuvant chemotherapy for stage III colon cancer has been the standard of care since 1990.[5] Unless there are factors associated with a high risk of recurrence (e.g., perforation, positive margins, adhesion to local organs, and/or obstruction), the current standard of care for stage II colon cancer is surgery alone, because the addition of adjuvant therapy has not borne an improvement in overall survival. If any of the previously noted risk factors that increase the potential of tumor recurrence are present, adjuvant therapy with a 5-fluorouracil (5-FU) and leucovorin (LV)–based therapy may be administered in stage II disease.[6] The use of adjuvant therapy in stage II colon cancer is considered controversial, and thus is best instituted in the context of a well-designed clinical trial.[6] Because of differences in the patterns of failure, adjuvant therapy for rectal cancer is different from that for colon cancer. The rectum lies below the peritoneal reflection, with an anatomically limited surgical field; thus, rectal cancer often recurs locally. Adjuvant radiation therapy with or without chemotherapy is rec-

ommended for stages I and II rectal disease because of the frequency of local recurrence. Colon cancer, on the other hand, has a wide anatomic surgical field and tends to recur within the peritoneal cavity, the liver, or the lungs, so a local modality such as radiotherapy has limited value. A systemic strategy with chemotherapy or immunotherapy is thus the appropriate modality for colon cancer. The following discussion on adjuvant therapy in colon cancer focuses on stage II and III disease.

Adjuvant Therapy in Colon Cancer

The mainstay of systemic chemotherapy for CRC is the thymidylate synthase (TS) inhibitor 5-FU. During the 1960s to 1990s, 5-FU was tested in the metastatic and adjuvant settings as a single agent, in combination with several chemotherapeutic agents, and with drugs felt to modulate its mechanism of action. The main adjuvant regimens incorporate 5-FU plus LV or levamisole.

ADJUVANT 5-FLUOROURACIL AND LEVAMISOLE

Based on the results of previous trials, the North Central Cancer Treatment Group (NCCTG) conducted an adjuvant therapy clinical trial comparing the combination of 5-FU and levamisole to levamisole alone to no further therapy postoperatively in patients with stage II and III CRC. At the time, levamisole, used by veterinarians to treat worms, was thought to have an immunomodulatory effect. After following patients for a median of 7 years, the NCCTG reported that adjuvant therapy with the combination of 5-FU and levamisole demonstrated a significant improvement in time to tumor progression and overall survival, specifically in patients with stage III disease.[7] This led to a confirmatory trial, which again showed an increase in disease-free and overall survival in patients with stage III CRC that were treated with 5-FU and levamisole.[8,9] Toxicities reported with the 5-FU and levamisole combination included myelosuppression; elevations in liver enzymes; alterations in taste, including a metallic taste; general body aches; neurotoxicity; and depression. These adverse events were mild and usually did not require the discontinuation of therapy.[10]

The results of these pivotal trials led a group of surgical, medical, and radiation oncologists plus gastrointerologists and the public to meet to discuss the role of adjuvant therapy. In 1990, both the National Institutes of Health (NIH) Consensus Development Conference on Adjuvant Therapy for Patients with Colon and Rectum Cancer and the Food and Drug Administration (FDA) pronounced 5-FU and levamisole the standard chemotherapeutic regimen in the adjuvant setting for stage III (Dukes' C) colon cancer.[5] This was the first time that a

postoperative therapy was recommended for this patient population. Even with long-term follow-up (i.e., a median follow-up of 7 years), the disease-free survival for adjuvant 5-FU and levamisole was 60% compared with 46% in the surgery alone arm. Because most postoperative recurrences occur within 5 years, the increased survival with the chemotherapy had dramatically changed the natural history of stage III colon cancer.[9]

ADJUVANT 5-FLUOROURACIL AND LEUCOVORIN

For years, 5-FU and levamisole remained the standard adjuvant therapy, until 5-FU and LV, the standard therapy for metastatic disease, recently challenged it. Because of years of research in the metastatic setting, there are a variety of 5-FU and LV dose and schedule strategies, as illustrated in Table 9.1. Adjuvant clini-

Table 9.1   Sample Doses and Schedules of 5-FU and LV Regimens

Nickname	Dose and Schedule
Bolus schedules	
"Mayo Clinic" or "loading dose" schedule	5-FU 450–500 mg/m² with LV 20 mg/m² IVB for 5 consecutive days every 28 days
"Roswell Park" or "weekly dose" schedule	5-FU 500–700 mg/m² with LV 20 or 500 mg/m² IV weekly for 6 weeks every 8 weeks
High-dose schedule	5-FU 1,000 mg/m² IV day 1, weekly × 12 weeks
Continuous Infusion	
Not applicable	5-FU 200–300 mg/m²/day CI for 28 days, every 6 weeks
"AIO German" schedule	5-FU 2,600 mg/m² CI over 24 hours with LV 500 mg/m² IV over 2 hours weekly for 6 weeks, every 8 weeks
"de Gramont" schedule	5-FU 300–400 mg/m² IVB with LV 200 mg/m² IV over 2 hours, followed by 5-FU 300–600 mg/m² CI over 22 hours days 1 and 2 each week, every 2 weeks
"Lockich" schedule	5-FU 300 mg/m² CI every day

IVB, intravenous bolus; CI, continuous infusion also CIV.

Source: Based on data from Chase JL, Hoff PMG, Pazdur R. Management of colorectal cancer. In: Berg DT, Chase JL, Clanton MS, et al., eds. Disease Management of Colorectal Cancer. Pittsburgh, PA: Oncology Education Services, 1998: 8–34 and Redmond K, ed. A Nurses' Guide to Colorectal Cancer. Brussels, Belgium: European Oncology Nursing Society and AstraZeneca UK Limited, 2000.

cal trials conducted in the early 1990s, using a number of different regimens, showed significant improvement in disease-free survival and overall survival with the combination of 5-FU and LV, as compared with surgery alone. The next generation of clinical trials was designed to directly compare various 5-FU and LV regimens, including 5-FU, LV, and levamisole, with standard 5-FU and levamisole. Collectively, these clinical trials supported the use of a 5-FU and LV–based therapy in the adjuvant setting. Moreover, the data suggested that 5-FU plus LV (given at low or high dose) administered for 6 months was equal in efficacy to 5-FU plus levamisole for 12 months. In addition, efficacy, disease-free survival, and overall survival were not significantly different between the various 5-FU and LV combinations used in these trials; therefore, all are considered appropriate regimens.[10] The data are unclear as to the role of the triple combination of 5-FU, LV, and levamisole in comparison to any of the doublet combinations, except that the triple combination caused more toxicity. Based on these data, 5-FU and LV–based therapy stepped into the forefront as the standard adjuvant therapy.[6]

Toxicity profiles were different between the various 5-FU and LV strategies but were as expected, based on data from the metastatic setting. 5-FU, LV, with or without levamisole, given daily for 5 days resulted in a higher incidence of stomatitis and leukopenia, while diarrhea was higher in the weekly schedule of 5-FU and LV.[10] Unexpectedly, women and patients over the age of 70 demonstrated a preponderance for developing stomatitis and leukopenia.[10] Older age (i.e., greater than 65 years at the time of diagnosis) is *not* a contraindication to adjuvant therapy, which has demonstrated benefits and acceptable toxicity profiles in this patient population.[11] In addition to toxicity data, these trials provided insight into the cost effectiveness of adjuvant therapy. The cost of 1 year of 5-FU and levamisole is less than $5,000 per year of life saved. Because the cost of 6 months

of 5-FU and LV is at least equal to, if not less than, 5-FU and levamisole, it, too, is considered a cost-effective therapy.[10]

What have we learned about adjuvant therapy for stage III colon cancer? Based on the available data, the National Comprehensive Cancer Network (NCCN) guidelines recommend a 5-FU and LV–based regimen for stage III colon cancer.[6] If perforation is present, they recommend the addition of radiation therapy to 5-FU and LV.[6] A patient's age alone also should not be an exclusion for adjuvant therapy, as elderly patients tolerate and benefit from therapy the same as younger patients with the same characteristics.[11] Therefore, adjuvant therapy is cost effective, and it should be offered to all patients with stage III disease who have undergone surgery with curative intent.

What have we learned about adjuvant therapy for stage II colon cancer? The role of adjuvant chemotherapy in stage II colon cancer, disease that has spread through the bowel wall but does not involve the nearby lymph nodes, remains unclear. In most cases, no postoperative therapy is required unless it is administered as part of a clinical trial investigating adjuvant therapy. For patients with risk factors associated with an increased risk of recurrence, as noted previously, 5-FU and LV either with or without radiation therapy may be administered.[6]

Future Directions in Adjuvant Therapy in Colon Cancer

IMMUNOLOGIC ADJUVANT THERAPY

The use of the patient's own immune system to destroy cancer cells continues to be an area of great interest. Levamisole (as previously discussed), interferon-alfa, interleukin-2, and bacillus Calmette-Guerin (BCG) have all been used as immunotherapeutic agents in this disease, mostly without great success. Another agent being tested in the adjuvant setting is the monoclonal antibody edrecolomab (Panorex, Mab17-1A). Edrecolomab is a murine monoclonal antibody that binds to the 17-1A tumor antigen, which is prevalent on the majority of adenocarcinomas. Interest in this antibody increased with reports from Riethmüller and colleagues that this agent demonstrated an increase in disease-free and overall survival in patients with stage III colon cancer when treated with edrecolomab postoperatively.[12] For reasons that are unclear, the decrease in relapse was due mostly to a decrease in distant metastasis, as compared with local relapses.[12] The toxicities of edrecolomab are usually mild and include an infusion-related hypersensitivity, anaphylaxis, low-grade fever, abdominal pain, flulike symptoms, nausea, vomiting, and diarrhea.[13] Two adjuvant trials using edrecolomab are under way. One trial, sponsored by Glaxo-Wellcome, is comparing single-agent edrecolomab alone or in combination with 5-FU–based chemotherapy in stage III colon cancer.[13] The second trial, led by the Cancer and Leukemia Group B (CALGB) cooperative group, is randomizing patients with stage II colon cancer to either edrecolomab alone or observation. (NB: Observation in stage II disease is the standard of care.[6])

SYSTEMIC CHEMOTHERAPY AGENTS

Once chemotherapeutic agents are shown to have activity in the metastatic setting, they are investigated in the adjuvant setting to evaluate their effectiveness in patients with earlier stage disease. Table 9.2 lists the agents currently undergoing investigation. One large phase III trial has been completed, and four others are ongoing in this patient population (see schemas in Figure 9.1). Two additional European phase III adjuvant trials are just being initiated. With the exception of edrecolomab (discussed previously), the nursing implications of these agents are discussed in detail in the section on treatment of metastatic disease.

COMPLETED TRIAL

The National Surgical Bowel and Breast Project (NSABP) has completed an adjuvant trial comparing UFT (uracil plus tegafur [Orzel]) with 5-FU and LV. The trial has completed accrual, but the data are not yet available. This trial is interesting because it compares an oral agent with the standard intravenous agents. Many patients, especially in the adjuvant setting, would prefer the convenience of taking oral therapy, which could be taken at home, as opposed to intravenous chemotherapy, which requires frequent trips to the doctor's office. It is hoped that in the next few years we will have the results as to whether this oral agent is effective in the adjuvant setting.

ONGOING TRIALS

The CALGB cooperative group is leading an effort in the United States and Canada comparing standard weekly 5-FU and LV either alone or in combination with irinotecan (see treatment details in Figure 9.1). The scientific rationale for this adjuvant study came from the results documented in a phase III trial in patients with chemotherapy-naïve metastatic CRC. In this later trial, patients treated with the combination

Table 9.2 Novel Agents Being Investigated in the Adjuvant Setting

Chemotherapeutic Agent	Trade Name	Mechanism of Action
Irinotecan (CPT-11)	Camptosar	Topoisomerase I inhibitor
Oxaliplatin	Eloxatine	Platinum derivative
Capecitabine	Xeloda	Oral fluoropyrimidine
UFT	Orzel	Oral fluoropyrimidine
Edrecolomab (Mab17-1A)	Panorex	Monoclonal antibody

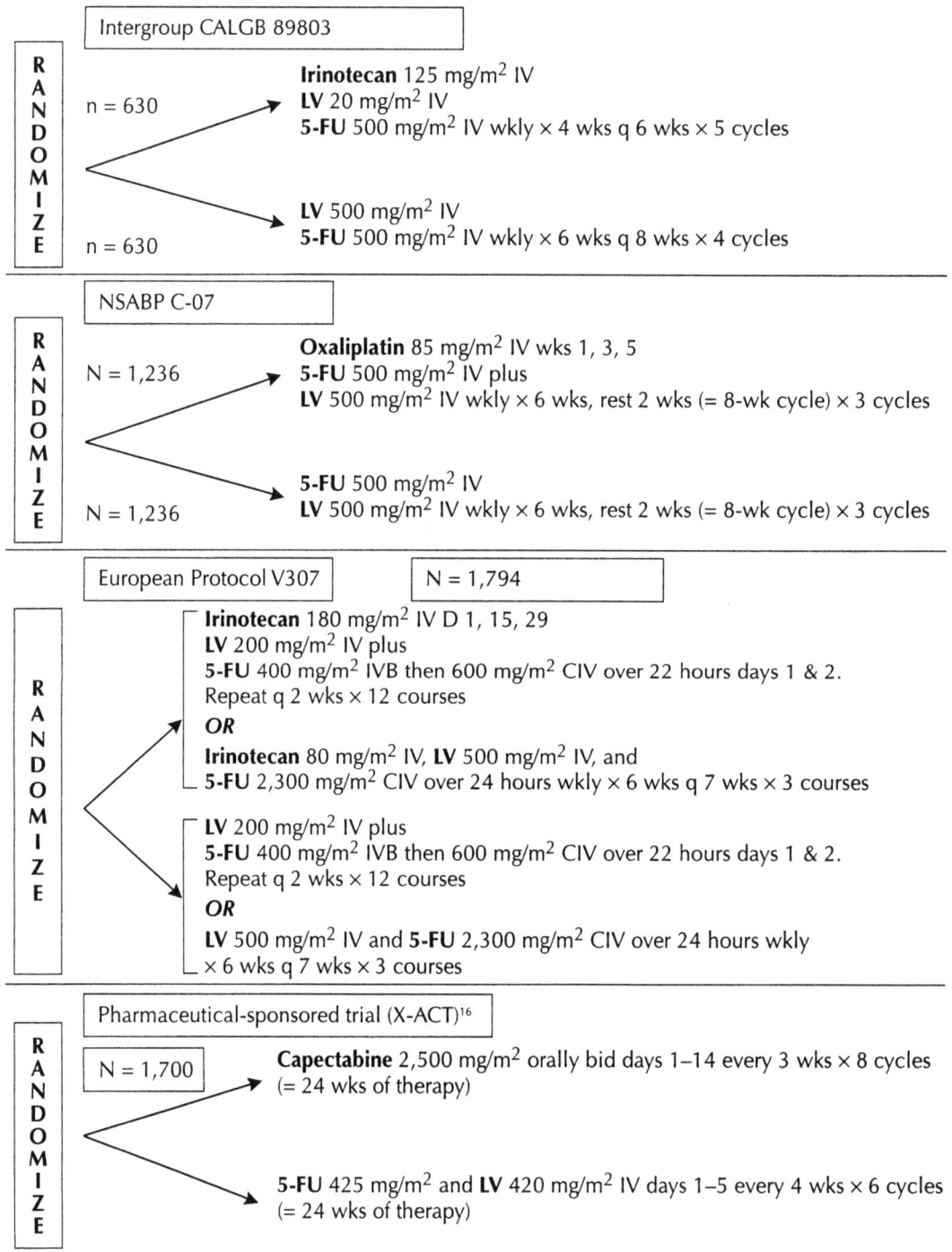

Figure 9.1   Ongoing phase III adjuvant trials for colon cancer.[15]

of irinotecan, 5-FU, and LV who had a normal performance status, few sites of metastatic tumor, and a relatively normal lactate dehydrogenase level (LDH), bilirubin, and white blood cell count (WBC)—that is, representing patients with a lower tumor burden—had a better outcome in terms of response and survival, raising the question of whether patients would benefit from the addition of irinotecan at an earlier point in the disease process.[14] Therefore, the primary goals of the adjuvant study are to investigate the efficacy, disease-free survival, and safety of irinotecan added to 5-FU and LV when given to patients with stage III CRC. In addition, this adjuvant study will prospectively assess several prognostic tumor markers (e.g., TS, *p53*, vascular endothelial growth factor [VEGF], the deleted-in-colon-cancer (*DCC*) gene, microsatellite instability [MSI], and topoisomerase I levels) and pathologic cellular features on recurrence and survival. Another interesting area being considered is the influence of diet and physical activity on toxicity, recurrence, and survival. A total of 1,260 patients will be accrued to this study.[15]

The NSABP is conducting another of the cooperative group phase III adjuvant trials. This trial randomizes patients with either stage II or III colon cancer to 5-FU and LV with or without oxaliplatin (see Figure 9.1 for treatment details). This trial is building upon data from trials conducted in Europe, which demonstrated a benefit for patients with metastatic CRC treated with the combination of oxaliplatin, 5-FU, and LV. With a total of 2,472 patients participating, the primary endpoints of the NSABP trial are efficacy, disease-free survival, and overall survival.[15]

The third adjuvant trial, the scientific rationale of which was also based on the success of a clinical trial in the metastatic setting, is the European study no. V307. This study has two treatment arms and two treatment schedules per arm (see treatment diagram in Figure 9.1). Similar to the CALGB study, this study compares

5-FU and LV with irinotecan, 5-FU, and LV, *but*, in this trial, the comparison is with infusional 5-FU. As in the CALGB, the primary endpoint of the European study is disease-free survival. At least 1,794 patients will be accrued and randomized in this study.

Hoffman-La Roche Pharmaceuticals is sponsoring two phase III trials of the same design—one in Europe and one in the United States, Canada, and Latin America—for patients with Dukes' C colon cancer. These trials compare capecitabine (Xeloda) to intravenous 5-FU and LV (see Figure 9.1 for details). The expected accrual is 1,700 patients from 100 centers. The primary endpoint is disease-free survival, with secondary endpoints of overall survival, toxicity, quality of life, and health economics. A subset of centers will also measure TS thymidine phosphorylase (TP), and dihydropyrimidine dehydrogenase (DPD) levels.[16]

As noted, there are two other European adjuvant trials being initiated. At the time this chapter was written, the details of these phase III trials were scant, but what was available is outlined here.

The United Kingdom Coordinating Committee on Cancer Research (UKCCCR, EU-99053) is comparing adjuvant 5-FU and LV to observation (details are not available on the specific patient population or the specific drug dosages). Approximately 2,500 patients will be accrued, with survival and tumor recurrence being the primary endpoints.[15] The study design is as follows:

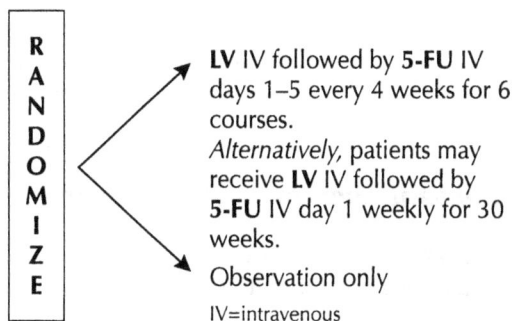

R A N D O M I Z E

→ **LV** IV followed by **5-FU** IV days 1–5 every 4 weeks for 6 courses. *Alternatively*, patients may receive **LV** IV followed by **5-FU** IV day 1 weekly for 30 weeks.

→ Observation only

IV=intravenous

```
R
A       ↗ LV IV followed by 5-FU IV days 1–5 every week for 6 courses
N
D
O         One of the following regimens stratified by institutional preference:
M         High dose 5-FU CIV over 48 hours every week for 8 weks. Repeated every 8
I         weeks for 3 courses.
Z         OR
E       ↘ LV IV over 2 hours followed by 5-FU CIV over 24 hours every week × 6.
          Repeated every 7 weeks for 3 courses.

          OR

          LV IV over 2 hours followed by 5-FU CIV over 22 hours on days 1 and 2.
          Repeated every 2 weeks for 12 courses.
```

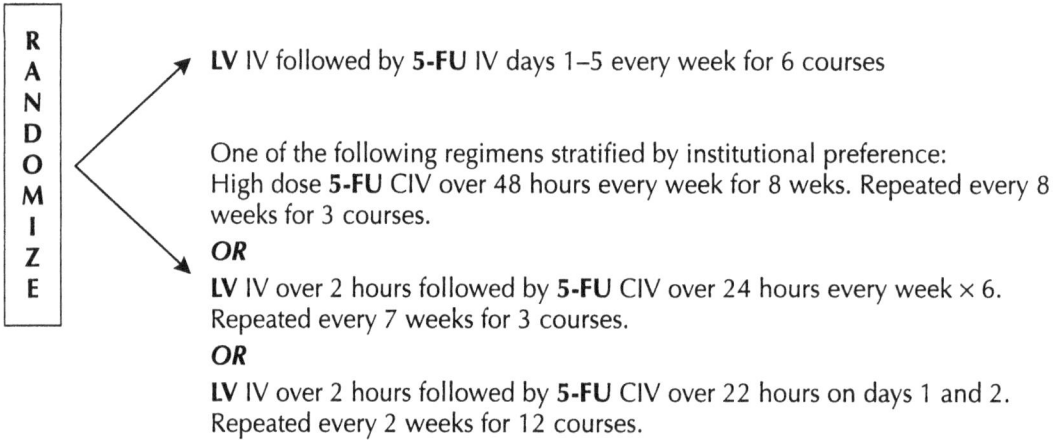

The European Organization for Research and Treatment of Cancer (EORTC) is conducting a Pan-European trial (EORTC-40963) comparing three different high-dose 5-FU regimens with or without LV with standard 5-FU and LV following radical curative resection. This trial is for patients with stage III colon cancer, but the specific doses of the three high-dose regimens are not available. Approximately 1,600 patients will participate in this clinical trial.[15] The design of this trial is shown above.

The outcome of the foregoing clinical trials, especially the trials conducted in the United States, will define the adjuvant chemotherapy offered to future U.S. patients with stage III colon cancer. In addition, outcomes of analyses on prognostic tumor markers, pathologic cellular features, and diet and their impact on recurrence and survival may provide patients with individualized answers about *their* optimal treatment.

Adjuvant Therapy in Rectal Cancer

There are two sets of issues relevant to adjuvant therapy in rectal cancer: whether to give the adjuvant therapy preoperatively or postoperatively and whether pelvic radiation therapy is given alone or with chemotherapy. The role of adjuvant therapy in rectal cancer is to decrease the risk of local recurrence and, if possible, to save the anal sphincter. Chemotherapy is given as a radiation sensitizer and to kill microscopic systemic disease. Because radiation therapy plays a pivotal role in the treatment of rectal cancer, the majority of the review of adjuvant therapy is discussed in the chapter on radiation therapy (see Chapter 8).

In 1990, the NIH Consensus Development Conference on Adjuvant Therapy for Patients with Colon and Rectum Cancer announced that combined adjuvant therapy with chemotherapy and pelvic radiation therapy was recommended for patients with stage II and III rectal cancer.[5] The recommended chemotherapy at that time was 5-FU and methyl CCNU. The recommended radiation dose was a total of 4,500 to 5,000 cGY given over approximately 5 to 6 weeks. Subsequently, in 1994, adjuvant continuous-infusion 5-FU during radiation therapy was found to increase the time to relapse and overall survival, as compared with the previous standard chemotherapy, resulting in a new standard regimen.[17]

Future Directions in Adjuvant Therapy in Rectal Cancer

Like colon cancer, novel agents are being used in the adjuvant setting in rectal cancer. To capitalize on the availability of oral agents that mimic the administration of continuous-infusion 5-FU, Brito and colleagues[18] reported on the use of UFT given with radiation therapy preoperatively to patients with resectable rectal cancer. The UFT and the radiation therapy were each given days 1 to 5 every week for 5 weeks. At the time of this report, the maximum tolerated dose for concomitant UFT and radiation therapy had not been reached, there had been one incidence of grade 3 diarrhea, and 7 of 9 patients with T3 or T4 rectal cancer had achieved an objective response.[18] Dunst and colleagues[19] conducted a similar trial to determine the maximum tolerated dose of capecitabine in combination with radiotherapy. The capecitabine was started 2 hours before initiating radiotherapy and continued twice a day for the duration of radiotherapy. At the time of this abstract, no dose-limiting toxicity had been documented, and the capecitabine dose had been escalated to 1,650 mg/m^2 day. Reported toxicities were as would be expected with the combined modality and are listed here in the order of reported frequency: mild to moderate leukopenia (67%), skin reaction to radiotherapy (50%), diarrhea (28%), constipation (28%), nausea (17%), and severe hand–foot syndrome (< 1%).[19] Of the five patients with locally advanced rectal cancer treated preoperatively, all five were successfully down-staged at the time of surgery.[19]

Current clinical trials regarding adjuvant therapy in rectal cancer also involve quality-of-life (QOL) issues such as chronic bowel dysfunction, sexuality, and sphincter-sparing oper-

ations. These trials are investigating the issue of preoperative versus postoperative adjuvant chemoradiotherapies, as they impact QOL, disease-free survival, and overall survival. Investigations of less invasive surgical procedures are also under way.

Therapeutic Options for Metastatic Disease

Not very long ago, the management of advanced CRC was very different than it is today. Because 5-FU was the only available chemotherapeutic agent, many physicians opted for a "watch and wait" approach, during which they watched patients until they developed symptoms due to progressive disease and only then started palliative therapy. This allowed physicians to observe an individual patient's natural disease course, which could vary from very slow growing tumors to rapidly progressing disease. This strategy allowed physicians to use the only available chemotherapy agent (i.e., 5-FU) when necessary, as the options after initial treatment failure were dismal and the therapy was palliative at best. Patients with rapidly growing tumors were treated immediately, while those with slow-growing tumors maintained their usual lifestyles until they developed cancer-related symptoms; then treatment was initiated. At the time of disease progression after treatment with 5-FU, physicians were faced with a quandary, as, until recently, there were no other active chemotherapy agents for advanced CRC. In the past few years, though, research in metastatic CRC has dramatically increased. The knowledge gained through these clinical trials has outlined a series of potentially promising interventions. The results of these new and important clinical trials have changed the treatment plan from "watch and wait" to early institution of treatment, whether it be a regional treatment or a systemic one. This chapter discusses systemic options, while regional treatment options are discussed in Chapter 11.

First-Line Systemic Therapeutic Options

With the results of a metaanalysis published in 1992, the combination of 5-FU and LV became the standard chemotherapy regimen for untreated advanced CRC. This analysis reported that the combination of 5-FU and LV improved the response rate, as compared with single-agent 5-FU (23% vs. 11%, respectively), with an overall survival of 11.5 months versus 11 months, respectively.[20]

As mentioned previously, there are several 5-FU and LV regimens. In general, in the United States, the 5-FU is given with low-dose LV daily for 5 days in a row, once a month or weekly, 6 out of 8 weeks, with either high- or low-dose LV. The exact dosages may vary slightly within these schedules (see Table 9.1). In Europe, the continuous-infusion schedule is common, but it is occasionally also used in the United States as a means to palliate symptoms. Continuous-infusion 5-FU is given in a variety of dosages administered over several different durations. The three common schedules noted here are considered comparable in efficacy, though the toxicity profiles differ, as noted in Table 9.3.[20]

IRINOTECAN (CPT-11)

In 1998, irinotecan (Camptosar) became the first new agent approved in almost 40 years for patients with advanced CRC. Irinotecan, an inhibitor of the enzyme topoisomerase I, has a mechanism of action different from that of 5-FU, which is a TS inhibitor. Irinotecan, a prodrug, must be converted to its active compound, SN-38, once inside the body. The conversion to SN-38 is completed by a series of enzymatic reactions catalyzed by hepatic en-zymes. Initially, irinotecan was approved by the FDA as a single-agent second-line therapy for patients with metastatic CRC after failure of a 5-FU–based regimen, but in 2000 it was also approved in combination with 5-FU and LV as the first-line treatment for metastatic CRC.

The rationale for the combination of irinotecan, 5-FU, and LV was based on the fact that 5-FU–based therapy has a minimal impact on survival, irinotecan has a novel mechanism of action, and single-agent second-line irinotecan improved overall survival. It was hoped then that if irinotecan were given early in the disease process, combined with standard 5-FU and LV, that this approach might further improve tumor control and survival. The FDA reviewed data on two independent multiinstitutional trials in which patients were randomized to receive irinotecan plus 5-FU and LV or 5-FU and LV alone. In one of the trials, patients were also randomized to receive irinotecan alone. The trial led by a U.S. group gave the 5-FU and LV daily for 5 consecutive days every 28 days (the specific schedule that the FDA considered the standard), while the irinotecan, 5-FU, plus LV combination and single-agent irinotecan were given weekly for 4 weeks every 6 weeks. The second trial, conducted in Europe, gave continuous-infusion 5-FU with or without irinotecan. Both studies found a statistically significant improvement in response rate, time to tumor progression, and overall survival for those patients treated with the combination of irinotecan, 5-FU, and LV arm when compared with 5-FU plus LV. In the U.S. trial, the response rates for the combination, 5-FU plus LV, and irinotecan alone were 39.4%, 20.8%, and 18.1%, respectively.[14] In the European trial, the response rates were 41% and 23%, respectively, for the combination and 5-FU/LV arms.[21] Overall survivals were 14.8 months, 12.6 months, and 12 months in the U.S. trial in patients treated in the combination arm, the 5-FU and LV arm, and the irinotecan-alone arm, respectively.[14] The median

Table 9.3 Common Side Effects of Selected Systemic Chemotherapeutic Agents

| | Thymidylate Synthase Inhibitors | | | | | | | |
	5-FU*	UFT	Capecitabine	Raltitrexed	Irinotecan	Oxaliplatin	C225	Thalidomide‡
Leukopenia or neutropenia	Common*	Reported	Common	Common	Common	Common		Reported
Thrombocytopenia	Common			Common	Common	Common		
Stomatitis	Common*	Reported	Common			Common†		
Diarrhea	Common*	Common	Common		Common	Common		
Constipation								Common
Hand–foot syndrome	Continuous-infusion schedules		Common			Common†		
Other skin reactions	Common				Alopecia	Alopecia†	Common Acne-like	Reported
Fatigue	Reported		Common	Common	Common	Common	Common	
Nausea, vomiting	Common	Common	Common	Reported	Common	Common	Common	
Abdominal cramping		Common	Common		Common	Common		
Elevated liver enzymes	Reported	Common		Common		Common†	Common	
Allergic reactions	Reported (leucovorin)	Common		Common			Common	
Peripheral neuropathy						Common		Common
Laryngeal dysesthesia						Reported		
Hypotension, dizziness								Common
Sedation								Common
Anemia	Common	Common	Reported		Common			
Thromboembolic events						Reported		Reported

*Side effects vary, based on dose and schedule.
†Side effect due to combination with 5-FU.
‡Also associated with severe teratogenicity.

Source: Based on data from Pazdur,[27] Pazdur et al.,[28] Van Cutsem,[34] Cohen et al.,[41] Nirenberg,[42] Whitley et al.,[43] Berg,[56] Berg,[59] Berg,[61] Pharmacia,[64] Roche Laboratories,[65] Timmerman,[66] Consumers' Guide,[69] Oncolink,[70] and Patient Self-Care Guides.[71]

survival was 17.4 months with the combination, compared with 14.1 months with the 5-FU and LV–alone arm in the European trial.[21] A combined analysis of these two trials, looking at the response rate, time to tumor progression, and overall survival, further confirmed the benefit of the addition of irinotecan to 5-FU and LV, with the following results[22]:

	Combination	5-FU/LV
Response rate	37%	21%
Time to tumor progression	6.9 mo	4.3 mo
Overall survival	15.9 mo	13.3 mo

In each individual study and in the combined analysis, the addition of irinotecan to a standard 5-FU and LV regimen achieved significant improvements in tumor control and survival without compromising the patients' QOL.[14,21,22] The results of the two phase III trials prompted the FDA to approve irinotecan, 5-FU, plus LV as the new first-line therapy in patients with newly diagnosed metastatic CRC.

The common toxicities in the trials were diarrhea and neutropenia. Treatment with irinotecan, 5-FU, and LV was associated with more severe diarrhea than with 5-FU plus LV, but less than with the irinotecan-alone arm.[14] Life-threatening diarrhea (e.g., diarrhea requiring hospitalization for supportive care) was infrequent in all three arms. Life-threatening neutropenia and neutropenic fever were almost half as frequent in either of the arms containing irinotecan as in the 5-FU plus LV arm. Fatigue and alopecia were more common in the treatments containing irinotecan.[14]

Second-Line Systemic Therapeutic Options

The approval of the addition of irinotecan to standard 5-FU and LV for newly diagnosed metastatic CRC has caused a quandary for physicians and patients. Before there was irinotecan, physicians frequently changed the method of 5-FU administration, building upon the possibility that it had a different mechanism of action with the different schedules. With the approval of irinotecan for second-line therapy, the need for the "watch and wait" approach for advanced CRC was challenged. Cunningham and colleagues[23] demonstrated that treating patients with metastatic CRC who had failed prior 5-FU with single-agent irinotecan, as opposed to best supportive care (BSC), significantly improved both overall survival and QOL.[23] BSC was determined by institutional standards and could include such therapies as antibiotics, pain medications, transfusions, palliative localized radiation therapy, and other symptomatic therapy (except irinotecan chemotherapy). The overall survival was 41% greater in the irinotecan arm, while patients noted significantly less fatigue, appetite loss, constipation, and a longer time to onset of pain, weight loss, and deterioration in performance status.[23] Patients did experience more diarrhea with irinotecan than with BSC. A second trial, reported by Rougier and colleagues,[24] demonstrated that additional infusional 5-FU after failure of a 5-FU–based regimen was inferior to single-agent irinotecan in terms of overall survival, although the QOL was equal in the two treatment arms. The overall survival was 10.8 months for irinotecan versus 8.5 months for infusional 5-FU.[24] In terms of cost effectiveness, although infusional 5-FU is a less expensive therapy, the higher cost of irinotecan is offset by the longer survival, thus making it as cost effective as other cancer treatments.[25]

These data provided strong evidence for the use of chemotherapy as a second-line antineoplastic therapy in metastatic CRC patients, instead of the "watch and wait" approach, and demonstrated that irinotecan provides a cost-effective survival advantage as second-line therapy. The problem, however, arose when the combination of irinotecan, 5-FU, and LV was approved as first-line therapy. Physicians were then left without a novel agent to use at the time of treatment failure. The current options noted by the NCCN consist of single-agent irinotecan, potentially at a dose and schedule different from that used in first-line therapy; continuous-infusion 5-FU; and a clinical trial with a novel agent.[6]

APPROVED SECOND-LINE CHEMOTHERAPY: IRINOTECAN

Irinotecan is approved as a single agent after treatment failure with a 5-FU–based therapy. There are two FDA-recognized dose and administration schedules: 125 mg/m^2 intravenously every week for 4 consecutive weeks in a 6-week cycle, and 350 mg/m^2 intravenously once every 3 weeks. The median response rate (15%–20%) and duration of survival (8–10 months) are comparable with both schedules. The toxicities are similar, though they may occur at different times during each treatment regimen. If patients have been treated with the combination involving irinotecan 125 mg/m^2 every week for 4 weeks in a 6-week cycle, physicians may decide to use single-agent irinotecan at an alternate dose and schedule at the time of tumor progression, though there have not been any clinical trials to document the effectiveness of this approach.[6]

SECOND-LINE CHEMOTHERAPEUTIC AGENTS AVAILABLE THROUGH CLINICAL TRIALS

Several analogues of 5-FU have been developed, though it is unclear whether these newer agents will prove to be superior to standard 5-FU.[26] An interesting group of TS inhibitors are the oral fluorinated pyrimidines, which are prodrugs of 5-FU. This means that these oral agents are absorbed intact and then must be metabolically converted to the substance 5-FU

either in the liver or in the tumor. The pharmacokinetics of the oral fluorinated pyrimidines mimic that of continuous-infusion 5-FU. Currently, two agents in this family have undergone U.S. clinical trials and are being reviewed by the FDA for widespread usage: UFT (Orzel) and capecitabine (Xeloda).[27]

UFT

UFT is the combination of uracil plus tegafur formulated in a 4 : 1 (uracil : tegafur) molar concentration. DPD is the main enzyme controlling the metabolism of fluorinated pyrimidines. Tegafur is a fluorinated pyrimidine. Uracil blocks both DPD and TS, thus increasing the bioavailability of tegafur for cytotoxicity. UFT is already available in Asia and Europe for colorectal, gastric, breast, and pancreatic cancers, though approval for CRC is pending in the United States.[27]

The NSABP has completed a trial in advanced disease, in which patients received either UFT plus LV or 5-FU plus LV. UFT was given at 300 mg/m^2/day tid with LV at 75 or 90 mg/d for 28 consecutive days every 35 days. The 5-FU plus LV regimen was the Mayo Clinic schedule (i.e., days 1–5 every 4 weeks). Statistically, both treatments were equal in terms of efficacy and survival.[28] Toxicity was significantly better in those patients treated with UFT plus LV, compared with those treated with 5-FU plus LV, with diarrhea, nausea, vomiting, and anemia being the most common UFT-related side effects.[28] These toxicities were reversible and easily manageable with dose delays, reductions, and symptomatic therapies. Mucositis, thrombocytopenia, and neutropenia occurred in both treatments but were significantly more frequent and more severe with intravenous 5-FU and LV.[28]

Capecitabine

Like UFT, capecitabine is a 5-FU prodrug. Unlike UFT, which is converted in the liver, capecitabine may be preferentially activated in tumors cells, because its conversion to 5-FU involves TP, an enzyme overexpressed in cancer cells. Capecitabine is commonly administered at a dose of 2,500 mg/m² PO for 14 days, followed by a 7-day rest period without treatment (i.e., a 21-day cycle), either with or without leucovorin.[27] Capecitabine, already approved for metastatic breast cancer, is being used in clinical trials for metastatic CRC, both as a single agent and in combination with other agents and modalities such as irinotecan and radiation therapy.[27,29,30] As is standard, the FDA is reviewing clinical trial data on this agent before deciding to expand its use to include metastatic CRC.

Two phase III trials comparing capecitabine with 5-FU and LV have been completed. Capecitabine was given at 2,500 mg/m² for 14 days every 3 weeks. 5-FU and LV were given at 425 mg/m² and 20 mg/m², respectively, days 1 to 5 every 4 weeks (Mayo Clinic schedule). Both trials reported a higher response rate with capecitabine but an equivalent duration of response and survival between the two treatments.[31,32] Patients treated with capecitabine experienced a better toxicity profile, with less neutropenia, stomatitis, sepsis, and need for hospitalization. Diarrhea, nausea, and vomiting were similar. Hand–foot syndrome and a clinically insignificant hyperbilirubinemia were more common with capecitabine. The investigators concluded that the convenience of this oral agent, which is at least equal to the Mayo Clinic regimen of 5-FU and LV, is better tolerated.[32]

Raltitrexed

Another TS inhibitor is raltitrexed (Tomudex). This agent is commercially available in Europe and Canada for the treatment of advanced CRC but has been available in the United States only as part of a clinical trial. This agent has an attractive administration schedule, that is, intravenously once every 3 weeks. Unfortunately, the efficacy data have been inconsistent, but are reportedly similar to those of 5-FU.[33,34] Toxicities are mild and include leukopenia, thrombocytopenia, fatigue, and a self-limiting elevation in liver enzymes. Clinical trials are investigating combining raltitrexed with a variety of agents, including both 5-FU and oxaliplatin.[33–35]

PLATINUM COMPOUNDS

Oxaliplatin (Eloxatine) is one investigational agent for metastatic CRC that is not a TS inhibitor. It has a mechanism of action similar to that of cisplatin and carboplatinum in that it forms intrastrand DNA cross-links, which inhibit DNA replication and transcription, resulting in cell death. Unlike the other platinum compounds, oxaliplatin has activity in CRC, and although still investigational in the United States, it is commercially available in Europe as both a first- and second-line therapy for patients with metastatic CRC.

Oxaliplatin is given either as a single agent or in combination with 5-FU and LV.[35,36] As outlined in Figure 9.2, it is also being combined with irinotecan in a cooperative group study looking at the treatment of metastatic disease. Oxaliplatin may be given in one of two dose schedules: 85 mg/m² every 2 weeks, or 130 mg/m² every 3 weeks. When combined with 5-FU, the oxaliplatin dose is as just given, and the specific 5-FU schedule is often one of those noted in Table 9.1; however, a lower dose of 5-FU may be needed due to the synergy between the two agents. Response rates with oxaliplatin vary, depending on whether it is given alone or in combination with 5-FU and whether it is given to previously treated or untreated patients. As a single agent, objective responses occur in approximately 10% to 18% of patients, with another 24% to 44% of patients experienc-

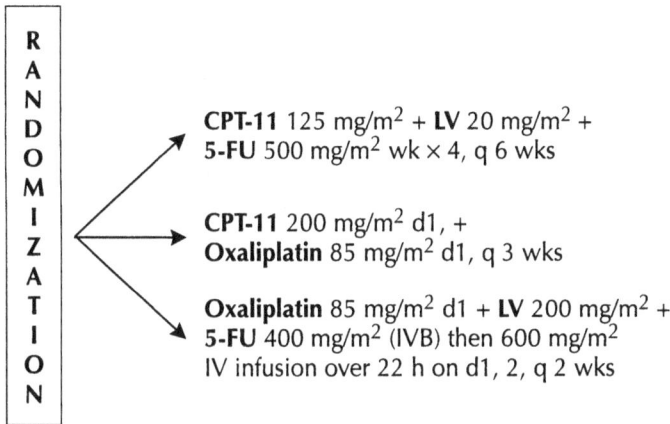

Figure 9.2 Intergroup Trial in Metastatic Colorectal Cancer.[15]

R
A
N
D
O
M
I
Z
A
T
I
O
N

CPT-11 125 mg/m^2 + **LV** 20 mg/m^2 +
5-FU 500 mg/m^2 wk × 4, q 6 wks

CPT-11 200 mg/m^2 d1, +
Oxaliplatin 85 mg/m^2 d1, q 3 wks

Oxaliplatin 85 mg/m^2 d1 + **LV** 200 mg/m^2 +
5-FU 400 mg/m^2 (IVB) then 600 mg/m^2
IV infusion over 22 h on d1, 2, q 2 wks

ing stable disease.[27,35,36] When oxaliplatin is combined with 5-FU and LV, objective response rates range from 7% to 55%, with higher responses seen in previously untreated patients.[27,35–37] Again, a significant number of patients experience a stabilization of their disease (20%–71%) with the combination therapy.[35]

AGENTS WITH NOVEL MECHANISMS OF ACTION

As addressed in great detail in Chapter 10, several agents with novel mechanisms of action are in clinical trials. Some of these are just being used to treat people for the first time, while others have completed phase II trials. Due to the emerging interest in these agents, C225 and thalidomide are briefly discussed in this section.

C225

C225 is an investigational biologic agent that attacks specific molecular targets, called epidermal growth factor (EGF) receptors, found on cancer cells. By blocking these targets, the cancer cell is unable to defend against the cytotoxicity of chemotherapy and radiation therapy.[38] C225 is being investigated in a variety of tumors, including lung, pancreas, breast, and

head and neck cancers, in addition to the disease at hand—CRC cancer.[38] Rubin and colleagues[39] report that the addition of this biologic agent may induce responses in patients who are refractory to prior therapies.

A phase II clinical trial combining C225 plus irinotecan in patients who were considered refractory to irinotecan has been conducted.[40] One hundred thirty-nine patients participated in this trial, in which C225 was administered weekly, starting with a loading dose of 400 mg/m^2 over 120 minutes, followed by weekly doses of 250 mg/m^2 over 60 minutes.[39–41] The irinotecan was administered at a weekly dose and schedule for 4 weeks on and 2 weeks off. Due to the potential for allergic reactions, a test dose of C225—a 20-mg/10 mL intravenous infusion over 10 minutes—was administered. If no allergic reaction occurred after a 30-minute observation period, the loading dose (noted previously) was infused.[41] Although specific details are pending, tumor shrinkage and slowing of tumor growth have been reported.[40] Toxicities directly related to C225 have been reported as mild to moderate and include allergic reactions, asthenia, fever, nausea, acne-like skin reactions, and increased serum alanine aminotransferase (ALT or SGPT). The allergic and skin reactions are the clinically significant toxicities.[41] A phase III trial in first-line metastatic CRC is planned.[40]

Thalidomide

Thalidomide is an investigational agent. Although its exact mechanism of action is unclear, it is believed to be an antiangiogenesis agent.[42] Antiangiogenesis agents block the development of the new blood vessels needed by cancerous tumors to grow. Its teratogenic effects are well known, but its role in cancer therapy is just being investigated. Thalidomide is being investigated in a variety of tumors, namely multiple myeloma, melanoma, and brain, breast, ovarian, prostate, and renal cell carcinomas. It is also being investigated in metastatic CRC.[42,43] A pilot study was initiated that combines thalidomide (400 mg/day PO at bedtime) with irinotecan (300–350 mg/m^2 every 3 weeks) in patients with advanced CRC.[44] During an interim analysis involving 11 patients, Govindarajan et al.[44] reported one incidence of grade 4 diarrhea with this combination. Two dose reductions were required: one for asthenia and the other for thalidomide-induced somnolence. No details are provided in the abstract about the incidence of grade 3 diarrhea, more common with irinotecan, or on the efficacy of this combination.[44] This preliminary work has led to a phase II clinical trial that will assess the toxicity and efficacy of this combination.[44] In addition to potential teratogenicity, sedation, constipation, peripheral neuropathy, deep vein thrombosis, pulmonary embolus, and skin rash are the side effects associated with thalidomide.[42]

Future Directions in Metastatic Colorectal Cancer

The availability of 5-FU, irinotecan, and oxaliplatin has led to an ongoing clinical trial in metastatic CRC (see Figure 9.2) to further test the efficacy of these agents when given in combination. Many other drug combinations are in the early stages of development (e.g., raltitrexed plus oxaliplatin; oxaliplatin plus either UFT or capecitabine; irinotecan, oxaliplatin, plus 5-FU and LV; capecitabine plus either oxaliplatin or irinotecan); the various combinations seem limitless. Finally, as discussed in Chapter 10, several novel compounds and a number of potentially new molecular targets have been identified that may lead to the development of new classes of drugs for CRC. Future clinical trials should help determine the optimal use of current agents, as well as the role of newer approaches in the treatment of CRC.

Nursing Implications of Systemic Therapy

Along with being responsible for the administration of systemic chemotherapy, oncology nurses are pivotal in patient education and symptom management. With each new agent entered into clinical trials and/or approved by the FDA, the nurse must become knowledgeable about the nuances of each specific agent, including the potential side effects and how best to manage them. Symptom prevention and management are vital skills for the nurse to master to ensure that the patient does not experience untoward side effects. Proactive nursing intervention is a priority with patients taking systemic chemotherapy. The nurse must:

- Educate the patient about the disease, therapy, expected side effects, and appropriate preventive and therapeutic measures.
- Assess the patient thoroughly at baseline and at regular intervals during therapy, either in person or, often, by telephone.
- Evaluate the symptom management strategies by maintaining regular contact with the

patient to ensure adequate symptom control and education.

Patient education materials must take into consideration the patient's literacy level, the patient's spoken language, the appropriateness of the information, and cultural sensitivity.[45,46] For specific patient populations, such as the elderly, special considerations also must be made for visual and hearing acuity along with other physiologic changes associated with aging, such as the potential for short-term memory problems.[47] Educational materials should include varying formats, such as written, oral, and video, because individual people learn best from different formats.[45,46,48] Assessment must be thorough and systematic. Simply asking the patient if a symptom is present or absent does not allow the clinician to fully characterize the side effect and thereby tailor the interventions.[49] The utilization of common criteria to describe side effects, such as the NCI Common Toxicity Criteria (CTC), can be invaluable. With a common language, clinicians can communicate effectively regarding specific patients and treatments.[50,52] Establishing a trusting relationship is also critical, so lines of communication must remain open.[51]

Patients receiving adjuvant therapy are newly diagnosed with their cancer and as such, need comprehensive education about their disease, treatment options, side effects, and symptom management strategies. Psychosocial support is also very important with a new diagnosis of cancer. Though adjuvant therapy is widely accepted as the standard of care for stage II and III rectal cancers and stage III colon cancer, some populations, such as the elderly, may not understand its importance in their overall care. In addition, many healthcare providers assume that elderly patients cannot withstand the rigors of chemotherapy and thus, even though they have undergone surgery, do not offer them chemotherapy.[51] Though the elderly are often underrepresented in clinical trials, there is a growing body of evidence that those with good performance status tolerate and benefit from adjuvant chemotherapy as well as do younger patients.[11,14,53,54] The oncology nurse can play a vital role in helping patients understand all their treatment options.

Selected Chemotherapy-Induced Side Effects

Diarrhea

Diarrhea is a common side effect of the chemotherapy agents used to treat CRC and has been labeled "the neglected symptom."[52] To initiate the appropriate intervention and to identify any change in status, a thorough assessment of the patient's bowel habits must start at pretreatment and continue throughout treatment.

Diarrhea may be managed differently, based on the underlying cause and the setting in which the patient is being treated.[52,55] It can be treated with pharmacologic interventions, dietary modifications, and, if indicated, chemotherapy dose modification or delay. The specific pharmacologic intervention is selected by its ability to relieve symptoms and according to the physician's preference. Additional factors are patient preference and ability to take oral medication, nurse preference, convenience, cost, patient age, and institutional standards.[55] The most common antidiarrheal medications prescribed are diphenoxylate hydrochloride with atropine sulfate and loperamide hydrochloride.[55] Adjunctive therapies are intravenous replacement of fluids and electrolytes and perineal or stomal skin care.[49] See Tables 9.4 and 9.5 for pharmacologic and dietary recommendations, respectively. Guidelines for chemotherapy dose modifications are outlined in the package insert for each chemotherapy agent.

Some patient populations may provide particular challenges to oncology nurses in terms of assessment and symptom management. Characteristics of such groups may include:

• Patients with a colostomy or ileostomy
• Patients experiencing chronic constipation
• Patients taking opioids or narcotics
• Stoic patients

Table 9.4 Summary of Diarrhea Management Strategies

	Recommended Treatment	Optional Treatments for Consideration
Irinotecan-induced cholinergic reaction	Prophylactic or therapeutic administration of atropine 0.25 to 1.0 mg IV or SQ[64]	Donnatal 5–10 mL orally every 4–6 hours PRN[49]
Irinotecan-induced late-onset diarrhea	Intensive loperamide (Imodium AD) regimen[64] • 4 mg at the first onset of late diarrhea and then 2 mg every 2 hours until the patient is diarrhea-free for at least 12 hours • During the night, may take 4 mg of loperamide every 4 hours	Diphenoxylate hydrochloride with atropine sulfate (Lomotil) 5 mg PO qid initially. Titrate to response.[72] Deodorized tincture of opium (DTO) 0.3–1.0 mL PO qid (maximum 6 mL/day)[72] or 5–10 drops (0.6 mL) after each stool (maximum 6 doses/day).[73] Octreotide acetate (Sandostatin) 100 µg bid or 150 µg tid SQ (standard dose).[73,74] Or 1,500 µg SQ tid (high dose).[75] Titrate to obtain response (range, 450–1,500 µg/day).[72] Sandostatin LAR Depot IM every month[76] Glutamine 10 g PO tid for 4–5 days starting the evening prior to the irinotecan infusion and continuing for 3–4 days after treatment.[77,78] Sucrose 100 mg and salt 2.5 g ("soup and Koolaid") regimen × 3 consecutive days (day of infusion + 2 days after): **Drink** Koolaid (unsweetened) mixed with 2 cups of sugar in 2 quarts of water or jello-tea (one package of jello mixed in warm/hot water) **plus** one can Campbell's soup (not low-salt variety) or 2 bouillon cubes desolved in water[73] (Oral comunication, December 6, 2000, Dr. Edith Mitchell)

(continues)

Table 9.4 *Continued*

	Recommended Treatment	Optional Treatments for Consideration
Diarrhea induced by other chemotherapy agents	Loperamide (Imodium AD) standard dose: 4 mg after the first loose stool, followed by 2 mg with each subsequent loose stool (maximum dose, 16 mg/day as directed by a physician)[72] Diphenoxylate hydrochloride with atropine sulfate (Lomotil) 5 mg PO qid initially. Titrate to response. Discontinue if not effective in 48 hours.[72] Deodorized tincture of opium (DTO) 0.3–1.0 mL PO qid (maximum 6 mL/day)[72] or 5–10 drops (0.6 mL) after each stool (maximum 6 doses/day)[73] Kaopectate 60–120 mL regular or 45–90 mL concentrated solution orally after each loose stool. Maximum duration of 48 hours.[72] Octreotide acetate (Sandostatin) 100 μg bid or 150 μg tid SQ (standard dose).[73,74] Or 1,500 μg SQ tid (high dose).[75] Titrate to response (range, 450–1,500 μg/day).[72]	Sandostatin LAR Depot IM every month[76] Glutamine 10 g PO tid for 4–5 days starting the evening prior to chemotherapy and continuing for 3–4 days after treatment[77,78]

Abbreviations: IV, intravenous; SQ, subcutaneous injection; IM, intramuscular; PRN, as needed; PO, orally; bid, twice a day; tid, three times a day; qid, four times a day, qHS, every night.

Source: Based on data from: Berg,[49] Pharmacia Oncology,[63] Wilkes et al.,[72] Viele,[73] Cascinu et al.,[74] Wadler et al.,[75] Novartis,[76] Savey,[77] and Savarese et al.[78]

- Elderly patients
- Culturally diverse patients

To assess whether the diarrhea has worsened in the patient with a colostomy or ileostomy, the patient's pretreatment volume of stool should be established. This may not be an easy task, depending on the patient's reliability to accurately report volume.[56] Furthermore, the ability to correlate volume with the severity of diarrhea also may be difficult, but it is essential. The new NCI CTC (version 2.0) has included criteria for assessing the severity of diarrhea in the patient with a colostomy, but the measures

Table 9.5   Dietary Recommendations for the Patient with Diarrhea

Dos	Don'ts
Fluids	
Force fluids (6–8 glasses daily)	*Drink* large volumes of fluid at one time
Drink a variety of liquids:	*Drink*
Water	Milk
Carbohydrate–electrolyte beverages	Liquids or nutritional supplements containing
Clear broth or bouillon	lactose
Uncaffeinated sodas	Alcohol
Oral rehydration solutions, e.g., Ricelyte and	Coffee
Pedialyte	Caffeinated beverages
Sports drinks (are controversial)	Specific fruit juices, e.g., prune and orange
	juice
Drink liquids at room temperature	*Drink* beverages that are very hot or very cold
Foods	
Eat small meals often	*Eat* large amounts of food at one time
Bland, low-fiber foods:	*Eat* diet high in roughage, including raw fruits,
B—bananas: replace nutrients	vegetables, whole grains, dried beans, popcorn
R—rice: easily digested, binding starch	*Eat* greasy, fatty, fried, seasoned foods, or sweet/
A—applesauce: sugars for energy	rich foods
T—toast: easily tolerated, binding starch	*Eat* gas-producing foods (beans, cabbage-family
	vegetables, onion, carbonated beverages)
Eat gelatins, yogurt, sherbet	*Eat* dairy products, including cheese, ice cream,
	pudding, chocolate
Cook all vegetables, meats, fish, and fruits	*Eat* raw or rare meat or fish
(cooked or canned)	
Cool to room temperature	
Eat more foods, such as pasta, boiled or baked	*Take* fiber supplements (Metamucil or Fibercon),
potatoes (no butter), baked chicken without	unless your doctor/nurse says it is all right, dur-
the skin, crackers, as the diarrhea resolves.	ing the diarrhea

Source: Adapted from Berg DT. Diarrhea. In: Yasko J, ed. Nursing Management of Symptoms Associated with Chemotherapy, 5th ed. West Conshohocken, PA: Meniscus Health Communications, 2001: 109–130.

are general (i.e., mild, moderate, or severe increase) and do not include any parameters for duration.[50] Patients on laxative therapy because of chronic constipation, possibly due to opioids or narcotics taken for pain, often hope for a balance between constipation and diarrhea. When adding a chemotherapy agent that can cause diarrhea to the equation, management becomes a challenge. Patients may fear constipation, and thus may underreport the incidence of diarrhea, or may fear that the antidiarrheal medication will induce constipation. It is im-

portant to carefully evaluate these patients and their laxative needs. Timely and accurate reporting of any incidence of diarrhea is important, so as not to jeopardize the success of diarrhea management.[56,57] "Stoic" patients, by definition, are indifferent to or are unaffected by positive and negative events. As such, they may underreport the incidence and severity of diarrhea. Without the appropriate level of intervention or with inappropriate compliance with the prescribed therapy, diarrhea may escalate and result in severe complications. Establishing a trusting relationship with the patient and their family may prove beneficial. Elderly patients and patients of diverse cultures may be uncomfortable talking about such an intimate, even taboo topic.[52] Moreover, there may be spoken language barriers, as well as differences in terminology as to the definition of *diarrhea*. This can make assessment and treatment difficult. Diarrhea also may be perceived, psychologically, as unimportant compared with all the other issues the patient is facing during the cancer experience.[52,57]

Nursing interventions are vital to ensure that the patient does not experience untoward side effects. Diarrhea often occurs at home, away from the clinical setting, so proactive education about when to start treatments, what specifically to take, when to stop the treatment, and, importantly, when to call for advice are all crucial. Standard and investigational options, as well as dietary recommendations to treat diarrhea, are noted in Tables 9.4 and 9.5.

Nausea and Vomiting

Nausea with or without vomiting is another common side effect of the chemotherapeutic agents used to treat CRC. Proactive interventions are very important for two main reasons: prevention of anticipatory nausea and vomiting, and maintenance of QOL. Nausea and vomiting may be acute, occurring during or shortly after treatment, or delayed, occurring more than 24 hours after treatment. As with diarrhea, a thorough assessment of the patient must start at pretreatment and continue throughout therapy so that the appropriate intervention can be instituted. Antiemetic agents are selected based on the emetogenic potential of the chemotherapy agent or regimen. Mildly emetogenic agents require different antiemetics than do severely emetogenic agents. The commercially available agents, 5-FU and irinotecan, are moderately emetogenic, while capecitabine has a low eme-

togenic potential.[51] See Table 9.6 for recommendations on specific antiemetic agents.

Bone Marrow Suppression

Bone marrow suppression is often the dose-limiting toxicity induced by chemotherapy. Given its frequent incidence and potential lethality, clinicians have become quite astute in managing patients with bone marrow suppression. The agents used to treat CRC do not often cause life-threatening bone marrow suppression, but the potential is there for severe neutropenia and, potentially, thrombocytopenia.

Three interventions are essential: monitoring the patient's complete white blood cell count (CBC) regularly; delaying the chemotherapy dose, as recommended, if there is marrow suppression; and modifying the chemotherapy dose in subsequent treatments, once there is marrow recovery. When monitoring the CBC, quantitating the absolute neutrophil count is very important. This is done by multiplying the total white blood cell count by the number of neutrophils (segmented plus banded neutrophils).[51] Supportive therapies such as colony-stimulating growth factors, antibiotics, transfusions, intravenous fluids, and the need for hospitalization are dictated by the patient's treatment regimen and the severity of the bone marrow suppression.

Fatigue

The symptom of fatigue is undergoing extensive research because the etiology is not well understood and the treatment recommendations are variable.[56] Fatigue is reported as the most prevalent side effect of chemotherapy.[58] Moreover, it may be debilitating and interfere with activities of daily living, thus decreasing QOL. Fatigue is reported, to some degree, with all chemotherapeutic agents and regimens used to treat CRC. Raltitrexed is associated with a higher incidence of fatigue, compared with the

Table 9.6   Antiemetic Recommendations for Chemotherapy

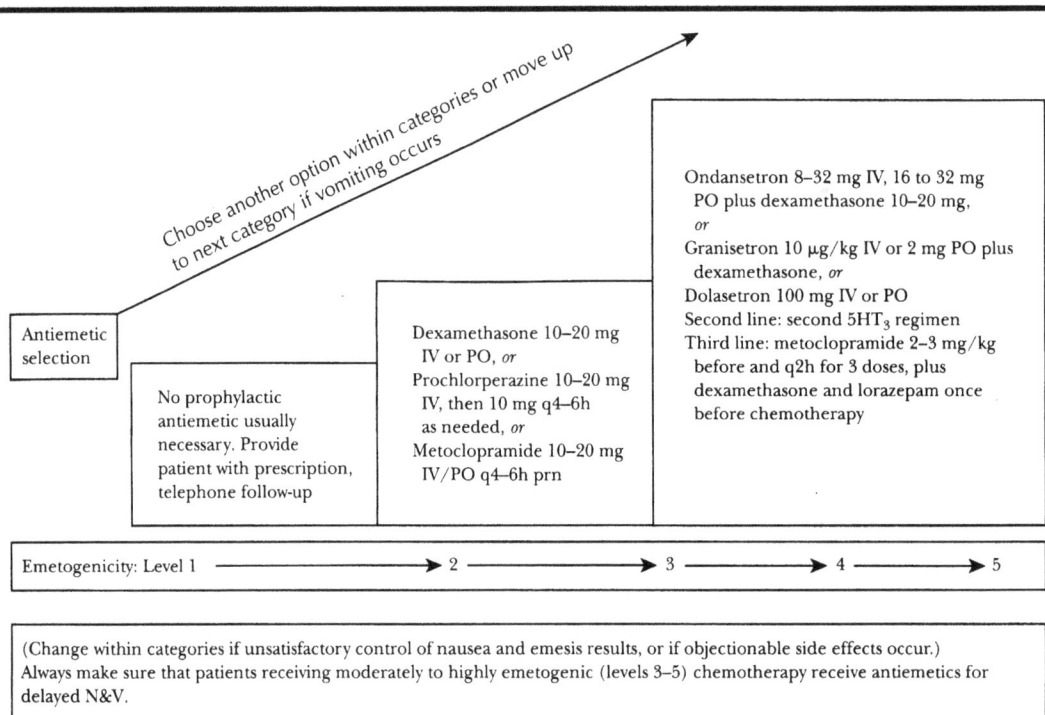

Choose another option within categories or move up
to next category if vomiting occurs

Antiemetic selection			
	No prophylactic antiemetic usually necessary. Provide patient with prescription, telephone follow-up	Dexamethasone 10–20 mg IV or PO, *or* Prochlorperazine 10–20 mg IV, then 10 mg q4–6h as needed, *or* Metoclopramide 10–20 mg IV/PO q4–6h prn	Ondansetron 8–32 mg IV, 16 to 32 mg PO plus dexamethasone 10–20 mg, *or* Granisetron 10 μg/kg IV or 2 mg PO plus dexamethasone, *or* Dolasetron 100 mg IV or PO Second line: second 5HT$_3$ regimen Third line: metoclopramide 2–3 mg/kg before and q2h for 3 doses, plus dexamethasone and lorazepam once before chemotherapy

Emetogenicity: Level 1 ⟶ 2 ⟶ 3 ⟶ 4 ⟶ 5

(Change within categories if unsatisfactory control of nausea and emesis results, or if objectionable side effects occur.) Always make sure that patients receiving moderately to highly emetogenic (levels 3–5) chemotherapy receive antiemetics for delayed N&V.

Source: Reprinted with permission from Wickham R. Nausea and vomiting. In: Yarbro CH, Frogge MH, Goodman M, eds. Cancer Symptom Management, 2nd ed. Sudbury, MA: Jones and Bartlett, 1999.

other agents that report mild to moderate fatigue.[59] In many instances, it is unclear whether the fatigue is due to the treatment or the disease itself.

Oncology nurses are in a pivotal role to help patients understand the fatigue and to manage it. The usual recommendations for fatigue management involve both nonpharmacologic and pharmacologic interventions, such as energy conservation strategies, exercise programs, and epoetin-alfa. Winningham and colleagues[60] have reported a pattern to fatigue; the severity of fatigue follows the pattern of bone marrow suppression. Helping patients understand and recognize this pattern can allow them to schedule activities around the time of heightened energy.

What have we learned, in general, about systemic chemotherapy symptom management? The common side effects associated with therapy for CRC are diarrhea, nausea, vomiting, bone marrow suppression, and fatigue. Pharmacologic and nonpharmacologic interventions are available for most of these side effects. Enlisting the assistance of patients and their caregivers is key to managing the side effects caused by chemotherapy agents. Most side effects occur at home; therefore, patients should be made aware of the need to remain vigilant concerning adverse events. For more detailed information about symptom management in the patient with CRC, see Chapter 14.

Nursing Management Issues with Specific Agents

Understanding the nuances of a chemotherapy agent is essential for the oncology nurse to ensure that the patient does not experience untoward side effects. The key to managing side effects, from any of the chemotherapy agents described, is to be watchful for side effects. Detailed nursing implications of the newer agents used to treat CRC—irinotecan, capecitabine, UFT, oxaliplatin, C225, and thalidomide—are discussed in this section (see Table 9.3 for a general overview).

Irinotecan

The cholinergic syndrome, late-onset diarrhea, neutropenia, and nausea and vomiting are the four primary irinotecan-induced toxicities that require astute nursing assessment and intervention.[61]

The signs and symptoms of the cholinergic syndrome may include one or any combination of the following symptoms: rhinorrhea, nasal congestion, lacrimation, salivation, diaphoresis, flushing, a sense of warmth, intestinal cramping, diarrhea, nausea, and vomiting. The symptoms usually occur during or shortly after administration of irinotecan, are often transient, and are infrequently severe. The cholinergic symptoms may be prevented or ameliorated with intravenous or subcutaneous atropine at a dose of 0.25 to 1.0 mg. The median time to the onset of cholinergic symptoms is 80 minutes (range, 17 minutes to 23.4 hours), and, with recommended treatment, the symptoms resolve within 10 minutes.[62]

Late-onset diarrhea is the most common, and often feared, toxicity associated with irinotecan.

As noted, diarrhea may occur as part of the cholinergic syndrome, but *late-onset diarrhea* is defined as diarrhea that occurs more than 24 hours after irinotecan administration. Patients experience a change in their usual bowel habits, such as watery stools, poorly formed or loose stools, an increase in bowel movements compared with their usual number of stools, or late abdominal cramping with or without diarrhea. There is a variation as to the onset and duration of irinotecan-induced diarrhea, based on the three common schedules[63]:

	Weekly	Every 3 Weeks	Combination
Median time to onset	~11 days	~5 days	~7 days
Duration	~3 days*	~9 days*	~2–4 days*

*In severe cases, diarrhea may last longer and may result in a severe sequela, such as dehydration.

The recommended treatment, an intensive dose of loperamide, and investigational options, used with anecdotal success, are noted in Table 9.4. Additional measures used to manage diarrhea involve dose delays or reductions, and dietary modifications. Doses of irinotecan, and 5-FU when using the combination, are decreased for an increase of 4 to 6 stools over baseline. If the patient is experiencing 7 or more stools per day, the irinotecan dose, and 5-FU dose in the combination regimen, are omitted until the treatment-related diarrhea has fully resolved. In addition to the omission of doses, the irinotecan dose and 5-FU dose, if appropriate, are reduced according to information provided by the manufacturer.[64] Dietary interventions are beneficial to not further irritate an already inflamed bowel, to reduce stool volume, to slow gastric emptying, and to increase intestinal transit time[49] (see dietary suggestions in Table 9.5).

As with diarrhea, neutropenia is a reason to decrease the dosage of irinotecan, with modifications made either during a course of therapy (if being given weekly) and/or at the beginning of the next cycle of therapy. Initial dose reductions should be considered in patients that were felt to be at high risk for neutropenia, that is, patients who had previously received pelvic or abdominal radiation therapy, are age $\geq$ 65 years, have a performance status of 2, or have increased bilirubin levels.[64] There is a variation as to the onset and duration of neutropenia, based on the three common schedules[23,24,63,64]:

	Weekly	Every 3 Weeks	Combination
Median time to nadir	~21 days	~8 days	~14 days
Duration	~7–14 days	~7–9 days	~9 days

Irinotecan is moderately emetogenic, and its effect can be acute or delayed. Premedication at least 30 minutes before the irinotecan infusion with dexamethasone plus an antiemetic agent is recommended. In light of the moderate emetogenic potential, the use of a 5-hydroxytryptamine type 3 [5-HT$_3$] blocker is often utilized. Some antiemetics are not recommended. Metoclopramide may contribute to diarrhea. Prochlorperazine, which is recommended for delayed nausea and vomiting, is not recommended on the same day as irinotecan because of an increased frequency of akathisia.[49,59,61]

A key point regarding the side effects of irinotecan given either alone or in combination with 5-FU and LV is that they are predictable and easily managed. To support oncology nurses in managing patients receiving irinotecan, the manufacturer of irinotecan has initiated a Nursing Consultation Telephone Line. Nurses can call and discuss, with experienced nurse clinicians, treatment issues such as dose modifications, symptom management, and other questions or concerns regarding various irinotecan-based regimens. At this time, the telephone line is available toll-free [(800) 289-5126, pass code 155399] on Tuesdays from 1:00 P.M. to 1:30 P.M. EST]. The patient education brochure, "Your Guide to Treatment," is also very helpful, as it provides both information about irinotecan and a "treatment tracker" for patients to document the frequency of their bowel movements and any other side effects. This brochure is available free of charge from Pharmacia Oncology.

Oral Fluorinated Pyrimidines

Compliance is a major concern with oral fluorinated pyrimidines. The medications must be taken as prescribed and stopped in light of developing severe toxicity. Educating the patient and family about the treatment plan, potential side effects, and self-care measures is extremely important. Reimbursement of oral therapies is also an issue for some patient populations. The Health Care Financing Administration (HCFA) has announced that "certain oral anti-cancer drugs," are covered by Medicare as of January 1, 1999. Nurses can use various resources to help the patient with reimbursement concerns; for example, Hoffman-La Roche Pharmaceuticals has a reimbursement hotline [(800) 443-6676] for assistance with capecitabine.

A benefit of the oral fluorinated pyrimidines is that their pharmacokinetics are similar to those of continuous-infusion 5-FU. Thus, in the future, CRC patients may never again have a need for implanted venous access devices and ambulatory pumps, because continuous-infusion 5-FU would be obsolete.

Capecitabine

The recommended dose of capecitabine is taken daily in two divided doses (approximately 12 hours apart) at the end of a meal for 2 weeks, followed by a 1-week rest period, given in 3-week cycles. The tablets should be swallowed with water.[65] In the package insert, the manufacture provides a dose-calculation table, recommending the number of tablets to be taken at each dose, based on body surface area and the two available tablet sizes, so as to allow equal morning and evening dosing.[65] (See Figure 9.3 for a sample patient diary to assist with capecitabine administration.)

The two most common side effects of capecitabine are palmar–plantar erythrodysesthesia (hand–foot syndrome) and diarrhea.[66] Stomatitis, nausea, vomiting, dyspepsia, anorexia, abdominal pain, constipation, fatigue, and transient hyperbilirubinemia are also reported.[31,66] Hair loss and bone marrow suppression are uncommon and, if they occur, are mild in nature.[65] Patients $\geq$ 80 years old reportedly experience a greater incidence of severe gastrointestinal side effects; therefore, caution should be exercised in monitoring the effects of capecitabine in the elderly.[65,66] Symptomatic measures, such as standard antidiarrheal or antiemetic treatments, are used to prevent and/or treat these side effects (see Tables 9.4, 9.5, and 9.6). The key intervention for capecitabine-related toxicities is to hold doses of capecitabine if toxicity reaches grade 2 or worse in severity until the toxicity has resolved.[66] The following definitions are provided to patients regarding when to stop therapy[65]:

Diarrhea: an increase of four or more stools each day or any diarrhea at night
Vomiting: two or more episodes in a 24-hour time period
Nausea: loss of appetite or a significant decrease in the amount of food eaten each day
Stomatitis: painful redness, swelling, or sores in the mouth or tongue
Hand–foot syndrome: painful swelling or

redness of hands and/or feet or any change that limits activities of daily living
Fever or infection: temperature $\geq$ 100.5°F or other sign of infection

Hand–foot syndrome is the dose-limiting toxicity and can be especially problematic. In the first stages, it is described as a tingling sensation, with mild erythemia, tenderness, rash, or dry/itchy skin on the palms of the hands and the soles of the feet. Without appropriate intervention, it may progress from these mild symptoms to desquamation or blistering.[59,61,66] It is important that the patient recognize any signs of progression, such as painful erythema, swelling of the hands and/or feet, and/or discomfort affecting the patient's activities of daily living (grade 2) or worse, such as, moist desquamation, ulceration, blistering, and severe pain (grade 3).[65] Once hand–foot syndrome is present, it may continue for the duration of treatment if only mild in nature.[66] For progressing or severe hand–foot syndrome, it is recommended that therapy be stopped until the toxicity has resolved, which may take 3 to 7 days.[66] Future dose recommendations are made by the physician, based on the severity of the side effect. Emollient lotions, creams containing lanolin, vitamin B_6, cotton gloves, and decreasing pressure to the palms and soles are symptomatic measures used to treat hand–foot syndrome.[61]

Several medications may interact with capecitabine and should thus be avoided. LV may increase the incidence and severity of gastrointestinal toxicity.[30] Maalox, or other antacids containing magnesium- and aluminum-hydroxides, may affect the absorption of capecitabine.[65,66] Careful monitoring is required in patients taking concomitant warfarin, coumarin-derivative anticoagulants, or phenytoin, due to reports of altered coagulation parameters and/or bleeding or phenytoin levels, respectively.[65,66] The manufacturer of capecitabine has initi-

Week 1	Week 2	Week 3 rest
am	am	am
pm	pm	pm
am	am	am
pm	pm	pm
am	am	am
pm	pm	pm
am	am	am
pm	pm	pm
am	am	am
pm	pm	pm
am	am	am
pm	pm	pm
am	am	am
pm	pm	pm

KEY: **D** = diarrhea   **N** = nausea   **V** = vomiting   **H** = hand-foot syndrome   **S** = stomatitis
F = fever   **O** = other symptoms   **R** = rest   **W** = withheld XELODA   **FG** = felt good !

Notes

_____

_____

_____

Figure 9.3   Sample patient treatment diary for capecitabine.

Source: Courtesy of Roche Pharmaceuticals at www.xeloda.com/patient/diary.html

ated a program called "Xtra" (Xeloda Therapy Reinforcement Access) to ensure that patients are comfortable taking capecitabine. This program provides extra support and education materials for patients starting therapy. Once enrolled, patients receive weekly telephone calls, for the first 12 weeks of therapy, from an oncology nurse and a Cancer Care, Inc. oncology social worker. More information about this program can be obtained by calling (877) XTRA-4-US (1-877-987-2487). "Frankly Speaking about Colorectal Cancer" is another patient education program cosponsored by The Wellness Community and the maker of capecitabine. An education kit created for patients and families provides information about the many issues, concerns, and questions experienced during and after therapy for CRC. The kit is available free of charge from The Wellness Community (1-888-793-WELL).

UFT

Common toxicities reported with UFT include diarrhea, nausea, vomiting, and elevations in bilirubin. Mucositis, neutropenia, neutropenic fever, thrombocytopenia, and hand–foot syndrome are uncommon.[28] As with capecitabine, the primary intervention for UFT-related toxicities is to hold doses of UFT if toxicity reaches grade 2 or worse in severity until the toxicity has resolved. Otherwise, standard symptomatic measures (e.g., antidiarrheal and antiemetic agents for the prevention and treatment of potential toxicities) are recommended.[27,61] More information on specific symptomatic measures may be available if UFT becomes commercially available.

Oxaliplatin

The side effects associated with oxaliplatin vary, depending on whether it is given as a single agent or in combination with 5-FU and LV. As was discussed previously, different 5-FU doses and schedules have different toxicity profiles; therefore, the specific 5-FU regimen greatly influences the toxicities of an oxaliplatin, 5-FU, and LV combination. Cold-induced peripheral sensory neuropathy and/or acute laryngopharyngeal dysesthesia, nausea, vomiting, abdominal cramping, neutropenia, thrombocytopenia, and fatigue are often common with an oxaliplatin-based regimen. Mucositis, hand–foot syndrome, alopecia, elevated hepatic enzymes, diarrhea, and myelosuppression are reported when oxaliplatin is combined with 5-FU.[27,35–37]

It should be noted that oxaliplatin-induced toxicities vary from those seen with other platinum compounds. Unlike other platinum compounds, the dose-limiting toxicity for oxaliplatin is neurologic. A cold-induced peripheral sensory neuropathy, characterized by numbness and tingling in the fingers and/or toes, with distal paresthesias and/or dysesthesias, is the primary toxicity.[61] This neuropathy may resolve before the next dose of oxaliplatin, but it tends to last longer with subsequent cycles. Because the neurologic toxicity can be cumulative, patients are at risk for functional impairment. Therefore, prior to each dose of oxaliplatin, the patient must be questioned and assessed for signs of neurologic toxicity (e.g., ability to pick up small objects, such as buttons, and to write their signatures). Patients and their caregivers must be aware that increasing difficulty with fine motor coordination may occur after multiple cycles and may adversely effect activities commonly performed by the patient. In general, when oxaliplatin is discontinued before severe impairment occurs, the sensory neuropathy is slowly reversible.[61]

An acute laryngopharyngeal dysesthesia, characterized as a sensation of tightness in the throat, is another neurotoxicity reported with oxaliplatin. Like the sensory neuropathy, this is cold-induced; therefore, it occurs in some

Table 9.7   Oxaliplatin Specific Neurologic Toxicity Scale for Clinical Trials

Toxicity Severity	Symptoms
Peripheral-Sensory Neuropathy	
Grade 1 (Mild)	Paresthesias and/or dysesthesias of limited duration; no interference with function; resolution before next cycle of therapy
Grade 2 (Moderate)	Paresthesias and/or dysesthesias lasting in-between cycles of therapy; no functional impairment
Grade 3 (Severe)	Alteration in activities of daily living with functional impairment, i.e., difficulty with buttoning
Grade 4 (Life-threatening)	Disabling or life-threatening paresthesias and/or dysesthesias
Laryngeal-Dysesthesias	
Mild	No description available
Moderate	No description available
Severe	No description available

Source: From Sanofi~Synthelabo. [Data on file], 1998, New York, NY.[80]

patients when they drink a cold beverage during the infusion or within several hours to days after their oxaliplatin infusion.[61] This sensation can be frightening to the patients, especially if they are not aware of its possibility and its association with cold. There are no recommended interventions because it often resolves spontaneously.[27,36] With the cold-induced neurotoxicities, patients need to be taught to avoid exposure to air conditioning, freezers, handling or drinking cold beverages, and so forth, especially within the first 48 to 96 hours of receiving oxaliplatin. A unique grading scale, developed for the clinical trials, provides criteria for assessing the intensity, duration, and functional status for the patient receiving oxaliplatin (Table 9.7).

C225

The side effects associated with C225 vary, depending on the concurrent chemotherapy agents being used for the specific tumor being treated (e.g., C225 plus irinotecan or cisplatin, doxorubicin, paclitaxel, gemcitabine, etc.).[41] The side effects directly associated with C225 are allergic reactions, asthenia, fever, nausea, skin reactions, and elevated SGPT. The allergic and skin reactions are the clinically significant toxicities and are discussed here.[41]

Due to the potential for allergic reactions, an initial test dose—20 mg/10 mL IV over 10 minutes—is administered, followed by an observation period of 30 minutes. If there is no reaction, the patient can continue with intravenous infusion of the full dose. If an allergic reaction occurs, the patient is treated according to institutional standards for anaphylactic reactions based on the severity of the particular reaction. All allergic reactions to date have occurred only during the test dose.[41] The reactions were severe in only 4% of patients, who then had further therapy discontinued. The remaining reactions (7% of patients) were mild or moderate, and therapy could be continued with prophylactic antihistamine treatment and prolonged intravenous infusion time.[41] Allergic reactions require close monitoring of the patient, both during the test dose and during the observation period. Patients need to be aware of this potential toxicity, so they can assist in reporting any untoward effects.

Over 80% of patients develop skin reactions, commonly seen as an acne-like rash or folliculitis on the face or trunk, especially the upper chest and/or back.[41] Additional descriptions of the skin reactions include redness, erythema, psoriasiform, maculopapular lesions, cellulitis, seborrheic dermatitis, oral aphthae, or paronychia. Nail bed changes also have been reported.[41] These reactions are dose-related, not dose-limiting, range from mild to severe in intensity, and are treated symptomatically with topical or systemic oral antibiotics, topical hydrocortisone, or topical retinoids without clear improvement. Dose delays also have been used in some patients.[41] The condition may be moderate in some patients with repeated therapy of C225. The skin reactions resolve once the therapy is discontinued.[41] This visible skin reaction can have an adverse emotional effect on the patient. The nurse must educate the patient and family prior to initiating the therapy, so they are aware of this possible reaction. Moreover, nurses can suggest symptomatic and cosmetic methods to treat the rash.

Thalidomide

The manufacturer of thalidomide has taken a proactive approach in preventing further adversity from severe teratogenicity. A program called S.T.E.P.S. (System for Thalidomide Education and Prescribing Safety) has been implemented. This program ensures that all prescribers, pharmacists, and patients are educated about thalidomide and its teratogenicity. The program details the required birth control measures: Women of childbearing age must have a negative pregnancy test each month of treatment and use two forms of birth control; men are required to use a latex condom during sexual intercourse with women of childbearing potential. To receive thalidomide, the patient must sign a required informed consent document and participate in periodic confidential surveys. In addition, only prescribers and pharmacies registered with the S.T.E.P.S. program can dispense thalidomide. A commitment to educate patients about risks, benefits, and contraceptive counseling is required of all prescribers.[42,43]

Thalidomide is associated with neurologic toxicities (sedation, peripheral neuropathy, and constipation), hypotension, peripheral edema, and, to a lesser degree, thromboembolic events, neutropenia, and skin rashes.[42,43] Education is key to the successful management of patients receiving this agent.

Sedation is a major side effect of thalidomide and one that can adversely affect the patient's QOL. Patients describe drowsiness, hangover, daytime sleepiness, dizziness, fatigue, weak-

ness, incoordination, shakiness, mood changes, confusion, and blurred vision.[43] Because sedation is dose dependent, a temporary dose reduction is often effective.[42] After 2 to 4 weeks of therapy, the sedation may moderate in some patients, although this is less likely in the elderly population.[43] Another suggestion is instructing the patient to take thalidomide at bedtime.[42] Patients should avoid other drugs that also cause sedation, such as alcoholic beverages, narcotics, antidepressants, and anxiolytics; therefore, nurses should interview patients regarding concomitant medications.[43]

Thalidomide-induced peripheral neuropathy is similar in mechanism to that caused by the taxanes, vincristine, and cisplatin.[43] It is characterized as a numbness and tingling of the hands and feet, which is often mild but can progress in severity. Assessing neurologic status at each visit is essential in diagnosing this side effect early, before there are any functional deficits. Discontinuation of therapy is the recommended treatment, due to the progressive nature of this toxicity.[43]

Prevention of constipation is key to the management of thalidomide therapy. Recommended interventions involve increased fluid intake, increased dietary fiber, regular exercise, and a bowel regimen starting with stool softeners or mild laxatives.[43] The bowel regimen can be altered, based on its effectiveness or lack thereof. Determining the patient's baseline bowel status is important in order to initiate appropriate measures.[42,43]

The nurse must assess the patient at each visit for signs and symptoms of other common side effects, such as hypotension, peripheral edema, neutropenia, and skin rashes. Bedtime dosing may alleviate daytime hypotension. Peripheral edema often does not require intervention, but, if needed, diuretics may be prescribed.[43] The incidence of neutropenia varies from 5% to 25%; thus, monitoring the patient's complete white blood cell count is important. If the absolute neutrophil count (ANC) is less than 750 cells/mm^3, therapy should be withheld and an evaluation of all concurrent therapies should be completed, with consideration for discontinuation, if appropriate.[43] In general, for skin rashes, symptomatic measures are appropriate if this side effect should develop, but if there are systemic symptoms, therapy should be discontinued.[43]

Given the results of completed phase II trials, research on the use of thalidomide in oncology is likely to expand; thus, the oncology nurse needs to be aware of the side effects and appropriate patient management strategies.

Conclusion

Over the past decade, we have seen the development of several new chemotherapeutic agents that may offer expanded systemic treatment options for patients with CRC. The oncologist no longer has only 5-FU to offer to patients. Irinotecan is now commercially available for patients for metastatic disease. Capecitabine and UFT may receive FDA approval for metastatic disease in the near future, thus creating a more convenient and better tolerated 5-FU therapy. Still in the clinical trial setting, oxaliplatin is offering patients another option. Novel agents, such as C225 and thalidomide, are increasingly being researched. There is optimism for treating patients with CRC that did not exist before.

With many exciting areas of investigation underway, the oncology nurse is also challenged to stay current with the various options. In the future, some of these options may be based on tumor-specific targets, which would be individualized to a specific patient. In addition, because these new investigations involve patient participation in clinical trials, the oncology nurse will need to educate patients about clinical trials in general. If the oral agents, such as UFT and capecitabine, prove beneficial, the nurse will be charged with assisting patients

with therapy compliance and managing side effects with the patients at home. Finally, research in the area of symptom management strategies is needed. There are many questions to be answered about the best way to manage irinotecan-induced diarrhea, capecitabine-induced hand–foot syndrome, and oxaliplatin-induced neurotoxicities, providing nurses with evidence-based interventions.

References

1. Greenlee RT, Murray T, Bolden S, et al. Cancer statistics 2000. CA Cancer J Clin. 2000; 50(1): 7–33.
2. Schatzkin AG. Colon and rectum. In: Harras A, ed. Cancer Rates and Risks, 4th ed. Bethesda, MD: National Institutes of Health, 1996: 129–135.
3. Guillem JG, Paty PB, Cohen AM. Surgical treatment of colorectal cancer. CA Cancer J Clin. 1997; 47(2):113–128.
4. National Comprehensive Cancer Network (NCCN) and American Cancer Society Colon and Rectal Cancer Treatment Guidelines for Patients. Atlanta, GA: Author, 2000.
5. National Institutes of Health consensus conference. Adjuvant therapy for patients with colon and rectal cancer. JAMA. 1990; 264(11): 1444–1450.
6. Engstrom PF, Benson AB, Choti MA, et al. National Comprehensive Cancer Network (NCCN) colorectal cancer practice guidelines. Oncology. 2000; 14(11A):203–213.
7. Laurie JA, Moertel CG, Fleming TR, et al. Surgical adjuvant therapy of large bowel carcinoma: An evaluation of levamisole and the combination of levamisole and fluorouracil: The North Central Cancer Treatment Group and the Mayo Clinic. J Clin Oncol. 1989; 7:1447–1456.
8. Moertel CG, Fleming TR, MacDonald JS, et al. Levamisole and fluorouracil for adjuvant therapy of resected colon carcinoma. N Engl J Med. 1990; 322:352–358.

9. Moertel CG, Flemining TR, MacDonald JS, et al. Fluorouracil plus levamisole as effective adjuvant therapy after resection of stage III colon carcinoma: A final report. Ann Intern Med. 1995; 122:321–326.

10. MacDonald JS. Adjuvant therapy of colon cancer. CA Cancer J Clin. 1999; 49(4):202–219.

11. Sargent D, Goldberg R, MacDonald J, et al. Adjuvant chemotherapy for colon cancer is beneficial without significantly increased toxicity in elderly patients: Results from 3351 patient meta-analysis. Proc Am Soc Clin Oncol. 2000; 19:933 (abstr).

12. Riethmüller G, Holz E, Schlimok G, et al. Monoclonal antibody therapy for resected Dukes' C colorectal cancer: Seven-year outcome of a multicenter randomized trial. J Clin Oncol. 1998; 16:1788–1794.

13. Fields LA, Nagy A, Schwartzberg L, et al. Edrecolomab (Panorex, 17-1a antibody) alone or in combination with 5-FU based chemotherapy in adjuvant treatment of stage III colon cancer: A safety review. Proc Am Soc Clin Oncol. 1999; 18:1676 (abstr).

14. Saltz LB, Cox JV, Blanke C, et al., for the Irinotecan Study Group. Irinotecan plus fluorouracil and leucovorin for metastatic colorectal cancer. N Engl J Med. 2000; 343(13):905–914.

15. National Cancer Institute Cancer Clinical Trials. Available at: Cancertrials.nci.nih.gov Accessed January 7, 2001.

16. Harstrick A. Future treatment options with Xeloda. Available at: www.roche.com.br/oncologia/xeloda/harstrick Accessed January 7, 2001.

17. O'Connell MJ, Martenson JA, Wieand HS, et al. Improving adjuvant therapy for rectal cancer by combining protracted-infusion fluorouracil with radiation therapy after curative surgery. N Engl J Med. 1994; 331(8):502–507.

18. Brito R, Lassere Y, Hoff P, et al. Schedule effect on maximum tolerated dose of Orzel® (UFT™ plus leucovorin). Proc Am Soc Clin Onc. 1999; 18:787 (abstr).

19. Dunst J, Reese T, Frings S. Phase I study of capecitabine combined with standard radiotherapy in patients with rectal cancer. Proc Am Soc Clin Oncol. 2000; 19:995 (abstr).

20. Fuchs CS, Mayer RJ. Colorectal cancer chemotherapy. In: Rustgi AK, ed. Gastrointestinal Cancers: Biology, Diagnosis, and Therapy. Boston, MA: Lippincott Williams & Wilkins, 1995: 423–442.

21. Douillard JY, Cunningham D, Roth AD, et al. Irinotecan combined with fluorouracil compared with fluorouracil alone as first-line treatment for metastatic colorectal cancer: A multicentre randomised trial. Lancet. 2000; 355: 1041–1047.

22. Saltz LB, Douillard JY, Pirotta N, et al. Combined analysis of two phase III randomized trials comparing irinotecan/5-fluorouracil/leucovorin versus 5-fluorouracil/leucovorin alone as first-line therapy of previously untreated metastatic colorectal cancer. Proc Am Soc Clin Oncol. 2000; 19:938 (abstr).

23. Cunningham D, Pyrhönen S, James RD, et al. Randomized trial of irinotecan plus supportive care versus supportive care alone after fluorouracil failure for patients with metastatic colorectal cancer. Lancet. 1998; 352(9138):1413–1418.

24. Rougier P, Van Cutsem E, Bajetta E, et al. Randomized trial of irinotecan versus fluorouracil by continuous infusion after fluorouracil failure in patients with metastatic colorectal cancer. Lancet. 1998; 352(9138):1407–1412.

25. Levy-Piedbois C, Durand-Zaleski I, Juhel H, et al. Cost-effectiveness of second-line treatment with irinotecan or infusional 5-FU in metastatic colorectal cancer. Ann Oncol. 2000; 11(2): 157–161.

26. Calvert H. Clinical Developments with Folate-Based Thymidylate Synthase Inhibitors. American Society of Clinical Oncology Education Book. Baltimore, MD: Lippincott Williams & Wilkins, 1998: 295–299.

27. Pazdur R. New Agents for Colorectal Cancers: Oral Fluorinated Pyrimidines and Oxaliplatin. American Society of Clinical Oncology Educa-

tion Book. Baltimore, MD: Lippincott Williams & Wilkins, 1998: 300–310.

28. Pazdur R, Douillard JY, Skillings JR, et al. Multicenter phase II study of 5-fluorouracil or UFT in combination with leucovorin in patients with metastatic colorectal cancer. Proc Am Soc Clin Oncol. 1999; 18:1009 (abstr).

29. Vanhoefer U, Mayer S, Harstrick A, et al. Phase I study of capecitabine in combination with weekly schedule of irinotecan as first-line chemotherapy in metastatic colorectal cancer. Proc Am Soc Clin Oncol. 2000; 19:1059 (abstr).

30. Van Cutsem E, Findlay M, Osterwalder B, et al. Capecitabine, an oral fluoropyrimidine carbamate with substantial activity in advanced colorectal cancer: Results of a randomized phase II study. J Clin Oncol. 2000; 18(6):1337–1345.

31. Cox JV, Pazdur R, Thibault A, et al. A phase III trial of Xeloda (capecitabine) in previously untreated advanced/metastatic colorectal cancer. Proc Am Soc Clin Oncol. 1999; 18:1016 (abstr).

32. Van Cutsem E. Phase III data on Xeloda® as first-line treatment in colorectal cancer: Experience from two large trials. Available at: www.roche.com.br/oncologia/xeloda/vancutsem Accessed January 7, 2001.

33. Cocconi G, Cunningham D, Van Cutsem E, et al. Open, randomized, multicenter trial of raltitrexed versus fluorouracil plus high-dose leucovorin in patients with advanced colorectal cancer. J Clin Oncol. 1998; 16:(9):2943–2952.

34. Van Cutsem E. Raltitrexed (Tomudex™). Exp Opin Investig Drugs. 1998; 7(5):823–834.

35. Cvitkovic E, Bekradda M. Oxaliplatin: A therapeutic option in colorectal cancer. Semin Oncol. 1999; 26(6):647–662.

36. Bleiberg H. Colorectal cancer—Is there an alternative to 5-FU? Eur J Cancer. 1997; 33(4): 536–541.

37. Giacchetti S, Perpoint B, Zidani R, et al. Phase III multicenter randomized trial of oxaliplatin added to chronomodulated fluorouracil-leucovorin as first-line treatment of metastatic colorectal cancer. J Clin Oncol. 2000; 18(1): 136–147.

38. C225: A new approach to cancer therapy. Available at: www3.mdanderson.org/focus/c225 Accessed October 5, 2000.

39. Rubin MS, Pasmantier M, Shin DM, et al. Monoclonal antibody IMC-C225, an anti-epidermal growth factor receptor (EGFR) used in the treatment of EGFR-positive tumors refractory to or in relapse from previous therapeutic regimens. Proc Am Soc Clin Oncol. 2000; 19:1860 (abstr).

40. ImClone's IMC-C225 shows promise in phase II colorectal cancer study. Reuters Medical News. Available at: Oncology.medscape.com/reuters/prof/2000/11/11.09/20001108drgd002.html Accessed November 15, 2000.

41. Cohen RB, Falcey JW, Paulter VJ, et al. Safety profile of the monoclonal antibody IMC-C225, anti-epidermal growth factor receptor (EGFR) used in the treatment of EGFR-positive tumors. Proc Am Soc Clin Oncol. 2000; 19:1862 (abstr).

42. Nirenberg A. Thalidomide: When everything old is new again. Clin J Oncol Nurs. 2001; 5(1): 15–18.

43. Whitley P, Nirenberg A, Mayorga J, et al. Thalidomide Nursing Roundtable Report. Stamford, CT: PharmaCom Group, Inc., 2000.

44. Govindarajan R, Zeitlin A, Seldis J, et al. Protective effect of thalidomide on gastrointestinal toxicity of CPT-11 (irinotecan). Proc Chemother Foundation Symp XVIII. 2000:32 (abstr).

45. Boyd MD. Colorectal cancer. In: Varricchio C, ed. A Cancer Source Book for Nurses. Atlanta, GA: American Cancer Society, 1997: 307–315.

46. Taoka KN, Itano JK. Cultural diversity among individuals with cancer. In: Yarbro CH, Frogge MH, Goodman M, et al., eds. Cancer Nursing Principles and Practice, 5th ed. Boston, MA: Jones and Bartlett, 2000: 100–134.

47. Polomano RC, McGuire DB, Scheidler VR. Management of pain. In: Yarbro CH, Frogge MH, Goodman M, et al., eds. Cancer Nursing Principles and Practice, 5th ed. Boston, MA: Jones and Bartlett, 2000: 657–690.

48. Padberg LF, Padberg RM. Patient education and support. In: Yarbro CH, Frogge MH, Goodman

M, et al., eds. Cancer Nursing Principles and Practice, 5th ed. Boston, MA: Jones and Bartlett, 2000: 1609–1631.

49. Berg DT. Diarrhea. In: Yasko J, ed. Nursing Management of Symptoms Associated with Chemotherapy, 5th ed. West Conshohockan, PA: Meniscus Health Communications, 2001: 109–130.

50. National Cancer Institute common toxicity criteria. Available at: www.ctep.info.nih.gov/ Accessed August 1, 2000.

51. Camp-Sorrell D. Chemotherapy: Toxicity management. In: Yarbro CH, Frogge MH, Goodman M, et al., eds. Cancer Nursing Principles and Practice, 5th ed. Boston, MA: Jones and Bartlett, 2000: 385–443.

52. Popescu RA, Norman A, Ross PJ, et al. Adjuvant or palliative chemotherapy for colorectal cancer in patients 70 years or older. J Clin Oncol. 1999; 17(8):2412–2418.

53. Grobovsky L, Kaplon M, Krozer-Hamati A, et al. Features of cancer in frail elderly patients (≥ 85 years of age). Proc Am Soc Clin Oncol. 2000; 19:2469 (abstr).

54. Engleking C, Rutledge DN, Ippoliti C, et al. Cancer related diarrhea: A neglected cause of cancer-related symptom distress. Oncol Nurs Forum. 1998; 25:859–860.

55. Rutledge DN, Engelking. Cancer-related diarrhea: Selected findings of a national survey of oncology nurse experiences. Oncol Nurs Forum. 1998; 25(5):861–872.

56. Berg DT. Toxicities and symptom management related to colorectal cancer chemotherapy. In: Berg DT, Chase JL, Clanton MS, et al., eds. Disease Management of Colorectal Cancer. Pittsburgh, PA: Oncology Education Services, 1998: 35–64.

57. Hogan CM. The nurse's role in diarrhea management. Oncol Nurs Forum. 1998; 25:879–886.

58. McDaniel RW, Rhodes VA. Fatigue. In: Yarbro CH, Frogge MH, Goodman M, et al., eds. Cancer Nursing Principles and Practice, 5th ed. Boston, MA: Jones and Bartlett, 2000: 737–753.

59. Berg D. Managing the side effects of chemother-

apy for colorectal cancer. Semin Oncol. 1998; 25(5):53–59 (suppl 11).

60. Winningham ML, Nail L, Barton-Burke M, et al. Fatigue and the cancer experience: The state of the knowledge. Oncol Nurs Forum. 1994; 21: 23–35.

61. Berg DT, Lilienfeld C. Therapeutic options for treating advanced colorectal cancer. Clin J Oncol Nurs. 2000; 4(5):209–216.

62. Petit RG, Rothenberg ML, Mitchell EP, et al. Cholinergic symptoms following CPT-11 infusion in the phase II multicenter trial of 250 mg/m^2 irinotecan given every two weeks. Proc Am Soc Clin Oncol. 1997; 16:953 (abstr).

63. Pharmacia Oncology. [Data on file]. Peapack, NJ: Author, 1999.

64. Pharmacia Oncology. Camptosar (irinotecan hydrochloride) [package insert]. Peapack, NJ: Author, 2000.

65. Roche Laboratories, Inc (2000). Xeloda (capecitabine) tablets [product insert]. Nutley, NJ: Author. Available at: www.xeloda.com/ XELODA_PI.html Accessed January 7, 2001.

66. Timmerman D. Capecitabine (Xeloda). Clin J Oncol Nurs. 2001; 5(1):36–37.

67. Chase JL, Hoff PMG, Pazdur R. Management of colorectal cancer. In: Berg DT, Chase JL, Clanton MS, et al., eds. Disease Management of Colorectal Cancer. Pittsburgh, PA: Oncology Education Services, 1998: 8–34.

68. Redmond K, ed. A Nurses' Guide to Colorectal Cancer. Brussels, Belgium: European Oncology Nursing Society and AstraZeneca UK Limited, 2000.

69. Consumers' Guide to cancer drugs. Available at: www.cancersource.com/resources/index.cfm Accessed January 7, 2001.

70. OncoLink Chemotherapy Drug Reference. Available at: www.oncolink.upenn.edu/ specialty/med_onc/chemo/drugs/reference Accessed January 1, 2001.

71. Patient Self-Care Guides. Available at: www .cancersource.com/resources/index.cfm Accessed January 7, 2001.

72. Wilkes GM, Ingwersen K, Barton-Burke M.

2000 Oncology Nursing Drug Handbook. Boston, MA: Jones and Bartlett, 2000: 717–725.

73. Viele CS. New developments and side effect management for colorectal cancer. Dev Support Cancer Care. 1999; 3(1):13–18.

74. Cascinu S, Fedeli A, Fedeli SL, et al. Octreotide versus loperamide in the treatment of fluorouracil-induced diarrhea: A randomized trial. J Clin Oncol. 1993; 11:148–151.

75. Wadler S, Haynes H, Wiernik PH. Phase I trial of the somatostatin analogue, octreotide acetate, in the treatment of fluoropyrimidine-induced diarrhea. J Clin Oncol. 1995; 13:222–226.

76. Novartis Protocol no. CSMS995US05 phase III randomized trial of octreotide in the prevention of diarrhea induced by irinotecan in patients with metastatic colorectal cancer. Available at: http://cancertrials.nci.nih.gov/ Accessed January 7, 2001.

77. Savey G. Enteral glutamine supplementation. Clin Rev Pract Guidelines. 1997; 12(6): 259–262.

78. Savarese D, Al-Zoubi A, Boucher J. Oral glutamine supplementation for treatment of irinotecan-associated late diarrhea. J Clin Oncol. 2000; 18:450.

79. Wickham R. Nausea and vomiting. In: Yarbro CH, Frogge MH, Goodman M, eds. Cancer Symptom Management, 2nd ed. Sudbury, MA: Jones and Bartlett, 1999: 228–263.

80. Sanofi~Synthelabo. [Data on file]. New York, NJ: Author, 1998.

CHAPTER 10 | Novel Agents in Colorectal Cancer

Marilyn Mulay, RN, MS, OCN

Introduction

History of Drug Development

For the past 40 years, the treatment for all solid tumor malignancies has mainly revolved around surgery, radiation, and the use of cytotoxic drugs. As the name implies, cytotoxic drugs work by attempting to destroy tumor cells through a variety of mechanisms. Unfortunately, while the tumor cells are attacked, the patient's normal cells also are attacked, causing many untoward side effects. Because cancer cells are genetically unstable, they are capable of mutation, which can produce drug-resistant cells. Many novel agents are thought to overcome traditional methods of drug resistance.

For the past two decades, researchers have been concentrating their efforts on determining what makes a tumor cell different from a normal cell; new drugs are being developed to target those differences. Because the new compounds attack properties unique to the cancer cells and not normal cells, they may be less toxic to the patient. Many of the drugs may not destroy tumor cells, but rather may interfere with properties that allow tumor cells to grow and spread. For this reason, many of the novel agents are thought to be cytostatic.

Cancer as a Chronic Illness

The idea that tumors may not be destroyed but stunted in their growth means that the cancer

191

may never be "cured." In fact, perhaps thinking about cancer treatment will change from the quest for cure to the acceptance of cancer as a chronic illness, such as diabetes or hypertension. Patients may need to take a medication every day of their lives, but they will die with the disease, not of it. This scenario raises the yet-unanswered questions about the long-term tolerability and side effects of these novel agents, as well as delivery methods that make chronic use acceptable. For example, a drug that must be administered intravenously every day, although perhaps prolonging a patient's life, would also negatively impact the quality of life.

Understanding Novel Agents

The term *novel agent* is derived from the fact that these drugs work by unique mechanisms, different than those that have traditionally been used in the treatment of cancer. Some of the newer ways to approach cancer treatment include a variety of new mechanisms. Angiogenesis inhibitor drugs, by stopping neovascularization, may limit tumor growth, and some may also lead to cancer cell death. Monoclonal antibodies (MoABs) target a specific antigen and may work in a variety of different ways, including boosting the patient's immune system or blocking cell growth factors. Vaccines, on the other hand, attempt to stimulate the patient's immune system to destroy cancer cells.

The term *signal transduction inhibitor* is associated with many novel agents, because, in addition to having the characteristics of an angiogenesis inhibitor or an MoAB, they work by blocking signals necessary to begin a cascade of events leading to cell division and multiplication. Most growth factors bind to transmembrane receptors, proteins that are localized to the cell membrane. The extracellular domain of each receptor forms a specific binding site for its ligand (i.e., growth factor). Once that

bond is formed, the intracellular domain of the receptor allows the receptor tyrosine kinase to begin a cascade of events leading to replication of oncogenes and cancerous cells (Figure 10.1).

Many new compounds are being tested in clinical trials, with some mixed responses. The following are questions remaining to be answered:

- Will it be necessary to combine cytostatic agents with cytotoxic drugs?
- When should cytostatic drugs be used: early or late in the disease?
- Are cytostatic drugs really cytostatic or just ineffective?
- How do we measure the success of cytostatic drugs when we might not be able to directly see tumor shrinkage on radiographic examination?
- Can we identify the antigens needed to develop effective vaccines?
- Are vaccines only useful in minimal disease settings?

Although many of these novel agents have been successful in the laboratory, whether these successes will translate to the clinic is yet to be determined.

Angiogenesis Inhibitors

In 1998, the popular press brought antiangiogenesis drugs to the media forefront in a story that heralded two drugs, endostatin and angiostatin, as cures for cancer within 2 years. What the public didn't realize was that these drugs were not yet ready to begin clinical trials, and approval, if they proved to be effective in humans, was years away.

Angiogenesis

Angiogenesis, also known as *neovascularization*, is the process by which new blood vessels

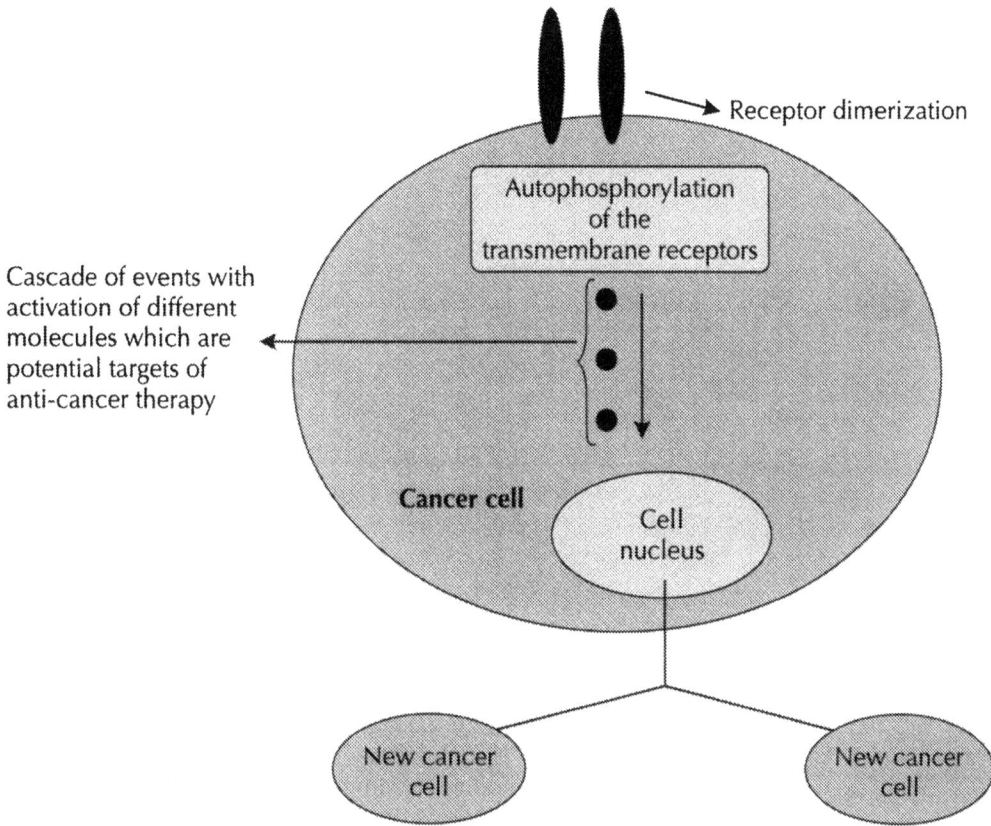

Figure 10.1 Cancer cell replication.

are formed. Angiogenesis occurs during pregnancy, infancy, and early childhood to support required growth. However, in the adult, angiogenesis normally does not occur except during menstruation and in pathologic states such as wound healing. The process is typically short-lived and will turn off after 1 to 2 weeks.

For cancer cells to grow beyond the size of a pinhead, they must recruit a new and larger blood supply. As a mass of cells outgrows its blood supply, the inevitable hypoxia, or lack of oxygen, causes a release of angiogenic factors that begins the cascade of cellular events called *angiogenesis*.[1] One protein that is currently thought to play a major role is vascular endothe-

lial growth factor (VEGF). Figure 10.2 is the author's conception of how this process works.

ANTIANGIOGENESIS DRUGS
Overall, there are four strategies being used to develop antiangiogenesis drugs:

- Inhibit proteins that stimulate the cascade (such as VEGF or fibroblast growth factor [FGF], the dominant angiogenic proteins).
- Block the transmission of signals via the receptors where various growth factors attach.
- Block the ability of endothelial cells to break down the surrounding matrix.

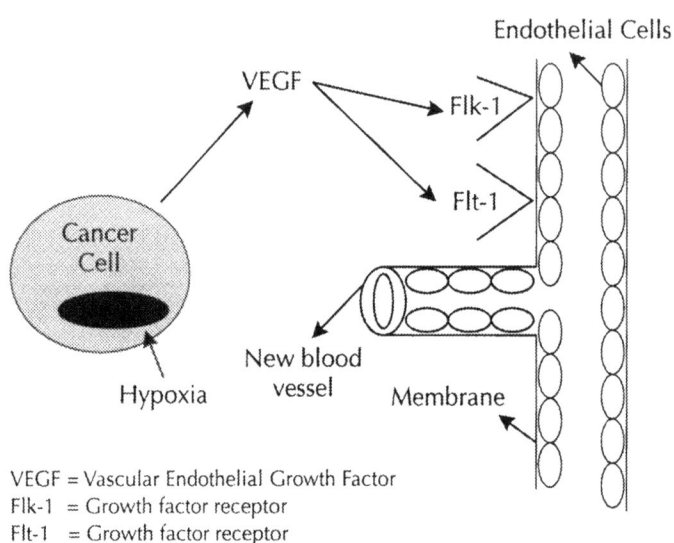

Endothelial Cells   **Figure 10.2**   Angiogenesis.

VEGF

Flk-1

Flt-1

Cancer
Cell

New blood
vessel

Hypoxia

Membrane

VEGF = Vascular Endothelial Growth Factor
Flk-1 = Growth factor receptor
Flt-1 = Growth factor receptor

- Block the action of integrins, molecules on the endothelial cell surface needed to form new blood vessels.[2]

Vascular Endothelial Growth Factor Inhibitors

Many of these angiogenic proteins have been identified, such as VEGFs. Although the cascade is increasingly better defined, we may only be at the beginning of understanding this process.

VEGF, secreted in response to tumor cells' hypoxia, can bind to receptors, called Flk-1 (fetal liver kinase) and Flt-1 (FMS-like tyrosine kinase), on the cell membrane. They attach to the surrounding membrane (extracellular matrix) and begin secreting enzymes that degrade the membrane. As the membrane is invaded, the endothelial vessels begin dividing and forming tubes, which become the blood supply for the mass.[1] This new and enriched blood supply provides the nutrients that can allow the mass to continue to grow and, perhaps, eventually to spread.

Angiogenesis also plays a significant role in metastasis. Tumors that have a higher density of blood vessels have been associated with early metastasis and can lead to poorer clinical outcomes. Also, the shedding of large numbers of tumor cells from the primary tumor may not begin until after the tumor has a network of blood vessels.[2] Cells in need of more blood vessels send out a signal to activate new blood vessel growth. VEGF and basic FGF (bFGF) are among the most dominant angiogenic proteins in sustaining new blood vessel growth.

SU5416

SU5416 is a synthetic small molecule that is currently in phase III testing in colorectal cancer. In a multicenter study, untreated metastatic colorectal patients are randomized to one of two arms of the study: 5-fluorouracil (5-FU) and leucovorin (LV) given weekly via the Roswell Park regimen (5-FU 600 mg/m^2 and LV 500 mg/m^2) with or without SU5416 given intravenously biweekly. In an earlier phase I/II study in which all patients were treated with

SU5416, 5-FU, and LV, no dose-limiting toxicities were attributed to the SU5416.[3] By early 2001, SU5416 will also be tested in a similar randomized trial including irinotecan in the treatment regimen, in accordance with the latest Food and Drug Administration (FDA) approval of 5-FU/LV/irinotecan as first-line therapy for colorectal cancer.

SU6668

A second-generation oral drug, SU6668, is in phase I clinical trials. SU6668 blocks not only the VEGF pathway involved in angiogenesis, but also bFGF, another angiogenic protein, and PDGF (platelet-derived growth factor). In so doing, not only are two major pathways of angiogenesis interrupted, but, theoretically, the drug may also have an anticancer effect through the PDGF receptor blockage.[4] In theory, that should make SU6668 more effective than its predecessor. However, as with all phase I trials, this drug is being tested as a single agent to determine the maximum tolerated dose and toxicities. Once that information is identified, the drug will proceed to phase II trials to determine efficacy.

Matrix Metalloproteinase Inhibitors

Recall that invasion of surrounding tissue must occur for the new blood vessels to form. Matrix metalloproteinases (MMPs) are degradative enzymes that are responsible for normal turnover and remodeling of the extracellular matrix, the membrane that holds cells together inside tissues.[5] By disrupting the cellular membrane, endothelial cells are mobilized in existing blood vessels and begin to form new blood vessels (see Figure 10.2).

Many MMP inhibitors are already in phase III clinical trials, such as Marimastat, Bay 12-95666, and AG 3340. Thus far, results have

been disappointing. It is not clear whether this is because the drugs simply are not effective in advanced disease or whether the studies had design flaws. To date, none are being tested in colorectal cancers.

Antiintegrins

As endothelial cells form into the tubular shape, they require a membrane to support the cells and become a blood vessel. Disruption of this process inhibits angiogenesis for existing cancer cells. Integrins are enzymes that are active in a cell-matrix interaction at the cell membrane. An antiintegrin drug, Vitaxin, is currently in phase I clinical trials. Vitaxin, an MoAB, targets $\alpha v \beta 3$, which is found in large amounts on endothelial cells.[6]

Thalidomide

Thalidomide was developed in the late 1950s and early 1960s to treat the nausea and vomiting associated with the first trimester of pregnancy. Its use resulted in devastating birth defects. The drug has now been reintroduced in the treatment of cancer because of its ability to interfere with blood vessel formation. Although thalidomide has not been formally tested in solid tumors, it is available by prescription to registered physicians so that patients can use it without securing a place in a clinical trial.

Because the most frequent adverse effect is somnolence, patients are often started at a low dose, with dose escalation determined by tolerability. Other side effects include constipation, peripheral neuropathy, neutropenia, and rash. As with most drugs, these side effects are reversed when the drug is withdrawn.

Thalidomide is being tested at the National Cancer Institute in a phase II clinical trial in patients with previously resected colorectal cancer. This study is a randomized, double-blind, placebo-controlled study of oral thalidomide for adjuvant therapy. The objectives of the study are to estimate disease-free survival probability and time to recurrence in this patient population, as well as pharmacokinetic information about the drug.[7]

Naturally Occurring Proteins

In all adults, there exists a finely controlled balance between factors promoting new vessel growth (angiogenic factors) and those inhibiting the growth (angiogenic inhibitors). These naturally occuring inhibitors can be manipulated to tilt the balance in one direction or the other. Collagen, estrogen, platelet factor 4, interleukin-12, and plasminogen are but a few proteins that may, in fact, be responsible for the observation that some tumors are slow-growing.

Some of the new drugs have been developed from the natural angiogenesis inhibitors. Angiostatin and endostatin are examples of naturally occurring inhibitors of angiogenesis. They are small fragments of collagen and plasminogen, respectively, and are currently in phase I clinical trials.[8]

Shark Cartilage

Cancer patients have used shark cartilage preparations for its presumed effect on angiogenesis. A trial to test efficacy was designed, giving 60 patients with advanced solid tumor malignancies 1 g orally in three divided doses daily. The results showed that shark cartilage as a single agent was inactive in patients with advanced-stage cancer.[9]

Drugs That Block Epidermal Growth Factor Receptors

C225

C225 is an MoAB that also works as a signal transduction inhibitor by blocking epidermal

growth factor (EGF) receptors[10] (Figure 10.3). A phase I study presented at the American Society of Clinical Oncology meeting in May 2000, showed that C225 may induce a response in heavily pretreated patients whose tumors express EGF.[11] Skin reactions (rash) and allergic reactions were the most clinically significant toxicities.[12] In the resulting phase II study, C225 was combined with irinotecan in patients who were already failing treatment with the drug. Irinotecan was given at 125 mg/m^2 weekly for 4 weeks, followed by a 2-week rest. C225 was administered intravenously weekly prior to the irinotecan, and on the rest weeks as well. The side effects were mainly attributed to the irinotecan, although some patients experienced a skin rash that waxed and waned without altering the treatment regimen. Overall, the C225 was well tolerated. Efficacy results are not yet available.[13] If the results are positive, this drug may continue into phase III trials.

Iressa

Iressa (tested under the name ZD1839) is an oral EGF inhibitor that blocks the EGF receptor from receiving the signal necessary to begin autophosphorylation and cell division (see Figure 10.3). In phase I trials with Iressa, 64 patients with advancing disease were treated with varying doses of the drug. Four patients experienced stable disease for 2 to 9 months.[14] Because of potentially significant antitumor ac-

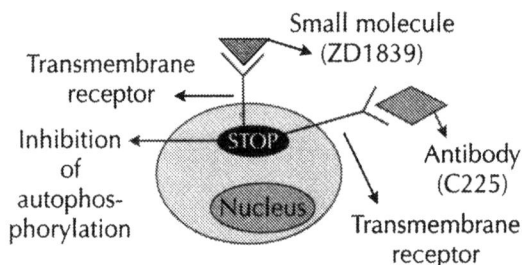

Figure 10.3   Signal blockage to EGF receptors.

tivity with only mild, reversible toxicity, a range of clinical trials are being launched, many in non–small lung cancer, where EGF is most active.[15]

Monoclonal Antibodies

MoABs, a form of immunotherapy, work on a specific antigen. MoABs can be utilized in a variety of ways in cancer treatment:

- React with specific types of cancer to enhance the patient's immune response to the cancer
- Act against cell growth factors
- Link to other anticancer drugs such as radioisotopes, biological response modifiers, or other toxins[16]

When used in antiangiogenesis therapy, they act against cell growth factors and thereby interrupt the process of new blood vessel formation.

Anti–Vascular Endothelial Growth Factor Inhibitors

Anti-VEGF antibody, as its name implies, is specific for VEGF. It is entering phase III studies that are designed to combine the antibody with cytotoxic drugs and compare the response with the same therapy without the antibody. Anti-VEGF antibody is starting phase III clinical trials in untreated metastatic colorectal cancer: one in combination with 5-FU and LV, using the Roswell Park regimen; and the other with 5-FU, LV, and irinotecan, using the Saltz regimen.

Panorex

Panorex is another MoAB that works by the same strategy that has been so successfully used in breast cancer with Herceptin and in lymphoma with Rituxan. Panorex is specific for the 17-1A antigen that is found on colon

cancer cells. Patients treated with Panorex following surgical resection of their disease were 30% less likely to experience a recurrence than were patients treated with surgery alone.[17] These dramatic results in clinical trials in Europe for Dukes' C colon cancer have led to the approval of Panorex in Germany. In the United States, studies comparing standard adjuvant chemotherapy (5-FU/LV), plus or minus Panorex, are awaiting final analysis.

Antisense Drugs

Unlike normal cells, cancer cells have a defect that allows them to replicate and grow in an uncontrolled manner. Cell division occurs as a result of replication of the DNA that is a double helix containing two complementary strands. One strand is called the *sense*, and the complementary strand is called the *antisense*. Antisense drugs interrupt that replication process by attaching to the complementary strand and preventing synthesis of faulty proteins and proliferation of the cancer cells.[18–20] The theory, although sound scientifically, must be subjected to clinical testing to verify the laboratory observations.

Farnesyl Transferase Inhibitors

Oncogenes encode specific proteins that have the ability to mutate and transform normal cells into malignant cells. Of these, *ras* is expressed in many cancer cells, including more than 50% of colon cancers.[21,22] *Ras* genes normally have the ability to turn on and off; however, in cancer, the *ras* gene becomes "stuck" in the *on* position. To inhibit the function of *ras*, drugs have been designed to block steps in the transmission of signals from the outside of the cell to the nucleus, where the *ras* gene is located. One such strategy is to block the enzyme farnesyl transferase, which appears to be necessary for *ras* to turn on. The drugs are, therefore, called farnesyl transferase inhibitors (FTIs).

R115777

R115777, an oral FTI, was recently tested in a phase I trial to determine dose and toxicities. The drug was given to 27 patients with various advanced cancers. One patient with metastatic colon cancer had a 46% decrease in carcinoembryonic antigen (CEA) levels and radiographically stable disease for 5 months.[23] Although interesting, caution must be exercised about this outcome, because such small numbers of patients do not provide statistically significant information.

FTI-277

Another FTI, FTI-277, was recently evaluated as a radiation sensitizer. In cells that expressed *ras*, this treatment led to increased apoptosis (death of cells) and deceased survival after radiation, when compared with cells that either did not express *ras* or were not exposed to the drug.[24] It is also of interest to note that, in this case, the FIT acted not only as a cytostatic drug, but also as a cytotoxic drug, because it did indeed cause death of cells. Interestingly, this class of drugs can also be effective in *ras*-negative tumors. Therefore, the search for the true mechanism of action is ongoing.

Vaccines

Vaccines are a biologic form of therapy currently under study in the treatment of human cancers. Unlike cytostatic drugs, vaccines attempt to confer *immunity* by injecting a weakened version of the disease into an individual (host). The host's immune system recognizes the antigen and develops antibodies against it, thereby establishing a safeguard against the disease. The vaccines for infectious diseases, such as tetanus and measles, work because the antigens that trigger the immune response are known. This is not necessarily the case in cancer.

To date, the effort to identify antigens that will trigger an immune response against cancer cells is ongoing. In the 1890s, William B. Coley observed that when patients developed infections in the vicinity of their cancer, they experienced a reduction in the size of their tumors.[25] However, cancer vaccines utilizing bacterial agents have proved ineffective.[26]

A newer approach to develop useful vaccines involves the use of tumor-associated antigens (TAAs). TAAs are proteins, enzymes, or carbohydrates that are present on tumor cells. In early studies, cells from a tumor were removed and crushed, rendered nonviable by irradiation or killing of the cancer cells, combined with a bacterial agent, and then injected into the patient. More recently, TAAs are utilizing normal protein structures that are secreted by some cancer cells. These vaccines can cause autoimmune responses in patients. Such responses have been demonstrated in vaccines used for the treatment of melanoma. Individuals who have a tumor response may also experience patches of depigmentation as the vaccine attacks melanosomes of normal skin cells.[25]

At the University of Cincinnati, an antiidiotype antibody vaccine using CEA was tested in 32 patients with completely resected Dukes' B, C, and D colorectal cancers and incompletely resected Dukes' D disease. Patients were injected every other week, for four injections, and then monthly until tumor regression or progression. Fourteen of the patients were also treated concurrently with 5-FU chemotherapy regimens. A cellular immune response was noted in all of the patients. Treatment with 5-FU did not affect the immune response. The vaccine is now in phase III clinical trials in patients with resected colon cancer.[27]

Dendritic cells (DCs), which are part of the

body's natural defense system, are also being utilized in an effort to trigger an immune response. DCs circulate, looking for foreign proteins (antigens). After the antigens are ingested by the DCs, they are then displayed on the cell membrane, triggering "killer T" cells to mobilize from the spleen and lymph nodes and attack the cells bearing the foreign antigen.[28] To prepare a vaccine, DCs are removed from the bloodstream, grown in the laboratory, and then exposed to a cancer antigen in culture. The primed DCs (vaccine) is injected subcutaneously into the patient to stimulate an immune response to the cancer cells bearing the antigen. Tumor shrinkage has been noted in animal studies with this approach, and vaccines are now in the early stages of clinical trials.[25]

Many questions remain unanswered about the use of cancer vaccines. It appears that they may be most useful in a minimal disease state, such as the adjuvant setting, or when there is only an elevation of CEA without radiographic confirmation of disease.

Assessing Response to Novel Agents

Traditionally, methods used to assess response to therapy may not be applicable to these new classes of drugs. Typically, when treating with cytotoxic agents, patients are restaged, using computerized tomography (CT) scans, after two or three cycles of therapy. However, because cytostatic drugs may work by stopping new growth, rather than by destroying existing tumor cells, new intervals and methods of assessing response may be needed. Consider the example of a patient who has a 3 × 3 cm liver lesion on CT scan prior to treatment, and who may, after 3 months of therapy with an angiogenesis inhibitor, have no change in the size of the lesion. Does having stable disease mean that the therapy *is* or *is not* working?

Assessment Intervals

Because drugs like angiogenesis inhibitors are believed to work slowly, traditional reassessment intervals may need to be redefined. Perhaps the standard 8- to 12-week restaging interval should be extended to 4 or 6 months, or is such a prolonged interval irresponsible if the drug is not working? Researchers are looking for surrogate markers to assess efficacy and to help determine the appropriate dose. When assessing response to novel agents, thought must be given to the mechanism of action and the anticipated response, to avoid stopping a potentially useful treatment prematurely.

Methods of Assessment

In looking at responses to new biologic agents, qualitative assessment methods may be better than traditional quantitative methods. To evaluate responses to antiangiogenic drugs, dynamic magnetic resonance imaging is being studied to assess blood flow. A baseline study would presumably show a well-vascularized tumor. Following treatment with an antiangiogenic agent, although the tumor may not have changed in size, it may appear pale in color and have a less dense network of blood vessels, indicating a compromise to its blood flow (Figure 10.4).

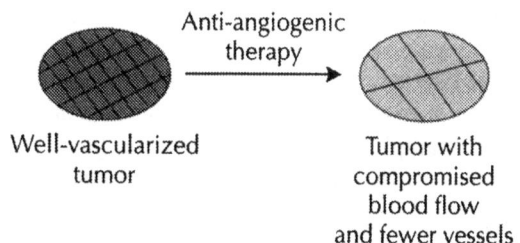

Figure 10.4 Tumor response to antiangiogenic therapy.

Positron emission tomography (PET) scans may be another useful method for assessing response to cytostatic agents. PET scans demonstrate intense signals of high metabolic activity, as in cancer cell proliferation. This is caused by an increased utilization of glucose in rapidly dividing cells. If, following cytostatic therapy, a follow-up scan shows decreased activity of the tracer molecule in the tumor area, it could mean a slowing or stopping of cellular activity.

Clearly, as biologic agents continue through clinical trials, assessment methods must also be studied. Great care must be exercised to evaluate potential responses as critically as possible.

Implications for Nurses

Today, patients are well-informed consumers who read articles, listen to talk shows, and surf the Internet for information about new therapies. Unfortunately, sometimes the information overload can lead to misconceptions and misunderstandings. Nurses play a significant role in helping patients and families sort through the information to gain a clear understanding of the facts and how they apply to a specific situation. For this reason, nurses must stay abreast of new developments in treatment.

Encouraging patient participation in clinical trials is yet another key role for nursing. For patients who have failed all known standard therapy, a clinical trial may offer treatment with a new agent years before it becomes commercially available. However, it is very important to provide balance through cautious optimism. The key word in clinical trials is *experimental*, and patients must understand the limitations. For example, in a phase I trial, the goal is to determine the safe dose and side effects. Some patients may receive subtherapeutic doses. After safe doses and treatment schedules are established, the drugs are then tested for efficacy in phase II trials. Just as with standard therapy, even if the drug is effective, not all

patients will respond. Patients must understand that *new* does not necessarily mean *better*. Nurses must help patients to understand the purpose of clinical trials and establish realistic expectations.

Information about current clinical trials can be obtained from a variety of sources. The National Cancer Institute maintains a database that provides a description of many clinical trials. It can be accessed through the Internet at http://cancertrials.nci.nih.gov/ or by calling 1-800-4-CANCER. Many of the pharmaceutical companies and comprehensive cancer centers also have web sites with information about current trials.

This is an exciting time in the battle against cancer. Research holds the promise of novel therapeutics to control cancer without sacrificing the patient's quality of life. The translation of technology from the basic science laboratory to the clinical setting is often difficult, if not impossible. Many of these novel agents may never reach the commercial market, due to intolerable side effects or lack of efficacy. Even when drugs prove safe and beneficial, completing clinical testing and receiving FDA approval can take from 8 to 12 years. Researchers remain optimistic about these and other novel agents, but caution must be exercised in raising unrealistic hopes in patients who are desperately seeking answers.

Acknowledgment

Many thanks to Fairooz Kabbinavar, MD, and Lee S. Rosen, MD, for their professional support.

References

1. Inhibitors of angiogenesis enter phase III testing. News release July 1998. J Natl Cancer Inst. 1998; 90(13):960.
2. Angiogenesis inhibitors in cancer research.

Press release on April 2, 1999, by the National Cancer Institute. Available at: http://rex.nci.nih.gov/massmedia/pressreleases/angio/html Accessed August 6, 2000.

3. Rosen PJ, Amado R, Hecht JR, et al. A phase I/II study of SU5416 in combination with 4-FU/leucovorin in patients with metastatic colorectal cancer. Proc Am Soc Clin Oncol. 2000; 19:5D (abstr).

4. Rosen L, Hannah A, Rosen P, et al. Phase I dose-escalating trial or oral SU006668, a novel multiple receptor tyrosine kinase inhibitor in patients with selected advanced malignancies. Abstract 708. Proc Am Soc Clin Oncol. 2000; 19:708 (abstr).

5. Nelson AR, Fingleton B, Rothenberg ML, et al. Matrix metalloproteinases: Biologic activity and clinical implications. J Clin Oncol. 2000; 18(5): 1135–1149.

6. Several angiogenesis inhibitors show potential in lab. News release April 5, 2000. J Natl Cancer Inst. 2000; 92(7):522.

7. Cancernet. Available at: www.cancernet.nci.nih.gov Accessed August 10, 2000.

8. Halim NS. Small molecules in large proteins: New class of angiogenesis inhibitors shows promise. Available at: http://www.the-scientist.com/yr2000/aug/research_000821.html Accessed August 22, 2000.

9. Miller DR, Anderson GT, Stark JJ, et al. Phase I/II trial of the safety and efficacy of shark cartilage in the treatment of advanced cancer. J Clin Oncol. 1998; 16:3649–3655.

10. Baselga J, Pfister D, Cooper MR, et al. Phase I studies of anti-epidermal growth factor receptor chimeric antibody C225 alone in combination with cisplatin. J Clin Oncol. 2000; 18(4): 904–914.

11. Rubin MS, Shin DM, Pasmantier M, et al. Monoclonal Antibody (MoAb) IMC-C225, an anti-epidermal growth factor receptor (EGFr), for patients with EGFr-positive tumors refractory to or in relapse from previous therapeutic regimens. Proc Am Soc Clin Oncol 2000; 19: 1860 (abstr).

12. Cohen RB, Falcey JW, Paulter VJ, et al. Safety profile of the monoclonal antibody (MoAb) IMC-C225, an anti-epidermal growth factor receptor (EGFr) used in the treatment of EGFr-positive tumors. Proc Am Soc Clin Oncol. 2000; 19:1862 (abstr).

13. Oncology: ImClone Systems and Merck KgaA initiate first international phase-III trial center for C225. Press release February 12, 1999. Available at: www.merck-ltd.co.uk/Corporate/c225.htm Accessed September 22, 2000.

14. New ways to attack cancer. (1999). Available at: www.abcnews.go.com Accessed September 22, 2000.

15. Kris M, Ranjson M, Ferry D, et al. Phase I study of oral ZD1839 (Iressa™), a novel inhibitor of epidermal growth factor receptor tyrosine kinase (EGFR-TK): Evidence of good tolerability and activity. Presented at AACR-NCI-EORTC International Conference on Molecular Targets and Cancer Therapeutics, Amsterdam, The Netherlands, November 1999.

16. Biological therapy: Using the immune system to treat cancer. Available at: www.icare.org/treatment/bt.htm Accessed August 10, 2000.

17. Panorex® (17-1A monoclonal antibody) is demonstrated to cure more patients with Duke's C colon cancer than surgery alone; and is the first monoclonal antibody to improve survival of patients with solid tumors. Lancet. 1994; 343: 1177–1183. Available at: http://webm93.ntx.net/TreatmentNewsUpdates/ColonCancerNews/ColonMay94.htm Accessed September 22, 2000.

18. Knight S. Antisense takes aim at cancer. (1999). Available at: www.qcwancer.com/Newsletter/develop_winter_99_antisense.htm Accessed July 23, 2000.

19. "Antisense" cancer treatment looks safe, promising. (1997). Available at: www.docguide.com Accessed August 10, 2000.

20. Cotter FE. Antisense therapy for malignancy. Proc Am Soc Clin Oncol. 2000; 19:338–348.

21. Barbacid M. *ras* Genes. Annu Rev Biochem. 1987; 56:779–827.

22. Bos JL. *ras* Oncogenes in human cancer: A review. Cancer Res. 1989; 49:4682–4689.

23. Zujewski J, Horak ID, Bol CJ, et al. Phase I and pharmacokinetic study of farnesyl protein transferase inhibitor R115777 in advanced cancer. J Clin Oncol. 2000; 18(4):927–941.

24. Bernard EJ, McKenna WG, Hamilton AD, et al. Inhibiting *ras* prenylation increases the radiosensitivity of human tumor cell lines with activating mutations of *ras* oncogenes. Cancer Res. 1998; 58:1754–1761.

25. Chang AE. Cancer vaccines: A primer about an emerging therapy. (2000). Available at: www.cancernews.com/vaccines Accessed August 10, 2000.

26. Harris JE, Ryan L, Hoover HC Jr, et al. Adjuvant active specific immunotherapy for stage II and III colon cancer with an autologous tumor cell vaccine: Eastern Cooperative Group Study E5283. J Clin Oncol. 2000; 18(1):148–157.

27. Foon KA, John WJ, Chakraborty M, et al. Clinical and immune responses in resected colon cancer patients treated with anti-idiotype monoclonal antibody vaccine that mimics the carcinoembryonic antigen. J Clin Oncol. 1999; 17(9): 2889–2895.

28. RNA-Dendritic cell combo shows promise as a universal cancer vaccine. Press release from Duke University, March 26, 1998. Available at: www.eurelaert.org/releases/rnadenclcmb.html Accessed November 15, 2000.

CHAPTER 11

Management of Hepatic Disease

Delores A. Saddler, RN, MSN, CGRN

Yvonne Lassere, RN, OCN, CCRP

Introduction

Patients with colorectal cancer comprise the majority of metastases to the liver from other organs. For most tumors, especially colorectal cancers, liver metastasis makes the patient essentially incurable.[1] Because the liver is the site of metastases from other organs, one of the major identified reasons may be its place as the first visceral organ that malignant cells of gastrointestinal origin encounter after release into capillaries, venules, and, finally, the portal circulation.[1] Of the more than 130,000 persons who develop colorectal cancer each year, half of these develop a recurrence at some point in their lifetimes, with the liver being the most common site of recurrence.[2] Fewer than 10% of patients who develop liver metastasis can undergo curative resection. At least half of those who do undergo this extensive surgery suffer a recurrence. Chemotherapy given systemically for metastasis results in only one-third of these patients receiving a partial response, with complete responses being almost nonexistent.[2] Systemic chemotherapy provides a median survival of only about 12 months, with a 5-year survival rate of 25% to 33%.[3] Noncolorectal cancers also cause metastasis to the liver, and some authors have suggested that these patients respond much worse after resection than those with colorectal metastases, and may be contraindicated for possible resection.[2,3]

Therefore, much of the survival data regarding liver metastasis include colorectal as well as noncolorectal cancers. While metastasis from tumors of the gastrointestinal tract comprise the highest amount of liver metastasis, and colorectal being the most frequent in this category, there are other sources of metastasis to the liver. These include melanoma; Wilms tumor; prostate, renal cell, testicular, breast, lung, gynecologic, and head and neck malignancies; adrenal tumors; soft-tissue and gastrointestinal sarcomas; and neuroendocrine tumors.[3] Approximately 25% of patients with colorectal cancer initially present with metastatic disease.[4,5]

Approximately 90% to 95% of primary liver cancer is hepatocellular, arising from the liver. Seven percent are cholangiocarcinoma, arising from the bile ducts, with the remainder being hepatoblastoma, angiosarcoma, or sarcoma. Fibrolamellare hepatocellur carcinoma primarily affects adolescent girls. Primary liver cancer and metastatic liver cancer cause the same or similar physiologic problems due to impairment of the liver itself and, as a result, utilize many of the same radiologic and surgical interventions.

In the United States, metastatic liver cancer is more common than primary liver cancer, while metatastic liver cancer is generally more amendable to surgical resection than primary liver cancer.[6] Before beginning any treatment, determination of whether the patient has primary or metastatic liver cancer is of utmost importance. This chapter focuses on treatment options for metastatic liver metastasis, with special interest on metastasis from cancers in the gastrointestinal tract, especially colorectal cancer.

Anatomy and Physiology

Liver

The liver is located in the right upper section of the abdomen and is surrounded by the stomach, gallbladder, and intestine (Figure 11.1). It is the largest organ in the body, weighing about 15 g.

It extends from the fifth intercostal space in the midclavicular line down to the right costal margin. The liver has two main anatomic lobes, which are further divided into caudate and quadrate lobes (Figure 11.2 on page 206). There are two sources of blood supply to the liver. The hepatic artery brings oxygenated blood to supply hepatocytes, and the hepatocytes process nutrients and detoxify harmful substances from the blood. The hepatic portal vein carries blood that is oxygen depleted but rich in materials from the digestive tract. Blood exits the liver through the hepatic veins, which empty into the inferior vena cava[7,8] (Figure 11.3 on page 207).

The liver is responsible for more than 400 functions in the body. These include processing of by-products of digested food; production of bile; metabolism of bilirubin; synthesis of coagulation factors; metabolism of fat, protein, and carbohydrates; storage of vitamins and minerals; detoxification; and regeneration. The right hepatic lobe is divided into four segments. The left lobe is divided into the left medial segment and two other segments. A capsule, referred to as Glisson's capsule, encompasses blood vessels, lymphatics, and nerves, and covers the liver.[6]

Two-thirds of the normal hepatic blood flow comes from the portal vein and, the other third from the hepatic artery. The hepatic artery branches into the abdominal aorta and supplies the liver with oxygenated blood from the systemic circulation. The portal vein supplies the liver with deoxygenated blood from the superior mesenteric and splenic veins. The portal vein further divides into two trunks as it enters the liver to supply blood to both lobes. The hepatic veins then drain into the inferior vena cava. The bile canaliculi carry bile, which has been produced by the hepatocytes and drain into the common bile duct. The common bile duct empties into the sphincter of Oddi, an opening into the duodenum. Bile transported from the liver is concentrated and stored in the gallbladder[6] (Figure 11.4 on page 208).

Figure 11.1   The digestive tract.

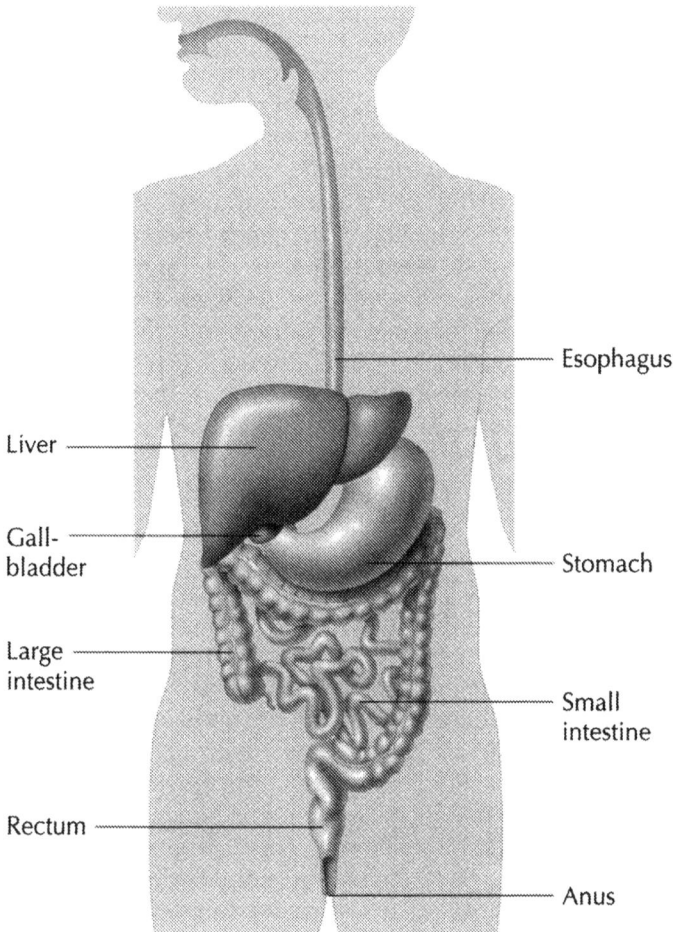

Esophagus

Liver

Gall-
bladder

Stomach

Large
intestine

Small
intestine

Rectum

Anus

Pathophysiology of Liver Metastasis

The liver is the site of metastases from many diverse and distant organ sites, especially the gastrointestinal tract. This is most likely due to its place as the first visceral organ that malignant cells of the gastrointestinal tract encounter after being released into capillaries, postcapillary venules, and, subsequently, the portal circulation.[1] While there is much information available regarding the development of primary colorectal cancer, little is known about the genetic alterations associated with its metastasis.

Metastasis is a very selective, nonrandom process that favors the survival of a minor subpopulation of metastatic cells that preexist within the primary tumor mass. These cells must then complete a sequence of interrelated steps in order to produce metastasis. An increased understanding of the molecular mechanisms mediating the metastatic process and the interaction between the metastatic cell and the host microenvironment are prime factors in developing treatment options for patients with liver metastasis. Another primary goal of cancer research is to identify patients likely to relapse following

Right lobe
of liver

Left lobe
of liver

Falciform
ligament

Inferior
border
of liver

Round
ligament

Inferior
border
of liver

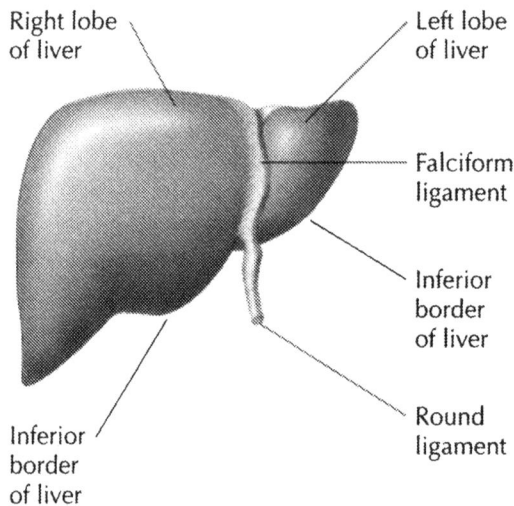

Figure 11.2   The normal liver.

surgery alone and to provide a foundation for preventive as well as new therapeutic treatment approaches.

The probability of developing metastasis depends on the stage of disease at the time of presentation, and patients diagnosed at a later stage are more likely to develop metastatic disease than patients who present with early-stage disease.[5] Of the 160,000 patients who develop colorectal carcinoma each year in the United States, half develop a recurrence at some point in their lifetimes, with the liver being the most common site.[2] Approximately 55% of colorectal cancers recur within 5 years. Despite surgery to remove the primary tumor, half recur regionally, and up to 80% produce distant metastasis.[1] It is now widely accepted that many malignant tumors contain heterogeneous subpopulations of cells. This heterogeneity is exhibited in a wide range of genetic, biochemical, immunologic, and biologic characteristics, such as growth rate, antigenic and immunogenic status, cell surface receptors and products, enzymes, karyotypes, cell morphologies, invasiveness, drug resistance, and metastatic potential.[9]

Nursing Implications

The diagnosis of hepatic metastasis creates anxiety and stress for the patient and family. Emotional support, multidisciplinary referrals for nutrition and care management, pain control, and symptom management are often the initiatives for the nurse. Patient education relative to the need for special scans or magnetic resonance imaging (MRI), lab work, angiography/arteriograms, and chemotherapy/surgical preparation should be done as soon as the patient is diagnosed or when the patient and family are emotionally ready to learn. The nurse should make a careful assessment of the patient's learning style and coping methods as well as the family dynamics and/or support system. A local physician should be involved in the planning and follow-up if the patient lives in another city. Patients should be made aware of the criteria used to determine surgery versus chemotherapy, and ample time should be allowed for questions regarding the planned treatment approach. Surgical resection with or without pre- and/or postoperative chemotherapy, cryosurgery, heat ablation (radiofrequency ablation [RFA], microwave, laser), liver transplantation, hepatic arterial infusion (HAI), and new approaches to treatment are areas with which the nurse should be familiar.

Surgical Resection of Metastatic Liver Lesions

If a tumor has not spread outside of the liver and is localized, surgery is the first recommended treatment option. Up to 75% of the liver can be removed, because it does regenerate if no cirrhosis or hepatitis is present. In some patients, a combination of resection and RFA (covered later in this chapter) may be used. During the resection of the tumor, patients may have an HAI pump placed to treat the liver with chemotherapy as an adjuvant therapy (covered

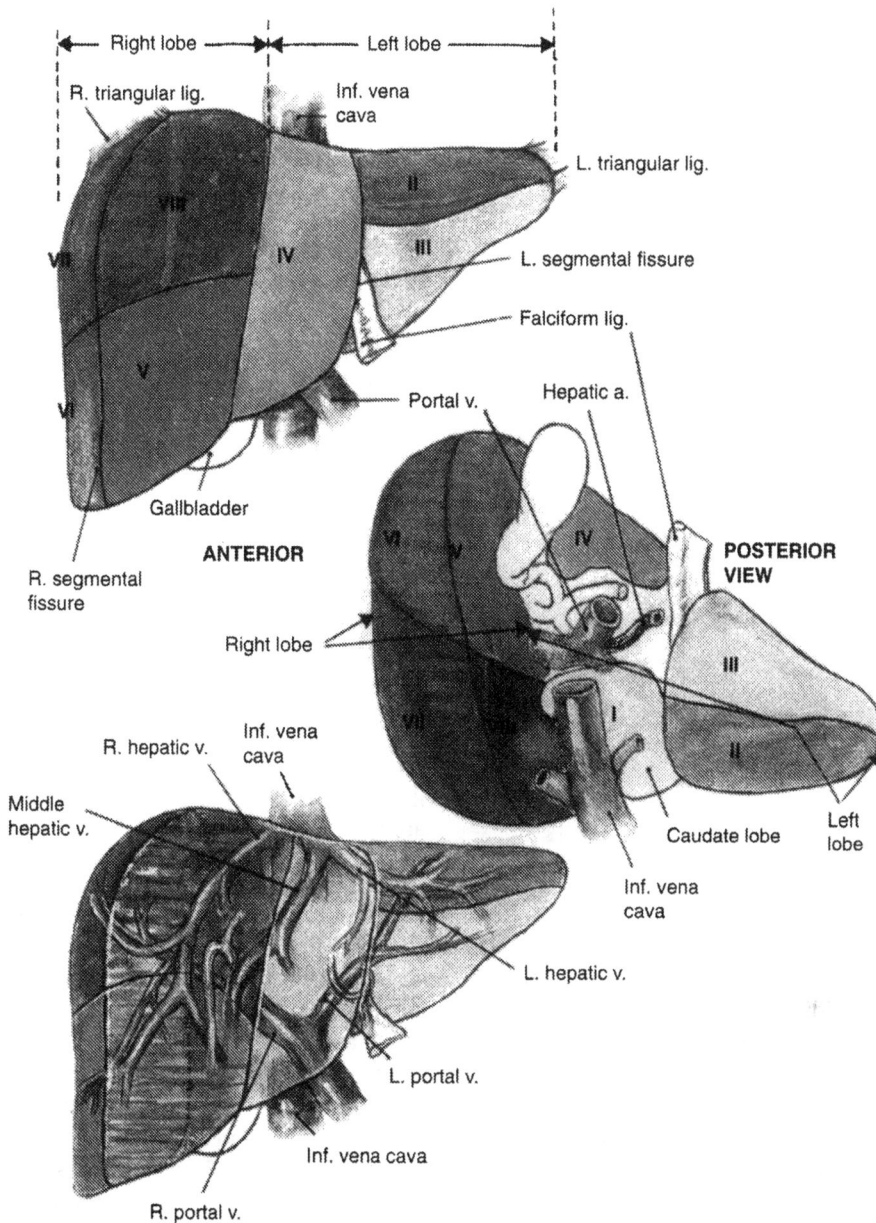

Figure 11.3 Normal anatomy of the liver.
Specific segments of the liver are referred to by their roman numeral. Top drawing is an anterior view. Center view is posterior and demonstrates the gallbladder system. The lower view is also an anterior view illustrating the rich vascular network.

Source: Reprinted with permission from Choti MA. The liver. In: Soidena JO, Schlossberg L, eds. The John Hopkins Atlas of Human Functional Anatomy, 4th ed. Baltimore. The John Hopkins University Press. 1997: 138.

Brachial artery
Aorta
Liver
Right hepatic artery
Common hepatic artery
Right gastric artery
Gastro-duodenal artery
Common iliac artery
Femoral artery

Carotid artery
Left hepatic artery
Spleen
Celiac artery
Left gastric artery
Splenic artery
Stomach
Duodenum
External iliac artery
Internal iliac artery

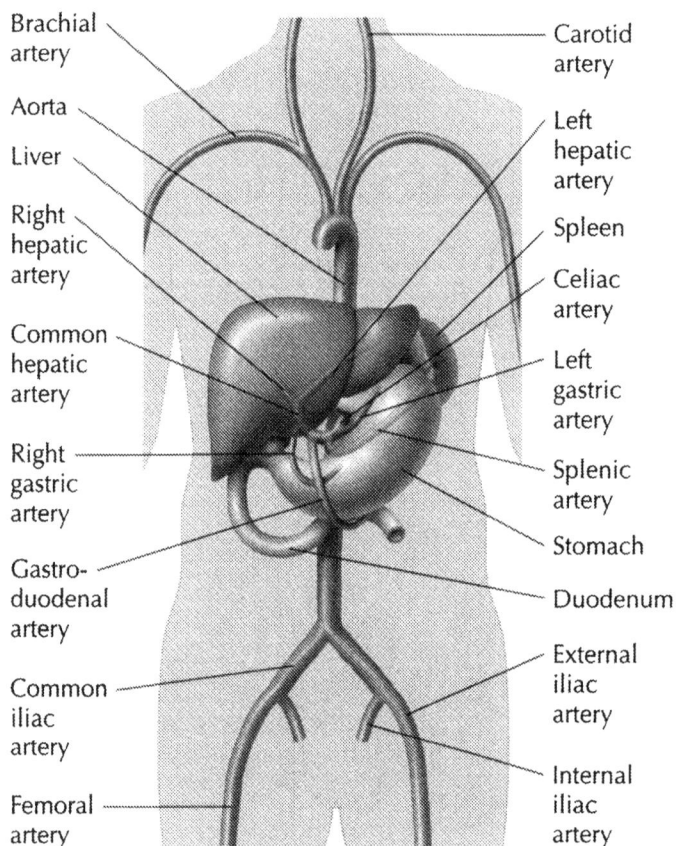

Figure 11.4   Diagram of principal arteries.

Source: Illustration reproduced with permission from The University of Texas M.D. Anderson Cancer Center.

later in this chapter). After the liver resection, patients are generally required to remain in the hospital for 2 or more weeks and generally require an additional month or two to recover before returning to routine activities.

Successful resection of colorectal cancer metastasis of the liver has evolved tremendously since the 1960s. In patients with liver-only disease, it provides long-term survival in a significant number of patients. Morbidity and mortality rates are low, long-term side effects seldom occur, and the immediate response is complete.[10] Patients treated with surgical resection only have had an approximately 33% 5-year overall survival rate and a 25% 5-year disease-free survival rate.[10]

Advances in computed technology, intraop-

erative ultrasonography (IOUS) and ultrasonic dissectors have been used in recent years to improve precision and control during the surgery. Surgeons who decide to perform hepatic surgery must have a very thorough understanding of the potential anatomic variations and the management of these variations. Because operating within a solid organ is much more difficult than working at its periphery, surgeons have only a few landmarks to use to guide them through the maze of intertwining hepatic and portal vessel branches below the surface of the liver.[10]

Patient Selection

Patient selection involves perioperative risk assessment, determining the technical feasibility and respectability of the liver metastasis, and evaluation of predictive prognostic criteria for long-term disease-free survival. Patients should be free of comorbid disease. If the associated conditions limit life expectancy more than the liver metastases, the patient is not a candidate for liver resection. Functional hepatic reserve and no cirrhosis, hepatitis B or C virus infection, or chronic alcohol abuse are comorbid conditions to consider. In the absence of cirrhosis, at least 20% of the normal hepatic parenchyma must remain following resection. Most patients tolerate a right or left hepatic lobectomy; however, a trisegmentectomy or resection of a patient with underlying chronic liver disease may create problems. The majority of patients may tolerate only segmental or wedge resections (Figure 11.5).

Resection is contraindicated in the presence of obvious tumor involvement of the portal vein bifurcation, hepatic vein confluence, or the inferior vena cava, as determined preoperatively. These resections are avoided because they impair vascular integrity to the remaining liver. Inferior vena cava resection is technically feasible but not indicated for the majority of patients with liver metastases, because adequate tumor-free resection margins cannot be obtained. Determining operative risk and technical feasibility is often more straightforward than determining the probability of long-term disease-free survival. Survival without treatment is generally easy to predict. That is, all untreated patients die within 5 years of diagnosis. Surgical resection of colorectal liver metastases improves 5-year survival from almost zero to 30% to 50%.[10] Surgeons must therefore individualize each situation before proceeding with resection. Wagner and colleagues[11] reviewed the data from the Mayo Clinic on survival in patients with untreated colorectal liver metastases and demonstrated the importance of the extent of hepatic involvement as a predictor of survival. Untreated patients with any extrahepatic metastasis or with liver-only disease replacing more

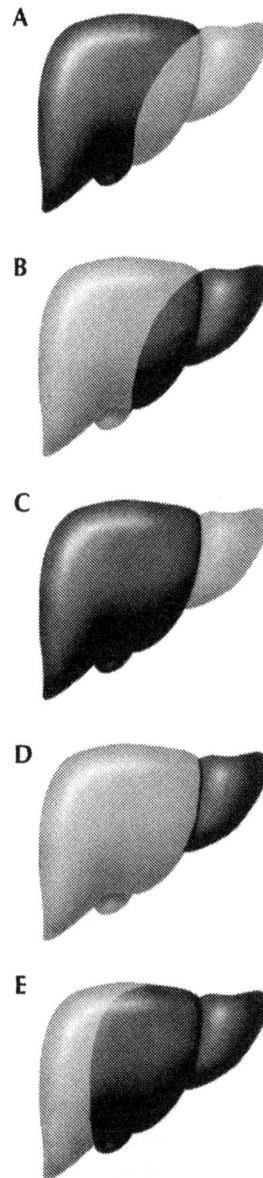

Figure 11.5 Common liver resections for metastatic colorectal cancer. **A:** Right lobectomy. **B:** Left lobectomy. **C:** Right trisegmentectomy. **D:** Left lateral segmentectomy. **E:** Left trisegmentectomy.

than 50% of the normal liver volume rarely survived more than 2 years. More than 20% of the patients with a solitary metastasis survived at least 3 years with no treatment. Patients with four or more liver metastases had a median survival of 10 months, compared with 24 months for patients with three or fewer metastases.[12] Patients with a solitary unilobar metastasis generally had a median survival of 21 months, compared with 15 months for patients with multiple liver lesions. Extrahepatic tumor recurrence is another indicator of poor prognosis, with a reduction in median survival from 18 months for liver-only disease to 9 months.

Selection criteria for patients have evolved over the past decade. The following are those that had absolute contraindications because of no long-term survival benefit:

• Portal lymph node metastases
• Coexistent extrahepatic recurrence
• The presence of four or more liver metastases
• Inability to preserve an adequate volume of functional hepatic parenchyma
• Inability to obtain at least a 1-cm tumor-free margin
• Hepatic vein confluence/inferior vena cava involvement by tumor
• Main portal vein bifurcation involvement by tumor

Mesenteric nodal metastases in the primary cancer resection specimen and a disease-free interval of less than 12 months were poor prognostic factors and relative contraindications.[10] Distribution of the metastases and the size of the lesions were not adversely effecting survival. Coexistent extrahepatic disease is contraindicated for liver resection, even if the disease is resectable. Adequate tumor-free surgical margins are imperative. Studies indicate a 60% 5-year survival rate for patients with tumor-free liver resection margins larger than 1 cm, a 30% rate if margins are negative but less than

1 cm from the liver metastases, and no 5-year survivors when margins are positive.[13]

Preoperative Preparation

Preoperative preparation involves an adequate assessment and patient selection. A computed tomography (CT) technique defining the extent of intrahepatic disease is used. The CT portography (liver protocol) is the most sensitive method for visualizing small lesions in the liver. A dynamic bolus intravenous contrast CT has also proved to be equally effective for evaluating the number and location of liver metastases. A chest x-ray is done and is usually sufficient, unless an abnormality is noted. Questionable lesions are further evaluated with chest CT or a biopsy, as indicated. Presacral changes seen on CT scans following low anterior and abdominoperineal resections for colorectal cancer must be fully evaluated to exclude pelvic recurrence and may involve monoclonal antibody scans, positron emission tomography (PET) scans, MRI, or biopsy. A repeat colonoscopy is indicated, especially if the disease-free interval is more than 2 years, if the entire colon was never completely evaluated.

Intraoperative ultrasonography (IOUS) is used to clarify marginal cases for resection by identifying small tumors not detected on preoperative CT scans or by demonstrating involvement of key vascular structures, precluding a margin-negative resection. Uncontrollable intraoperative bleeding or excessive transfusion requirements may result from the inability of the surgeon to apply the basic principle of vascular surgery: inflow and outflow control. The liver is very vascular and receives approximately 20% of the cardiac output. Hepatic arterial anatomy is variable. Preoperative angiography is usually not required for anatomic definition unless a pump is being considered. Portal venous anatomy is more predictable, with the most common hazard being the posterior branch of the right portal vein, which often exits within 1 cm of the main portal vein bifurcation and courses almost directly posterior. Brisk hemorrhage may occur during isolation of the main right portal vein branch if the posterior branch is entered inadvertently.[10] The hepatic veins are the source of most of the intraoperative blood loss during hepatic resection. The portal triad inflow vasculature is relatively easy to control prior to parenchymal transection, but the hepatic veins cannot always be controlled extrahepatically. Therefore, the relevant hepatic veins must be ligated during parenchymal transection; failure to do so results in excessive back-bleeding. Variations in the pattern of hepatic venous drainage are often present, primarily of the right lobe. IOUS of the liver is helpful for identifying the intrahepatic course of the hepatic veins.

Surgical Procedures

The surgical procedure can be described as having three components: determination of resectability, inflow and outflow vascular control, and parenchymal dissection. Liver resection for colorectal metastases requires excellent exposure of both the upper abdomen and pelvis, because the surgeon must search for other sites of recurrence and have adequate exposure of the liver and suprahepatic vena cava. After completing the manual and visual exploration of the abdomen, pelvis, liver, and lymph node–bearing areas, the liver is completely mobilized by dividing the ligaments for a more thorough hepatic evaluation. IOUS is used again at this point to make sure no lesions have been missed and to assess the proximity of the metastases to vascular and ductal structures. The extent of the hepatic resection correlates with the amount of portal dissection. A segmental or wedge resection of the liver can be safely accomplished with total portal inflow occlusion. The actual surgical technique requires expertise on behalf

of the surgeon and frequent use of the IOUS as an intraoperative diagnostic tool. The final aspect of the resection involves ensuring homeostasis and preventing bile leakage from the cut edge of the liver. The cut edge of the liver parenchyma is extensively coagulated, and a portion of the greater omentum is mobilized and secured over its surface. Closed suction drains are placed in a dependent area around the operative site to evacuate any residual blood or bile that may accumulate during the first few days.

Postoperative Care

Postoperative care focuses mostly on intravascular volume management and prevention of pulmonary complications. When the closed abdominal suction catheter drainage becomes serous and the volume increases, it signals the onset of fluid mobilization and the need to reduce intravenous fluid infusion rates. Postoperative ileus is usually short-lived and resumption of medications, fluids, and nutrition within 48 hours of surgery can occur. Drains are removed 48 to 72 hours after surgery in the absence of a biliary leak. A large number of patients may develop a pleural effusion, which is usually asymptomatic and does not require drainage. The development of intra- and extrahepatic recurrences after liver resection for colorectal metastases indicates that postmetastectomy programs must address both the liver and extrahepatic sites. Trials evaluating regional and systemic chemotherapy are under way, and further refinement of patient selection for resection leading to true survival benefit is being addressed. Individuals with hepatic lesions not initially amenable to surgical excision may undergo neoadjuvant chemotherapy to reduce tumor bulk. This is done in order to convert the patient to a surgical candidate. However, no benefit in survival has been demonstrated with this approach using fluorouracil, oxaliplatin, and folinic acid.[6] Among patients with colorectal cancer who have undergone a prior liver resection for metastases, approximately 50% to 60% of recurrences occur within the liver. Repeat hepatectomy is possible, because the liver regenerates almost to its original mass within 4 to 6 weeks. Repeat resection on metastases is technically more difficult secondary to adhesions and to the cut surface of the previous resection to neighboring organs. Regeneration also changes the shape of the organ, and vascular structures create a more difficult resection. Operative mortality is relative to initial hepatic resection, although the morbidity rates are higher.

Hepatic resection for metastases other than colorectal cancer has not been clearly defined or studied. Adenocarcinomas from gastrointestinal sites such as pancreas, gallbladder, and stomach frequently metastasize to the liver. Ocular melanoma is a rare tumor but has an increased rate of metastases to the liver. In contrast, the liver is infrequently the site of metastases from prostate cancer. Despite the high incidence of hepatic metastases at death, fewer than 5% of cancer patients have disease confined to the liver.[3] Patients with metastatic hepatic lesions, which demonstrated more than 50% reduction in tumor volume in response to preoperative chemotherapy, had a significantly improved disease-free survival compared with those who did not respond.[3] A short course of preoperative chemotherapy allows time for extrahepatic micrometastasis to become clinically detectable, thereby sparing the patient from an extensive, unnecessary surgery. Preoperative chemotherapy is also given to reduce the tumor volume in order to improve the likelihood of obtaining tumor-free margins at resection. Postoperative adjuvant chemotherapy is considered for patients with tumors responsive to preoperative chemotherapy. Some clinicians are more inclined to administer adjuvant chemotherapy to patients who have never received

it. Patients who have not had chemotherapy for more than a year prior to hepatic metastases are also given chemotherapy to improve survival. Investigations regarding the administration of regional chemotherapy, systemic chemotherapy, or both, are being done.

Neuroendocrine tumors are slow-growing, and the patient may survive many years despite advanced metastatic disease. These patients make up the largest group of survivors after resection of noncolorectal liver metastases. The results of liver transplants are generally disappointing due to the fact that most patients with primary as well as metastatic hepatic malignancies develop early tumor recurrence.[14,15] While neuroendocrine tumors are generally more indolent and transplantation may be effective for significant palliation, the unacceptable high recurrence rate has not justified the utilization of the few available donor organs.

Nursing Implications for the Postoperative Patient

After hepatic resection, potential complications include hemorrhage, biliary leak or biloma, subphrenic abscess, infection, pneumonia, pleural effusion, transient metabolic consequences, portal hypertension, clotting defects, and hepatic failure. To better care for these patients postoperatively, the nurse must have knowledge of the potential complications, signs of impending problems, and how to manage them. Liver function tests generally rise initially after surgery but return to normal a week or so afterward. High liver function tests may represent an injury to the vascular inflow or outflow in the remaining liver, and a Doppler ultrasound should be done to rule out portal vein thrombosis. The patient's glucose level should be monitored to prevent hepatic failure. When outflow tapers off, drainage tubes are removed. If ascites develops, nutritional intake and ventilation may occur. To prevent this, sodium must be restricted to 1,000 to 1,500 mg per day, and water to 1,500 mL per day. A loop diuretic in addition to spironolactone should help to decrease the patient's weight. The potassium, BUN, and creatinine should be monitored closely, and potassium may need to be replaced if ascites develops and a diuretic is used therapeutically.[6]

The first 24 hours are critical, and the patient should be monitored for complications (Table 11.1). Hemorrhage, biliary leak or biloma, infection, subphrenic abscess, portal hypertension, hepatic failure, clotting problems, pneu-

Table 11.1 Postoperative Nursing Care

Complications	Signs and Symptoms
Hemorrhage	Hypotension, tachycardia, increased abdominal girth, decreased hemoglobin and/or hematocrit
Bile leak or biloma	Pain, fever, increased abdominal girth
Subphrenic abscess	Low-grade fever, sharp, piercing right upper quadrant pain
Portal vein thrombosis or obstruction	Jaundice, increased liver function tests, abnormal flow from drains
Portal vein hypertension	Jaundice, increased liver function tests, abnormal flow from drains
Hepatic failure	Jaundice, increased liver function tests, hyperbilirubinemia, mental confusion, increased ammonia
Infection	Fever, redness or swelling of incision
Clotting problems	Abnormal bleeding, abnormal coagulation profiles
Pneumonia	Abnormal breath sounds, difficulty breathing
Pleural effusion	Abnormal breath sounds, difficulty breathing

monia and pleural effusion, and transient metabolic consequences are potential postoperative problems.[6] Hypotension, tachycardia, increased abdominal girth, and a decrease in the hemoglobin and hematocrit are signs of hemorrhage. Assessment of urine and stool should also be done, as well as frequent checks of the surgical incision site. Wound drains are typically placed to prevent bile accumulation. In case of a leak or if no drains are placed, a collection of bile, called biloma, may develop. Pain, fever, and a distended abdomen are signs of a leak or biloma. A percutaneous drainage may be needed if a leak develops. A subphrenic abscess may occur if a perihepatic infection or necrosis of the remaining liver occurs. A sharp, piercing pain in the right upper quadrant and a low-grade fever may be signs of an abscess. Chest auscultation should be done routinely, unless the abscess occurs late in the postoperative process. If patients have cirrhosis, they are at increased risk for infection after hepatic resection, due to the decrease in protein storage. The mortality rate with this complication is high for these patients. Assessment of vital signs, wound healing, and patency of drains is very important. Pneumonia and pleural effusions are common after a liver resection, especially after a right hepatectomy. An aggressive pulmonary toilet, with deep breathing and coughing and incentive spirometry, is required postoperatively. The nurse should stress frequent ambulation, along with instructions for deep breathing and coughing prior to the surgery. If the patient becomes jaundiced in the face of increasing liver function tests and demonstrates signs of hepatic failure, a portal vein thrombosis and/or obstruction should be ruled out. Portal hypertension may result from the rerouting of the portal venous flow. Fortunately, the liver has a great potential for increasing blood flow if it has enough time to compensate. Bleeding from the wound site or the cavity and/or changes in the central venous pressure should be reported to the surgeon immediately. Severe coagulation defects may occur postoperatively and may require treatment with fresh-frozen plasma. Assessing abdominal girth, urine, and stool, and monitoring the wound site should help prevent life-threatening situations. Hepatic failure can occur as a result of portal vein thrombosis or insufficiency in the hepatic parenchyma. This is especially prone in patients with cirrhosis. Increasing bilirubin and liver function tests will occur if hepatic failure is eminent. The patient may develop mental confusion and increased ammonia levels in the face of impending liver failure.

In summary, careful monitoring of mental status, vital signs, laboratory values, urine and stool output, and observation of the surgical wound site are major areas on which the nurse should focus postoperatively.

Hepatic Arterial Infusion Chemotherapy

Regional chemotherapy via HAI is generally used for unresectable hepatic colorectal metastases. HAI provides a higher concentration of drug to the tumor, whereas the normal liver tissue is exposed to proportionately less drug owing to its dual blood supply provided by the portal vein and hepatic artery.[16] Depending on the drug utilized, the concentration of drug that can be delivered to the liver exceeds the dose that can be given systemically, due to the fact that certain drugs are extracted by the liver at a high rate.[2] As a result, high doses of chemotherapy are directed into the hepatic artery, exposing the tumor to increased concentrations of the drug while limiting systemic exposure and toxicity.[17,18] Drug administration is given every 2 weeks and may include floxuridine (FUDR) and 5-fluorouracil (5-FU) with or without leucovorin (LV) calcium. These cycles of chemotherapy may alternate with cycles of a maintenance solution of heparinized saline.[5]

Preoperative Evaluations

A preoperative angiography, with selective injection of the celiac and superior mesenteric arteries, should be done before the hepatic pump is placed. The anatomy should be consistent with the common hepatic artery arising from the celiac artery. The common hepatic artery then gives rise to the gastroduodenal artery (GDA) and separates into two branches 2 cm or more distally into the right and left hepatic arteries.[19] Variant anatomy may be noted and includes the common hepatic artery dividing into three branches, a replaced right or left hepatic artery, or the common hepatic arising from the superior mesenteric artery.[19]

Surgical Procedure

The surgeon performs an exploratory laparotomy via a right subcostal incision and explores the abdomen to make sure there are no extrahepatic metastases. If extrahepatic metastases are located and malignancy is confirmed histologically by frozen section, placement of HAI devices is contraindicated.[2] The implantable pump is placed in a subcutaneous pocket on the lower abdominal wall. A separate right-sided transverse incision is made inferior to the subcostal incision for the placement of the pump. The pocket is created in the subcutaneous fat with a thin flap (4–6 mm) overlying the pump. A thick flap makes palpation of the access diaphragm difficult or impossible. The pocket is made entirely caudad to the incision, because it may migrate upward, causing the wound to overlay the access ports. The pump is positioned so that access ports are inferior to the transverse incision, with the bolus access port between the 3 and 6 o'clock positions. To avoid hematoma formation and to decrease infection, complete hemostatis in the pocket is essential.

After the pump is placed in the pocket, the catheter is brought through the fascia and the peritoneum of the abdominal wall. The pump is then fixed in the pocket with several nonabsorbable sutures placed through the suture loops on the pump[2] (Figures 11.6 and 11.7). Another approach includes attaching the catheter to a subcutaneous implanted port; however, this is not widely advocated because of the high risk of device-related complications.[20,21] The GDA is ligated and then used for cannulation. Injection of a fluorescein solution is done through the pump bolus access port or the port chamber. A Wood's light, with an ultraviolet lamp, is then used to determine adequate perfusion of both lobes of the liver, as well as any misper-

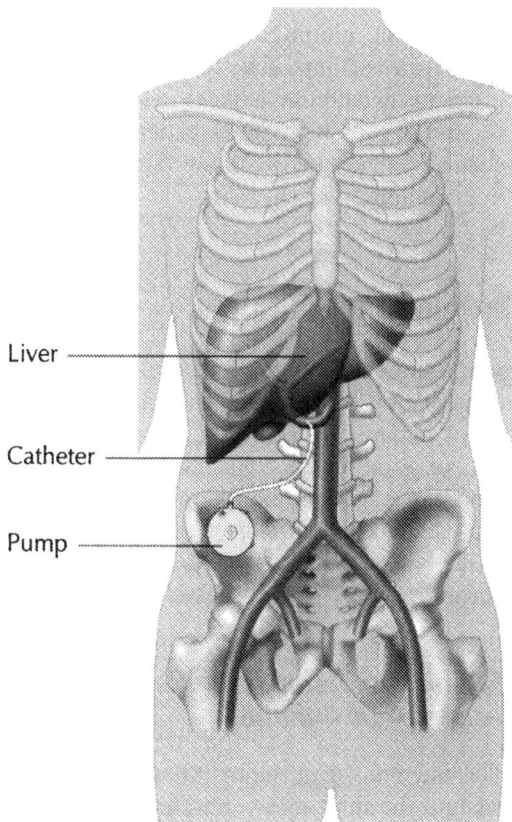

Figure 11.7 Top view of the IsoMed Constant-Flow Infusion Pump.

Source: Reprinted with permission from Medtronics, Inc. © Medtronics, Inc. 2001.

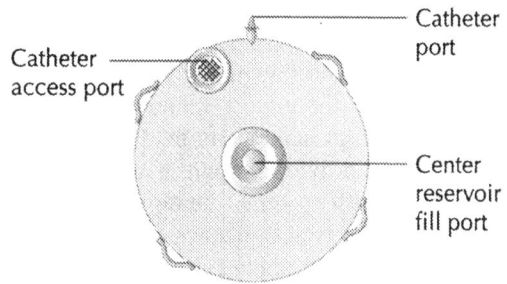

Figure 11.6 HAI therapy delivers concentrated doses of chemotherapy directly into the liver's hepatic artery, where it is most effective.

Source: Reprinted with permission from Medtronics, Inc. © Medtronics, Inc. 2001.

fusion. A cholecystectomy may be routinely performed at the time of pump placement. Postoperatively, a nuclear scan is used to assess pump perfusion. Extrahepatic perfusion must be ruled out and bilobular flow must be documented before the surgery is completed. Gastroduodenal ulceration and inadequate liver perfusion are potential complications if the pump is placed incorrectly. Sclerosing cholangitis is a postchemotherapy complication and requires the oncologist to carefully determine the need for decreased dosages versus discontinuation of therapy. Successful implantation of HAI pumps requires the coordinated efforts of the surgeon, invasive radiologist, operating room staff, and nuclear medicine radiologist.[2]

Complications related to HAI include partial or complete thrombosis of the hepatic artery, leakage of infusion from the artery, occlusion or displacement of the catheter, acalculous cholecystitis, and chemical hepatitis. Increasing bilirubin and bile duct strictures may indicate biliary sclerosis, which may require a biliary stent. A cholangiography should be done to determine the cause of the biliary obstruction (stricture or nodes).

HAI chemotherapy can also be given as adjuvant therapy following hepatic resection for metastases from colorectal cancer. Combined therapy (systemic and regional) has a potential benefit following liver resection for metastatic colorectal cancer. Hepatectomy, however, is rarely performed following intraarterial chemotherapy unless the tumor volume has been reduced enough to make it surgically resectable. HAI therapy provides response rates that exceed those with systemic therapy for patients with colorectal cancer metastases confined to the liver; however, studies are still under way to validate an improved survival with this methodology versus systemic therapy. HAI is used for patients who have failed systemic therapy or have an intolerance to systemic therapy. The role of HAI therapy in adjuvant treatment is still undefined.[2]

Nursing Implications for Hepatic Arterial Infusion Therapy

The importance of a multidisciplinary team is magnified with the HAI approach to liver metastasis therapy. The knowledge and skill of the surgeon is critical. The invasive radiologist must know hepatic arterial anatomy to assist the surgeon in the preoperative and intraoperative management of the patient. The medical and surgical oncologist has to be able to recognize and treat complications promptly. The pharmacist must know drug dosages and administration, pharmacokinetics, and potential complications. The nurse must be able to educate the patient on the preoperative studies required, the preoperative instructions, and recognition of potential complications following surgery and during chemotherapy treatment, and must coordinate the other disciplines so that the entire process is less stressful for the patient. Education of the patient by the nurse and/or pharmacist is important in evaluating the need for prophylactic therapies such as H_2 blockers to prevent gastroduodenal irritation and gastric ulcers.[5] The nurse or pharmacist gives instructions to the patient regarding situations that may alter flow rates, such as exercise

or temperature changes. The patient is given information to carry at all times relative to the placement and model number of the pump, in case it is needed, such as at the airport, or in the presence of metal detection devices, or when experiencing complications requiring medical care while away from home. In many instances, the nurse may be responsible for refilling the pump with chemotherapy and heparin solution. Pumps may be left in place once they are no longer used. They may be removed electively or emergently, as in the event of an infection in the pocket. The nurse should be aware of potential complications, including gastritis, duodenitis, bleeding, infection, pump inversion, malfunction, clotting, disconnection, perforation, extravasations, dislodgement, or perfusion problems, in addition to those listed previously. A careful assessment of the patient's complaint should alert the nurse to the need for appropriate interventions.

Intralesion Therapy

Intralesion therapy may be used alone or in combination with other forms of treatment. It is still under investigation and can only be used to treat specific areas, thus missing any micrometastases. The intralesion therapies being investigated—ethanol injections, percutaneous acetic acid injections, RFA, chemoembolization, and cryotherapy—are discussed in this section.

Ethanol Injections and Percutaneous Acetic Acid Injections

The injection of absolute ethanol, percutaneously or during surgery, into hepatic lesions is an alternate treatment for liver metastasis. The alcohol dehydrates the tumor cells and causes cell death. Only tumors less than or equal to 3 to 4 cm are treated.[22] There is generally pain related to the injection, and to reduce the pain, the needle should be left in place up to 30 seconds and then withdrawn slowly. Alcohol intoxication is a potential complication and could occur after a single treatment with large volumes of alcohol.[6] Changes in liver function tests are due to hepatic necrosis, hemolysis, and localized thrombosis. Contraindications to this procedure include activated partial thromboplastin times less than 40% and platelets less than 40,000; advanced cirrhosis; extrahepatic disease; thrombosis of the main vein or portal branches; and biliary tree dilatation.[23] Combination therapy may include Lipiodol arterial embolization with the alcohol injection. Percutaneous acetic acid injection may be used to treat small lesions. It works by dissolving lipids and extracting collagen, to cause death of the tumor cells.[24] Injection of hot saline is another treatment option.[25]

Nursing Implications for Injections

The primary role of the nurse in these treatment modalities is patient education and support. Information relative to the actual procedure and potential side effects, and assessment of pain management are the key initiatives.

Radiofrequency Ablation

RFA is a localized thermal technique designed to destroy tumor tissue. By heating the tumor tissue to temperatures that exceed 60°C, a direct coagulate necrosis occurs in the treated tissue. This treatment is perfomed on patients who have unresectable liver cancer or liver metastasis.

The Leveen needle is a specially designed, sterile electrode used to perform the RFA. It is designed such that it has multiple individual electrode arms that deploy from the distal end of the insulated 15-gauge delivery cannula. The Leveen needle is attached to a radiofrequency current generator, the Radiotherapeutics RF 2000, designed to provide monopolar and bipolar radiofrequency output.[26] The generator pads are attached to the patient's thighs, and an exploratory laparotomy and intraoperative ultrasound are done to guide the surgeon in locating and verifying the size and number of tumors in the liver. The generator settings are adjusted during the procedure, starting with 50 watts and increasing by 10 watts at 1-minute intervals up to a maximum of 90 watts, or until roll-off occurs. Roll-off is the point at which power output falls precipitously because of a marked increase in tissue impedance.[26] Immediate complications may include bleeding at the needle insertion site and/or thermal damage to adjacent organs. The patient remains in the hospital 4 to 7 days, during which time liver and renal functions are monitored. Dynamic CT is important in the posttreatment evaluation to identify any nonenhancing foci that may demonstrate tumor necrosis.

Nursing Implications for Radiofrequency Ablation

Due to the fact that this procedure is still undergoing evaluation, a research nurse is generally involved in the presurgical, intraoperative, and postoperative management of patients undergoing this treatment. Presurgical tests, instructions, and consents for treatment are obtained by the research nurse. Preoperative teaching includes bowel prep (i.e., two bottles of magnesium citrate following a clear liquid diet the day prior to surgery and an antibiotic the night before surgery), pulmonary toilet, pain management, wound care, and postoperative ambulation. The inpatient and outpatient nurse assesses the patient for postoperative complications, and removes the staples upon the postoperative visit. If lesions are found to be too large or there is extrahepatic disease noted during the surgery, the procedure is aborted. In these cases, the nurse is available to provide support and education about chemotherapy or other therapy, as indicated.

Some patients may develop a postablation syndrome. This may present as flulike symptoms with a low-grade fever, accompanied by general malaise up to 72 hours after the procedure. The syndrome may last up to a week after the procedure. Serious complications are few but have been reported.[27]

Chemoembolization

Chemoembolization is a local regional approach used as a treatment option. Because a majority of tumors receive blood supply from the hepatic artery, while the normal liver receives its blood supply from the portal vein, a catheter is placed into the hepatic artery and chemoembolization is administered into the hepatic artery. This modality is primarily used to treat hypervascular tumors such as hepatocellular carcinomas and neuroendocrine tumors rather than colorectal metastases, which are often hypovascular tumors with no demonstrated benefits from this method of treatment.[6] When used for metastatic disease, this procedure allows the metastases to be treated with high concentrations of chemotherapy.[5]

Nursing Implications for Chemoembolization

Nursing care is directed to the management of symptoms and potential side effects. These include abdominal pain, nausea or vomiting, and fever.

Cryosurgery (Cryotherapy)

The use of cryosurgery dates back to 1845.[28] It involves direct freezing of lesions, which then undergo coagulation necrosis. It causes tissue destruction and cell death by several mechanisms. The direct cellular damage is a result of the physiochemical effects of intracellular ice formation, extracellular ice formation, and solute-solvent shifts, causing cell dehydration and rupture. The indirect cell damage results from a loss of structural integrity as well as vascular channel and small vessel obliteration, with resulting hypoxemia.[28] Most patients treated with cryosurgery have multiple colorectal cancer metastases. Cryosurgery also may be used to freeze the margin of the resected tumor. Five-year survival rates of approximately 22% have been reported with this procedure.[29]

Intraoperatively, the patient is placed in the supine position. Large-caliber central venous lines are used, and a pulmonary artery catheter monitoring device is placed. The patient's upper or lower extremities are covered with forced-air heating blankets to prevent hypothermia. The patient's core temperature is monitored continuously during the procedure. A right subcostal incision is made. The abdominal cavity is then explored to exclude extrahepatic disease and nodal deposits. A second incision is made in the left subcostal area. The liver is then mobilized and fully assessed both by intraoperative ultrasound and visually. Using IOUS, the transducers are placed strategically. An echogenic 18-gauge needle is placed in the tumor. A guidewire is placed through the needle, and the dilator and sheath introducer cannula are placed. The guidewire and dilator are then withdrawn, and the cryoprobe is placed through the cannula into the tumor. One or more of the probes are inserted into the target lesions and cooled in sequence; then maximum cooling power is applied so that freezing occurs as rapidly as possible. The maximal freeze cycle is initiated by circulating liquid nitrogen at $-196°C$ through the cryoprobe. Ultrasound is used to monitor the freezing. Each lesion is frozen for 15 minutes, followed by a 10-minute natural thaw period without active rewarming and a second 15-

minute freeze (Figure 11.8 on page P-8 of insert). Some centers routinely place an HAI catheter via the gastroduodenal artery and subcutaneous reservoir for postoperative chemotherapy. Cholecystectomy and ligation of the right gastric artery may be performed routinely to prevent cytotoxic cholecystitis and peptic ulceration. At the end of the procedure, homeostasis is checked and the wound closed. Suction drains may be placed above and below the liver.

A number of complications are associated with this procedure. These include death, hypothermia, biliary fistulas, bleeding, thrombocytopenia, liver surface cracking fracture, consumptive coagulopathy, cryogenic shock, iatrogenic cryoprobe injuries, electrolyte disturbances, nitrogen embolism, intrahepatic abscess, subphrenic abscess, pleural effusions, acute renal failure, acute tubular necrosis, myoglobinuria, transient elevation of liver enzymes, pyrexia, and hypoglycemia.

Nursing Implications for Cryosurgery (Cryotherapy)

As with the other surgical procedures, preoperative teaching of these patients is a must. A detailed description of the procedure and potential postprocedure side effects is necessary to reduce anxiety. Assessment of the patient for treatment side effects should be ongoing. Part of the follow-up includes serial clinical examinations, CT scans, chest x-rays, serial liver function tests, and carcinoembryonic antigen (CEA) levels. The CEA levels and CT scans are used to evaluate response to treatment.

Other Treatments

Hepatic Artery Ligation

A form of vascular ablation, hepatic artery ligation (HAL) is a surgical procedure in which the proper hepatic artery, or a lobar branch distal to the take-off of the gastroduodenal artery, is ligated. This is only a temporary procedure, as collateral blood vessels usually form rapidly, often in less than a week. Therefore, HAL or more extensive dearterialzation procedures have not demonstrated any impact on patient survival and are not routinely recommended.[30] This concept and the concept for hepatic arterial embolization and chemoembolization are based on the fact that the liver has two sources of vascular inflow (portal vein and hepatic artery). Normal hepatocytes receive most of their blood supply from the portal vein, while hepatocellular tumors derive nearly all of their influx from the hepatic artery.

New Therapies

Many of the new therapies are targeted at primary hepatoma but may eventually be useful in the management/treatment of metastatic disease. The nurse should be aware of these new developments and be a resource for the patients. The following are some of the new therapies under investigation[8]:

Gene therapy: involves the manipulation of genes to make cancer cells vulnerable to treatment modalities. At this time, the primary focus is on the *p53* gene. Approaches include correcting defects, altering the immunogenicity of a tumor, interjecting cytokines into the tumor, introducing a suicide gene to increase sensitivity to chemical agents, and modifying tumor-infiltrating lymphocytes.

Biotherapy: involves the use of biologic agents to activate the immune system.

Antiangiogenic therapy: targets the independent blood supply of malignant tumors. These agents inhibit VEGF. Other antiangiogenic strategies use protease inhibitors and inhibitors of endothelial proliferation and migration (e.g., angiostatin and endostatin).[31]

Apoptosis: involves cell death that affects single, scattered cells while sparing adjacent cells. Current studies focus on the mechanism of apoptosis and the way in which anticancer therapies induce anti-apoptosis and tumorgenesis in liver tumors.[32]

Conclusion

Treatment of patients with hepatic metastasis involves standard as well as investigative procedures. Resection of part or most of the liver and alternative surgical options require a complete preoperative evaluation of the patient to make sure the patient is a good surgical candidate. The use of special CT scans and IOUS technology has greatly increased the effectiveness of these procedures and decreased morbidity and mortality for these patients. A multidisciplinary approach to the evaluation and care of these patients provides optimal care and support. The nurse's primary role involves patient education, assessment of potential complications, evaluation of symptoms, side-effect management, support, and pain management. Careful monitoring of laboratory values and frequent observation of the vital signs, abdominal girth, urine and stool output, ascites, itching, bleeding, and mental status are an ongoing part of the immediate postoperative care, assessment, and follow-up. Referrals to support services and reinforcement of nutritional requirements and basic care needs are done routinely in the ambulatory setting. In addition, the oncology nurse must be aware of advances in treatment options and research efforts underway for patients with hepatic metastasis.

References

1. Chul HC, Radinsky R. Biology of colorectal cancer liver metastasis. In: Curley S, ed. Liver Cancer. New York, NY: Springer, 1998: 212–229.

2. Ellis L, Chase J, Patt Y, et al. Hepatic arterial infusion chemotherapy for colorectal cancer metastasis to the liver. In: Curley S, ed. Liver Cancer. New York, NY: Springer, 1998: 150–172.

3. Tuttle T. Hepatectomy for non-colorectal liver metastases. In: Curley S, ed. Liver Cancer. New York, NY: Springer, 1998: 201–211.

4. Guillem JG, Paty PB, Cohen AM. Surgical treatment of colorectal cancer. CA Cancer J Clin. 1997; 47(2):113–128.

5. Berg DT, Lilienfeld C. Therapeutic options for treating advanced colorectal cancer. J Clin Oncol Nurs. 2000; 4(5):209–216.

6. Rychcik J. Liver cancer: Primary and metastatic disease. In: Yarbro CH, Goodman M, Frogg M, et al., eds. Cancer Nursing: Principles and Practice, 5th ed. Boston, MA: Jones and Bartlett, 2000: 1269–1297.

7. Seeley RR. The digestive system. In: Seeley RR, Stephens TD, Tate P, eds. Essentials of Anatomy and Physiology. St. Louis, MO: Mosby, 1995: 425–459.

8. Barber FD, Nelson J. Liver cancer. Am J Nursing. 2000; (April):41–46.

9. Kerbel RS. Growth dominance of the metastatic cancer cell: Cellular and molecular aspects. Adv Cancer Res. 1990; 55:87.

10. Shumate C. Hepatic resection for colorectal cancer metastases. In: Curley S, ed. Liver Cancer. New York, NY: Springer, 1998: 136–149.

11. Wagner J, Adson M, Van Heerdon J, et al. The natural history of hepatic metastasis from colorectal cancer: A comparison with resective treatment. Ann Surg. 1984; 199(5):502–508.

12. Goslin R, Steele G, Zamcheck N, et al. Factors influencing survival in patients with hepatic metastasis from adenocarcinoma of the colon or rectum. Dis Colon Rectum. 1982; 25:749.

13. Cady B, Stone M, McDermott W, et al. Technical and biologic factors in disease free survival after resection for colorectal cancer metastasis. Arch Surg. 1992; 127:561.

14. Penn I. Hepatic transplantation in primary and metastatic cancer of the liver. Surgery. 1991; 110:726.

15. Lang H, Oldhafer K, Weimann A, et al. Liver transplantation for metastatic neuroendocrine tumors. Ann Surg. 1997; 225:347.

16. Coia L, Ellenhorn J, Auyoub JP. Colorectal and anal cancers. In: Pazdur R, Coi L, Haskins W, et al. Cancer Management: A Multidisciplinary Approach. Melville, NY: PRR, 2000: 273–299.

17. Watkins E, Khozie AM, Nahra KS. Surgical basis for arterial infusion chemotherapy of disseminated carcinoma of the liver. Surg Gynecol Obstet. 1970; 130:581–605.

18. Lin G, Lunderguisht A, Hagerstrand I, et al. Postmortem examination of the blood supply and vascular pattern of small liver metastasis in man. Surg. 1984; 96(3):517–526.

19. Campbell KA, Burns RC, Setzmann JV, et al. Regional chemotherapy devices: Effect of experience and anatomy on complications. J Clin Oncol. 1993; 11:822–826.

20. Curley S, Chase JL, Roh MS, et al. Technical considerations and complications associated with the placement of 180 implantable hepatic arterial infusion devices. Surgery. 1993; 114: 928.

21. Fordy C, Burke D, Earlam S, et al. Treatment interruptions and complications with two continuous hepatic artery floxuridine infusion systems in colorectal liver metastases. Br J Cancer. 1995; 72:1023.

22. Lencioni R, Bartolozzi C. Nonsurgical treatment of hepatocellulare carcinoma. Cancer J. 1997; 10(1):17–23.

23. Taavitsainen M, Velmas T, Kauppila R. Fatal liver necrosis following percutaneous ethanol injections for hepatocellular carcinoma. Abdom Imaging. 1993; 18:307–359.

24. Livraghi T, Giorgio A, Marin G, et al. HCC and cirrhosis in 746 patients: Long-term results of percutaneous ethanol injection. Radiology. 1995; 197:101–108.

25. Yeltri A, Martina C, Bonenti G, et al. Therapy of malignant hepatic tumors using percutaneous hot saline injections: Feasibility study and preliminary results. Radiol Med. 1995; 90: 463–469.

26. Melliza D, Woodall M. Radiofrequency ablation of liver tumors: The complementary roles of the clinic and research nurse. Gastroenterol Nurs. 2000; 23(5):210–214.

27. McGahan J. Radiofrequency ablation of hepatocellular carcinoma. Pract Gastorenterol. 2000; 24(11):21–34.

28. Gagne D, Roh M. Cryosurgery for hepatic malignancies. In: Curley S, ed. Liver Cancer. New York, NY: Springer, 1998: 173–200.

29. Henderson CA. Therapeutic options for the treatment of colorectal cancer following 5-fluorouracil failure. Semin Oncol. 1998; 25:29–30 (suppl 11).

30. Wagman LD, Hoff PM, Robertson J, et al. Liver, gallbladder, and biliary tract cancers. In: Pazdur R, Coia L, Haskins W, et al., eds. Cancer Management: A Multidisciplinary Approach. Melville, NY: PRR, 2000: 255–271.

31. Bergsland EK, Warren RS. Antiangiogenic agenic agents in the treatment of liver tumors. In: Clavien P, Malden M, eds. Malignant Liver Tumors: Current and Emerging Therapies. Oxford, UK: Blackwell Science, 1999: 258–269.

32. Cusack JC. Induction of apoptosis in liver tumors. In: Clavien P, Malden MA, eds. Blackwell Science, 1999: 270–276.

CHAPTER 12 | Quality-of-Life Issues for Individuals with Colorectal Cancer

Cynthia R. King, PhD, NP, MSN, RN, FAAN

Introduction

Problem

Colorectal carcinoma is a significant problem for individuals in the United States. It is a common malignancy that accounts for a large portion of all cancer-related morbidity and mortality. It is the fourth most common nonskin malignancy.[1] Colorectal cancer is the second leading cause of cancer-related mortality and the fourth most prevalent malignant disease in the United States.[2] Colorectal cancer affects 1 of every 18 Americans. If caught early, it can be cured, but 25% present with metastatic disease.[3] Overall survival rates range between 55% and 75% for patients undergoing curative surgery resection, while 5-year survival rates range from 27% to 69% for people with node-positive cancer.[4] Colorectal cancer is the only major disease in the United States that affects men and women almost equally.[4] It was anticipated that in 2000 there would be 130,700 new cases of colorectal cancer and 56,300 deaths.[1] Additionally, there are 1.24 million survivors of colorectal cancer currently. Consequently, colorectal cancer significantly affects the quality of life (QOL) of many individuals in the United States. Despite the large number of individuals affected by colorectal cancer, there is relatively little information about QOL issues for individuals with this disease.

Surgery continues to offer the best chance for curing colorectal cancer, but newer therapies have also been developed. These include chemotherapy, cryosurgery, radiotherapy, biotherapy (immunotherapy), and other investigative therapies.[5] Yet, an objective tumor response

223

does not necessarily mean that the individual experiences freedom from distress and suffering and a decrease in QOL.

In past years, the standard outcome measures in cancer clinical trials were tumor response, survival, time to disease progression, and treatment-related toxicity. These outcome measures are still important, but there is an increasing need to assess the impact of the disease and its treatment in patients' and families' QOL. As with any cancer, individuals with colorectal cancer may suffer numerous physical symptoms (pain, nausea, fatigue), other demands of illness (poor body image, work-related and financial issues, changes in roles and relationships), and decrease in quality of life.[6–15] With recent advances in the treatment of colorectal cancer and the increased interest in QOL issues for cancer patients in general, it is crucial that healthcare providers begin to evaluate the impact of this disease and its treatment on individuals and their families.

Controversial Issues Related to Quality of Life

Despite the progress made in the research related to QOL issues for cancer patients, there remain numerous controversies among experts. No single definition of QOL exists. There are controversies over the number and type of dimensions that make up the concept of QOL, experts continue to debate whether QOL is a unidimensional or multidimensional concept, and there are controversies related to measuring QOL in research. Some of these issues are discussed throughout this chapter. This will help nurses to understand why it has been difficult to develop a significant amount of knowledge concerning QOL in individuals with colorectal cancer.

Definition of Quality of Life

There is currently no one universally accepted definition of QOL. However, most experts describe QOL as being a multidimensional concept, which is subjective, dynamic, and encompasses perceptions of both negative and positive aspects. The World Health Organization defines QOL as "individuals' perceptions of their position in life in the context of the culture and value system in which they live and in relation to their goals and standards and concerns."[16] Padilla and Grant[17] stated that QOL refers to "that which makes life worth living and connotes the caring aspects of nursing, because nursing is concerned not only with survival and decreased morbidity, but with the whole patient." Unfortunately, many healthcare providers fail to define QOL, because they believe there is an accepted meaning or the term is too ambiguous to describe. When discussing the term of QOL, it is also important to distinguish it from other related concepts (e.g., well-being, life satisfaction, hope). In the future, experts may decide that one definition may not be adequate to describe QOL throughout the disease trajectory, or the meaning and importance of QOL may be defined as discipline-specific or population-specific.[11]

Dimensions of Quality of Life

There is also significant controversy regarding the exact number of dimensions of QOL. There has been little theoretical basis for the dimensions proposed in the literature.[18,19] Possible dimensions may include physical aspects, symptoms, psychological/emotional aspects, social aspects, cognitive aspects, and/or spiritual aspects. Most experts agree that QOL is multidimensional and composed of at least four to five dimensions.[11,20] The physical dimension is the one that is easiest to understand and approximates the outcome measures traditionally used. Questions designed to measure this dimension usually ask about strength, ability to perform activities of daily living, and self-care. This may correlate with the healthcare providers' estimate of functional status.[18,21,22] Psychological status is usually measured by anxiety, fear, or depression and by instruments developed for healthy subjects. Thus, healthcare professionals may be poor evaluators of psychological well-being.[18,21,22] The social dimension of QOL involves how individuals continue their relationships with family, friends, colleagues, and other individuals.[18,21,22] Spiritual well-being involves the perception that an individual's life has purpose and meaning.[18,21,22]

A conceptual model (Figure 12.1) developed by Drs. Grant and Ferrell at the City of Hope Medical Center is frequently used in QOL research. This QOL model has four dimensions: physical well-being, psychological well-being, social well-being, and spiritual well-being. This model emphasizes the need for a multidimen-

sional definition of QOL. Each of the four dimensions consists of generic themes of concern for all cancer populations, as well as items specific to particular types of cancer or treatment. This model has been validated in many research studies in different cancer populations.[17,19,23–27] This model is based on the assumptions that QOL is subjective, based on the patient's self-report, always changing, and a multidimensional concept. These dimensions are used throughout this chapter to refer to QOL for individuals with colorectal cancer.

Measurement Issues

Several measurement issues remain controversial. These include (1) the use of generic versus specific measurement tools, (2) the use of a single QOL instrument versus a battery of tools, (3) the use of dimension scores versus a total score, (4) the use of self-administered tools versus those of proxies, (5) quantitative versus qualitative tools, (6) measurement at one time

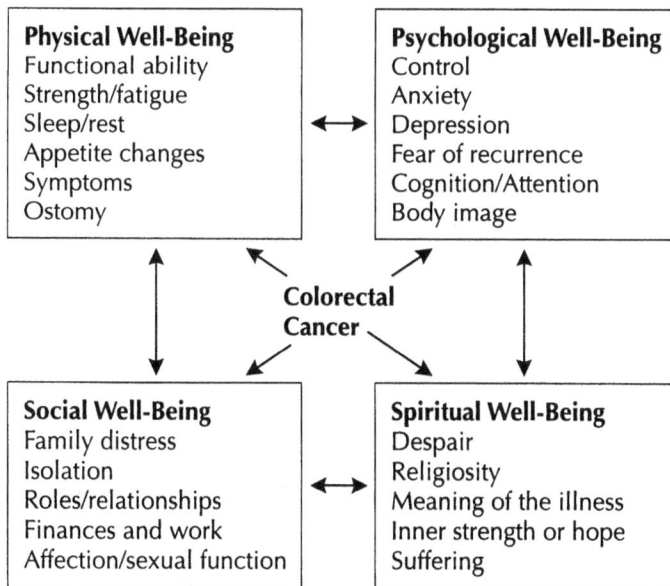

Physical Well-Being	**Psychological Well-Being**
Functional ability	Control
Strength/fatigue	Anxiety
Sleep/rest	Depression
Appetite changes	Fear of recurrence
Symptoms	Cognition/Attention
Ostomy	Body image

Colorectal Cancer

Social Well-Being	**Spiritual Well-Being**
Family distress	Despair
Isolation	Religiosity
Roles/relationships	Meaning of the illness
Finances and work	Inner strength or hope
Affection/sexual function	Suffering

Figure 12.1 Quality-of-life model for individuals with cancer.

Source: Adapted from research by Dr. Marcia Grant and Dr. Betty Ferrell (Ferrell et al.,[23] Ferrell et al.,[24] Padilla et al.,[25] Padilla and Grant,[17] Padilla et al.,[26] Padilla et al.,[19] Padilla et al.[27]).

point versus multiple occasions, and (7) whether tools are culturally sensitive.

There are differences between generic tools and specific tools to measure QOL. Generic tools are used to measure the entire spectrum of dimensions related to QOL and include health profiles and utility measures. Health profiles are often lengthy and measure different aspects of QOL in a wide variety of conditions. They are not specific to a disease or treatment. Examples are the Sickness Impact Profile (SIP),[28] the Medical Outcomes Study Short Form-36 (MOS SF-36),[29] the Demands of Illness Inventory,[30] and the Functional Assessment of Cancer Therapy Scale (FACT-G).[31] These generic tools provide a common database for comparing results, allocating resources, and developing health policy.[20] Specific instruments evaluate specific diseases (cancer, arthritis), populations (individuals with colorectal cancer), certain dimensions (spiritual), or particular conditions (nausea and vomiting). These tools may be more responsive but are not as comprehensive and cannot be used to compare different diseases or dimensions.[18,20,22,32] Table 12.1 displays examples of generic versus specific QOL instruments.

There is an ongoing debate among experts as to whether one instrument is better to measure QOL, or a battery of tests. There is no correct answer. Rich data on multiple dimensions of QOL may be obtained with a battery of tests, but scores cannot be combined from the tests. Additionally, analyzing change across time and small sample sizes may be problems with using a battery of tests.[22] Whether a QOL instrument should provide scores for each dimension or a total score is yet to be determined. Some tools even provide dimension scores as well as a total score. The number and variation in tools used to measure QOL is enormous. There continues to be a lack of consensus on the best instruments to measure this concept. However, recently, investigators have suggested that a "core

Table 12.1 Examples of Generic versus Specific Quality-of-Life Tools

Generic Questionnaires
  The Beck Depression Inventory (BDI)
  Demands of Illness Inventory (DOII)
  Functional Assessment of Cancer
    Therapy–General Scale (FACT-G)
  Symptom Distress Scale
  Medical Outcome Study Short-Form General
    Health Survey (MOS)
  The Nottingham Health Profile
  Profile of Mood States
  Quality of Life Index by Padilla et al.[19] (QLI)
  Quality of Life Index (QL-Index)
  The Sickness Impact Profile
Cancer-Specific Questionnaires
  Breast Cancer Chemotherapy Questionnaire
  Cancer Rehabilitation Evaluation System
    (CARES)
  City of Hope Medical Center Quality of Life:
    Bone Marrow Transplant
  European Organization for Research and
    Treatment of Cancer (EORTC) Quality of Life
    Questionnaire (QLQ-C30); additional
    modules for disease such as lung, colorectal,
    and bone marrow transplant
  Functional Assessment of Cancer Therapy
    Scale (FACT-G); additional modules for head
    and neck, breast, prostate, lung, and
    colorectal cancer
  Functional Living Index: Cancer (FLIC)
  Southwest Oncology Group Quality of Life
    Questionnaire

Source: Adapted from Haberman MR, Bush N. Quality of life: Methodological and measurement issues. In: King CR, Hinds PS, eds. Quality of Life: From Nursing and Patient Perspectives: Theory, Research and Practice. Boston, MA: Jones and Bartlett, 1998:117–139 and Cella D. Quality of life as an outcome of cancer treatment. In: Groenwald SL, Frogge MH, Goodman M, et al., eds. Cancer Nursing: Principles and Practice, 4th ed. Boston, MA: Jones and Bartlett, 1997: 203–213.

plus module" tool might provide an acceptable answer. This involves using a global QOL tool, which measures multiple dimensions of QOL as the core tool. Then a smaller module can be added to measure a specific disease, population, or condition. An example of this is the European Organization for Research and Treatment of Cancer (EORTC) QOL Questionnaire (QLQ-C30).[18,33–35]

Although tools vary, most are developed to be self-administered. If the patient is unable to answer questions, then a "proxy" may be used. If physicians serve as proxies, the data often emphasize physical well-being, while nurses and families tend to emphasize psychological well-being. Research has begun to demonstrate that proxy respondents tend to underestimate the patients' QOL and to be biased by the observer's own internal standards of what constitutes a desirable QOL.[20,22,36,37] Thus, it is generally recommended that a self-report be obtained directly from the patient.

Quantitative instruments are frequently used to measure QOL. These tools tend to use closed-question formats and categorical scaling. They often are less time consuming and less burdensome for the patients. However, qualitative instruments often stress the importance of the patient's perspective and provide rich data. This approach utilizes more open-ended questions and may be more time consuming. Another approach to QOL research involves combining both quantitative and qualitative methods. Each method provides a different type of outcome data.[20,22]

Initially, QOL research was performed at one time point during the disease trajectory. As experts learned more about QOL, they realized that this did not provide a thorough understanding of QOL or how to improve outcomes throughout treatment and survival. Thus, it has been recognized that multiple measurements are needed in order to evaluate improvements over time. Additionally, researchers have discovered the need for assessments and measurements of QOL to be culturally sensitive. This involves the need to translate QOL instruments into multiple languages, conducting studies to examine cross-cultural applicability, and determining the impact of cultural variables on perceived QOL.[11,38]

There are numerous instruments available to measure QOL and related constructs. However, many of these are either not multidimensional or not specific to colorectal cancer. The EORTC has constructed a colorectal cancer–specific QOL module (QLQ-CR38).[39] This tool was developed to evaluate disease symptoms and side effects related to treatment modalities (e.g., surgery, radiation, chemotherapy), and QOL aspects affected by treatments (e.g., body image and sexuality). This tool incorporates two functional scales (body image and sexuality) and seven symptom scales (micturition problems, symptoms in the area of the gastrointestinal tract, chemotherapy side effects, problems with defecation, stoma-related problems, male and female sexual problems). The remaining single items evaluate future perspective and weight loss. All items are rated on a scale of 1 (not at all) to 4 (too much). The items have a 1-week time frame. The QLQ-CR38 has been tested with 117 colorectal cancer patients on several occasions. The time points were prior to treatment with radiation or chemotherapy, during treatment, and 3 months following the second assessment. This instrument has been shown to be reliable and valid.[39]

Ward et al.[40] also developed an instrument for colorectal patients called the Functional Assessment of Cancer Therapy–Colorectal (FACT-C) Questionnaire. It is a self-report tool, which includes specific concerns related to colorectal cancer and concerns common to all cancer patients (assessed by the FACT-G). The FACT-C questionnaire was shown to be reliable and valid and sensitive to changes in functional status.

Overall, measuring QOL for any individual with cancer, and specifically individuals with colorectal cancer, can be difficult but important. Successful assessments and measurements should be brief and easy to understand, easy

Table 12.2   Recommendations for Quality-of-Life Research with Individuals with Colorectal Cancer

---

Self-administered if possible
Use multidimensional tools if possible.
Use easy-to-read tools.
Use tools that are not lengthy.
Use tools that are sensitive to changes in QOL.
Use tools that are culturally sensitive.
Use tools that are reliable and valid.
Include global questions about cancer experience and specific questions about colorectal cancer.
Define when the initial measurement will be performed (preferably baseline).
Repeat measurements at intervals.
Research an aspect of QOL in which you expect a substantial difference in outcome.
Evaluate the potential burden on the subjects.

---

to score and prepare for analysis, and not be excessively burdensome for patients. Table 12.2 provides recommendations to consider when conducting research with individuals with colorectal cancer.

Why Is Quality of Life Important to Colorectal Cancer Patients?

Why should oncology nurses and other healthcare practitioners be concerned with QOL issues for individuals with colorectal cancer? At the patient level, data gained concerning QOL can help inform newly diagnosed patients regarding common concerns and reactions to cancer and treatment. QOL assessment also provides a valued perspective of the patient's experience beyond clinical measures of the disease, treatment, and survival. Additionally, this information can be used to help individuals with cancer to make medical decisions. At the level of the healthcare provider, information regard-

ing QOL for patients can lead to changing treatment regimens or stopping treatment. At a national level, QOL information can be used to assess the benefits of alternative interventions and establish priorities for resource allocation.[41] Thus, QOL is an important concept when assessing cancer care at all levels (e.g., individual, healthcare practitioner, and national healthcare policy).

What Have We Learned about Quality of Life in Colorectal Cancer Patients?

There is currently less QOL information available regarding individuals with colorectal cancer than regarding individuals with other types of cancer.[42] However, colorectal cancer patients have been reporting that cancer and treatment have affected their QOL.[43] QOL assessments have been performed with colorectal patients. These studies have mostly described the impact of the problem on physical and psychological well-being in the course of the disease trajectory.[8,26,44]

More recently, researchers have begun to incorporate QOL measures into randomized clinical trials to evaluate the effectiveness of different treatments (in which the cost of the survival gain is weighed against the quality of the gain). Specifically randomized trials have shown that chemotherapy improves survival and QOL in advanced colorectal cancer.[45–50] A median survival of 5 months for supportive care versus 11 months for patients randomized to receive chemotherapy ($p = 0.006$) was shown by Scheithauer and colleagues.[46] Glimelius and associates[48] randomized patients with metastatic gastrointestinal carcinoma to chemotherapy plus supportive care versus supportive care alone. Not only was survival longer in the chemotherapy group, but twice as many patients in the chemotherapy group had favorable QOL outcomes. In two randomized trials, patients previously treated with metastatic colorectal cancer were treated with irinotecan or best supportive care in one trial, and irinotecan or infusional 5-fluorouracil (5-FU) in the second trial.[50] In both trials, overall survival was significantly longer in patients treated with irinotecan. QOL was also significantly superior in patients treated with irinotecan compared with best supportive care, yet equal to those patients treated with infusional 5-FU. The impact on survival and QOL changed clinical practice, in that irinotecan became the standard treatment for patients that had failed on 5-FU.[50] A triple-drug combination of irinotecan, 5-FU, and leucovorin was recently shown to be superior in terms of response, duration of response, and overall survival relative to standard 5-FU and leucovorin in previously untreated patients.[51,52] The QOL analysis showed that, overall, there was no significant difference between the two treatments, though there was less fatigue, anorexia, pain, and a better ability to perform activities of daily living in patients treated with the triple-drug combination. In other words, the addition of another cytotoxic agent benefitted patients with metastatic colorectal cancer in terms of efficacy without being detrimental to their QOL.[51] Although a study by Anderson and Palmer[53] did not demonstrate the expected advantages of increased QOL in advanced colorectal cancer patients receiving chemotherapy, a number of important issues were identified. For example, it was determined the QOL tool must address disease-related symptoms and toxicities of the treatment under evaluation that have an impact on QOL. The tool must also be completed frequently enough to detect difference, but not be burdensome to the patient. Also, the timing of the measurement of QOL in relation to the administration of treatment (e.g., chemotherapy) must be considered. It is possible that the ideal frequency of QOL mea-

surements would be daily, but this would indeed be burdensome for the patient.

Jonker and associates[49] performed a meta-analysis of randomized controlled trials to specifically estimate the benefit of chemotherapy in prolonging survival and QOL for individuals with metastatic colorectal cancer. QOL was measured by a variety of tools in the different studies. Several of the tools used included the FLIC,[46] the Rotterdam checklist, and the Hospital Anxiety and Depression Scale.[47] The meta-analysis showed that chemotherapy does result in a significant survival advantage compared with supportive care or nonchemotherapy management. This benefit appeared consistent for a variety of different chemotherapy regimens and regardless of the route of administration. Unfortunately, the authors do not directly address the QOL issues in this metaanalysis.

In 1999, Bernhard et al.[54] evaluated whether colon cancer patients undergoing surgery with or without adjuvant chemotherapy change their internal standards on which they base QOL assessment and, if so, whether this "reframing" changes the interpretation of QOL findings. Patients underwent radical resection of adenocarcinoma of the colon and perioperative chemotherapy and then were randomized to one of three arms: (1) observation only, (2) 5-FU and levamisol, and (3) 5-FU alone. QOL was measured by linear analogue self-assessment indicators. QOL was measured before surgery, after surgery, before adjuvant treatment, at the beginning of chemotherapy/observation, and 2 months after beginning therapy. One hundred eighty-seven patients participated. When asked about presurgery QOL after surgery was completed, patients rated their QOL significantly lower than before. Moreover, when asked about their preadjuvant QOL while under treatment or observation, they also rated QOL as lower than at the beginning.

Unfortunately, some studies have evaluated cancer patients with different diagnoses (e.g., colorectal, prostate, and lung) and measured multiple dimensions of QOL (e.g., physical and psychological) all in one study. For example, Hwang and associates[55] assessed fatigue (physical), depression (psychological), symptom distress, QOL, and survival in male cancer patients with different diagnoses. These researchers did not analyze the data for colorectal cancer patients separately.

Overall, there has been little global information about QOL for individuals with colorectal cancer. Additionally, there is little information about how colorectal patients view their physical well-being, psychological well-being, social well-being, and spiritual well-being during their disease trajectory. Some healthcare professionals may assume that colorectal cancer patients have similar concerns in each of these dimensions of QOL as other cancer patients; however, these assumptions may lead to inappropriate interventions.

Physical Well-Being

Healthcare professionals have learned that colorectal cancer and its treatment can significantly affect the individual's physical well-being. For example, physical well-being was affected when patients suffered from frequent or irregular bowel movements, diarrhea, constipation, gas, or urinary problems.[43] Specifically, surgery can cause short-term pain and tenderness in the area of the operation. Temporary constipation or diarrhea also may result after surgery for colorectal cancer. Individuals who have a colostomy may develop irritation of the skin around the stoma. Although individuals without a stoma may fare better than those with one, the former groups of individuals may also suffer from physical impairments of bowel and genitourinary function as a result of sphincter-saving procedures.[56] Surgeries involving extensive rectal resection may require the interruption of the hypogastric sympathetic nerves or

the pelvic parasympathetic sacral splanchnic plexus and, thus cause bladder and sexual dysfunction.[57]

Chemotherapy also may cause physical side effects, such as nausea, vomiting, hair loss, mouth sores, diarrhea, fatigue, infection, or bleeding.[57] Physical effects from radiation may include skin changes, fatigue, loss of appetite, nausea, diarrhea, intestinal obstruction, or bleeding through the rectum.[57] Biotherapy (or immunotherapy) may cause the individual to suffer flulike symptoms, such as chills, fever, weakness, or nausea. What is known is that all individuals with colorectal cancer may suffer physical effects while undergoing treatment. These side effects or symptoms ultimately can negatively affect QOL.

Vordermark et al.[58] found that 22 colostomy-free survivors of anal cancer treated with radiation therapy or chemotherapy had QOL scores similar to those found in patients with less severe, benign anorectal disorders. In general, it appears that individuals with colorectal cancer who have damage to the internal and external sphincters tend to have a lower QOL.[59]

Psychological Well-Being

From recent research it has been discovered that psychological well-being in colorectal cancer patients is often compromised by high levels of generalized forms of distress and negative body image. There was a higher incidence among women and younger patients.[43] The literature supports the fact that having an ostomy after surgery can negatively affect psychological well-being and sexuality. Men may have erectile dysfunction and ejaculatory difficulties, while women may have dyspareunia. And certainly an ostomy can alter an individual's body image.[60] Different treatments for colorectal cancer can cause various short- or long-term changes psychologically (e.g., depression, anxiety, fear of recurrence). In the research performed by Whyness and Neilson,[61] individuals with colorectal cancer demonstrated statistically significant improvement emotionally/psychologically at 3 months after surgery.

Social Well-Being

As shown previously in the QOL model developed by Drs. Grant and Ferrell, the social well-being of individuals with cancer may suffer due to the disease and treatment. Among colorectal cancer patients, it has been demonstrated that social well-being may be affected adversely, including work, relationships with family and friends, and leisure activities. Additionally, the sexual functioning of male patients may be impaired (e.g., erectile or ejaculatory functioning, sexual activity), as was the sexual functioning of the female patients (e.g., dyspareunia, cessation of intercourse).[43]

A study was performed by Ramsey and colleagues[42] with 173 individuals with colorectal carcinoma. The subjects completed two self-administered questionnaires: the Functional Assessment of Cancer Therapy Scales for Colorectal Cancer (FACT-C) and the Health Utilities Index (HUI) Mark III. In the first 3 years after diagnosis, the QOL was lower and varied among subjects, while after 3 years, respondents reported a high level of QOL. Specifically pain, ambulation, and social well-being were most adversely affected across all stages and times from diagnosis. Low income status was also associated with worse outcomes and poorer QOL. Thus, even though individuals with colorectal cancer may have an increase in QOL several years after diagnosis, they may continue to suffer in several areas, particularly in social well-being.

Spiritual Well-Being

Few, if any, QOL studies of individuals with colorectal cancer have examined the impact of the disease and treatment on the individual's spiritual well-being. However, research has shown that this is an important aspect of QOL of individuals with cancer. Studies have demonstrated that a decrease in physical status can cause an increase in awareness of personal mortality and heighten the individual's spiritual needs.[62–65]

Clinical Nursing Implications

The information learned from QOL research is valuable for oncology nurses. The goals of oncology nursing are to provide holistic and supportive care to patients and families throughout the trajectory of their illness. Nurses have known for decades that the impact of the diagnosis of cancer, and specifically colorectal cancer, affects the physical, psychological, social and spiritual well-being of patients. Thus, QOL issues are important to clinical nurses. With information gained from QOL research, nurses can provide valuable guidance to newly diagnosed or previously treated colorectal cancer patients.

Table 12.3 displays some recommendations for oncology nurses to improve the QOL for individuals with colorectal cancer. These recommendations include simple tips, such as being present with the patient, to more complex recommendations, such as assessing and managing symptoms and long-term effects of treatment that can negatively affect QOL.

Future Research Related to Quality-of-Life Issues in Colorectal Cancer Patients

From this chapter it can be seen that there is a need for further research regarding the QOL of individuals with colorectal cancer. The research needs to involve a multidimensional assessment

Table 12.3   Recommendations to Improve Quality of Life for Individuals with Colorectal Cancer

Be present and listen to patient's concerns.

Assess the patient's view of QOL (physical, psychological, social, and spiritual).

Help patients and families identify what makes their QOL better or worse.

Encourage patients to participate in activities that improve QOL.

Be respectful and honest.

Serve as an advocate.

Ask about body image and sexuality issues.

Ask about and help with any concerns if the patient has an ostomy.

Provide education and information (concentrate on concrete objective information).

Help the patient derive hope.

Help the patient to accomplish goals.

Assist with religious and/or spiritual issues.

Care for the family as well as the patient.

Encourage support from the patient's family and friends.

Provide support groups for patients and families.

Be aware of and manage symptoms and potential long-term effects of treatment and the impact on QOL.

Provide appropriate skin care if the individual is receiving radiation therapy.

---

of outcomes, gathered from the view of the individual with colorectal cancer. Although a variety of generic or colorectal-specific QOL questionnaires can be used, researchers are encouraged to use both qualitative and quantitative methods, depending on available resources. Qualitative research can add a richness that is unattainable with quantitative methods. Research needs to concentrate on dimensions other than physical well-being (e.g., psychological, social, and spiritual well-being). Oncology nurses will have important roles in conducting this research as well as encouraging patients with colorectal cancer to enroll in studies that examine QOL outcomes. The results of this future research will ultimately be used by consumer advocates, insurance companies, and healthcare policymakers to allocate limited cancer care resources. But more importantly, the information from future research can be used by oncology nurses in the clinical setting to help improve the QOL of individuals with colorectal cancer.

Conclusion

As massive changes in healthcare continue to increase the demand for the evaluation of QOL outcomes, as well as physical and medical outcomes, oncology nurses will play a key role in QOL and its relationship to practice, education, and research. Despite the fact there are still controversial issues related to QOL research with cancer patients, oncology nurses can and will learn more about how to improve the QOL for individuals with cancer, and specifically with individuals with colorectal cancer. Both clinical practice and education can be guided by what is currently known regarding the QOL of individuals with colorectal cancer, and cancer survivors in general. However, oncology nurses will need to continue to adapt practice and education in the future as we expand our knowledge base and nursing skills related to caring for individuals with colorectal cancer.

References

1. Greenlee RT, Murray T, Bolden S, et al. Cancer statistics. CA Cancer J Clin. 2000; 50:7–23.
2. American Cancer Society. Cancer Facts and Figures 2000. Atlanta, GA: Author, 2000.
3. Berg DT, Lilienfeld C. Therapeutic options of

treating advanced colorectal cancer. Clin J Oncol Nurs. 2000; 4(5):209–216.

4. Jessup JM, Menck HR, Frengen A, et al. Diagnosing colorectal carcinoma. Clinical and molecular approaches. CA Cancer J Clin. 1997; 47: 70–92.

5. Klemm P, Miller MA, Fernsler J. Demands of illness in people treated for colorectal cancer. Oncol Nurs Forum. 2000; 27(4):633–639.

6. Courneya KS, Friedenreich CM. Relationship between exercise pattern across the cancer experience and current quality of life in colorectal cancer survivors. J Altern Complement Med. 1997; 3(3):215–226.

7. Ferrell BR, Grant M, Funk B, et al. Quality of life in breast cancer. Part 1: Physical and social well-being. Cancer Nurs. 1997; 20:398–408.

8. Forsberg C, Cedermark B. Well-being, general health and coping ability: 1-year follow-up of patients treated for colorectal and gastric cancer. Eur J Cancer Care. 1996; 5:209–216.

9. Frost MH, Brueggen C, Mangan M. Intervening with the psychosocial needs of patients and families. Perceived importance and skill level. Cancer Nurs. 1997; 20:350–358.

10. Houston D. Supportive therapies for cancer. Chemotherapy patients and the role of the oncology nurse. Cancer Nurs. 1997; 20:409–413.

11. King CR, Haberman M, Berry DL, et al. Quality of life and the cancer experience: The state of the knowledge. Oncol Nurs Forum. 1997; 24: 27–41.

12. McClement SE, Woodgate RL, Degner L. Symptom distress in adult patients with cancer. Cancer Nurs. 1997; 20:236–243.

13. Schag CAC, Ganz PA, Wing DS, et al. Quality of life in adult survivors of lung, colon and prostate cancer. Qual Life. 1994; 3:127–141.

14. Sullivan T, Weinert C, Fulton RD. Living with cancer. Self-identified needs of rural dwellers. Fam Commun Health. 1994; 16(2):41–49.

15. Woods NF, Haberman MR, Packard, NJ. Demands of illness and individual, dyadic, and family adaptation in chronic illness. West J Nurs Res. 1993; 15:10–30.

16. World Health Organization, Division of Mental Health. WHO-QOL Study Protocol: The Development of the World Health Organization Quality of Life Assessment Instrument (MNG/PSF/93.9). Geneva, Switzerland: WHO, 1993.

17. Padilla GV, Grant MM. Quality of life as a cancer nursing outcome variable. Adv Nurs Sci. 1985; 8(1):45–60.

18. Aaronson NK. Quality of life research in cancer clinical trials: A need for common rules and language. In: Tchekmedyian NS, Cella DF, eds. Quality of Life in Oncology Practice and Research. Williston Park, NY: Dominus Publishing Company, 1991: 33–42.

19. Padilla GV, Presant C, Grant M, et al. Quality of life index for patients with cancer. Res Nurs Health. 1983; 6:117–126.

20. Haberman MR, Bush N. Quality of life: Methodological and measurement issues. In: King CR, Hinds PS, eds. Quality of Life: From Nursing and Patient Perspectives: Theory, Research and Practice. Boston, MA: Jones and Bartlett, 1998: 117–139.

21. Schipper H, Clinch J, Powell V. Definitions and conceptual issues. In: B. Spilker, ed. Quality of Life Assessments in Clinical Trials. New York, NY: Raven Press, 1990: 11–24.

22. King CR. Overview of quality of life and controversial issues. In: King CR, Hinds PS, eds. Quality of Life: From Nursing and Patient Perspectives: Theory, Research and Practice. Boston, MA: Jones and Bartlett, 1998: 23–34.

23. Ferrell BR, Grant M, Schmidt GM, et al. The meaning of quality of life for bone marrow transplant survivors. Part I: The impact of bone marrow transplant on quality of life. Cancer Nurs. 1992; 15(3):153–160.

24. Ferrell BT, Hassey Dow K, Leigh S, et al. Quality of life in long-term cancer survivors. Oncol Nurs Forum. 1995; 22(6):915–922.

25. Padilla GV, Ferrell B, Grant MM. Defining the

content domain of quality of life for cancer patients with pain. Cancer Nurs. 1990; 13(2): 108–115.

26. Padilla GV, Grant M, Lipsett S, et al. Health-related quality of life and colorectal cancer. Cancer. 1992; 70(5):1450–1456.

27. Padilla GV, Grant M, Ferrell BR, et al. Quality of life-cancer. In: Spilker B, ed. Quality of Life and Pharmacoeconomics in Clinical Trials, 2nd ed. Philadelphia, PA: Lippincott-Raven, 1996: 301–308.

28. Bergner M, Bobbitt RA, Carter WB, et al. The sickness impact profile: Development and final version of a health status measure. Med Care. 1981; 19:787–806.

29. Stewart AL, Greenfield S, Hays RD, et al. Functional status and well-being of patients with chronic conditions. Results from the medical outcomes study. JAMA. 1989; 262:907–913.

30. Haberman MR, Woods NF, Packard NJ. Demands of chronic illness. Reliability and validity assessment of a demands-of-illness inventory. Hol Nurse Pract. 1990: 5(1):25–35.

31. Cella DF, Tulsky DS, Gray G, et al. The functional assessment of cancer therapy scale: Development and validation of the general measure. J Clin Oncol. 1993; 11(3):570–579.

32. Guyatt GH, Jaeschke R. Measurements in clinical trials: Choosing the appropriate approach. In: Spilket B, ed. Quality of Life Assessments in Clinical Trials. New York, NY: Raven Press, 1990: 37–46.

33. Aaronson NK, Ahmedzai Bergman B, Bullinger M, et al., for the European Organization for Research and Treatment of Cancer Study Group on Quality of Life. The European Organization for Research and Treatment of Cancer QLQ-C30; a quality of life instrument for use in international clinical trials in oncology. J Natl Cancer Inst. 1993; 85:365–376.

34. Aaronson NK, Bakker W, Stewart AL, et al. Multidimensional approach to the measurement of quality of life in lung cancer clinical trials. In: Aaronson NK, Beckman JH, eds. Monograph

35. Series of the European Organization for Research and Treatment of Cancer. New York, NY: Raven Press, 1987: 63–82.

35. Aaronson NK, Bullinger M, Ahmedzai S. A modular approach to quality of life assessment in cancer clinical trials. Recent Results Cancer Res. 1988; 111:231–249.

36. King CR, Ferrell BR, Grant M, et al. Nurses' perceptions of the meaning of quality of life for bone marrow transplant survivors. Cancer Nurs. 1995; 18:118–129.

37. Sprangers MAG, Aaronson NK. The role of health care providers and significant others in evaluating the quality of life of patients with chronic disease: A review. J Clin Epidemiol. 1992; 45:743–760.

38. Campos SS, Johnson TM. Cultural considerations. In: Spilker B, ed. Quality of Life Assessments in Clinical Trials. New York, NY: Raven Press, 1990: 163–170.

39. Sprangers MAG, te Velde A, Aaronson NK. The construction and testing of the EORTC colorectal cancer-specific quality of life questionnaire module (QLQ-CR38). Eur J Cancer. 1999; 35:238–247.

40. Ward WK, Hahn EA, Mo F, et al. Reliability and validity of the functional assessment of cancer therapy-colorectal (FACT-C) quality of life instrument. Qual Life Res. 1999; 8(3):181–195.

41. Spilker B. Introduction. In: Spilker B, ed. Quality of Life Assessments in Clinical Trials. New York, NY: Raven Press, 1990: 3–9.

42. Ramsey SD, Andersen MR, Etzioni R, et al. Quality of life in survivors of colorectal carcinoma. Cancer. 2000; 88(6):1303.

43. Sprangers MAG. Quality of life assessment in colorectal cancer patients: Evaluation of cancer therapies. Semin Oncol. 1999; 26(3):691–696.

44. Ulander K, Jeppson B, Grahn G. Quality of life and independence in activities of daily living preoperatively and at follow-up in patients with colorectal cancer. Support Cancer Care. 1997; 5:402–409.

45. Nordic Gastrointestinal Tumor Adjuvant Ther-

apy Group. Expectancy of primary chemotherapy in patients with advanced asymptomatic colorectal cancer: A randomized trial. J Clin Oncol. 1992; 10:904–911.

46. Scheithauer W, Rosen H, Komek GV, et al. Randomised comparison of combination chemotherapy plus supportive care alone in patients with metastatic colorectal cancer. BMJ. 1993; 306:752–755.

47. Allen-Mersh TG, Earlam S, Fordy C, et al. Quality of life and survival with continuous hepatic-artery floxuridine infusion for colorectal liver metastases. Lancet. 1994; 344:1255–1260.

48. Glimelius B, Hoffman K, Graf W, et al. Quality of life during chemotherapy in patients with symptomatic advanced colorectal cancer. Cancer. 1994; 73:556–562.

49. Jonker DJ, Maroun JA, Kocha W. Survival benefit of chemotherapy in metastatic colorectal cancer: A meta-analysis of randomized controlled trials. Br J Cancer. 2000; 82(11):1789–1794.

50. Cunningham D. Setting a new standard-irinotecan (Campto) in the second-line therapy of colorectal cancer: Final results of two phase II studies and implications for clinical practice. Semin Oncol. 1999; 26(1):1–5 (suppl 5).

51. Saltz LB, Cox JV, Blanke C, et al. Irinotecan plus fluorouracil and leucovorin for metastatic colorectal cancer. N Engl J Med. 2000; 343(13): 905–914.

52. Douillard JY, Cunningham D, Roth AD, et al. Irinotecan combined with fluorouracil compared with fluorouracil alone as first-line treatment for metastatic colorectal cancer: A multicentre randomised trial. Lancet. 2000; 355: 1041–1047.

53. Anderson H, Palmer MK. Measuring quality of life: Impact of chemotherapy for advanced colorectal cancer. Experience from two recent large phase III trials. Br J Cancer. 1998; 77: 9–14 (suppl 2).

54. Bernhard J, Hurny C, Maibach R, et al. Quality of life as subjective experience: Reframing of perception in patients with colon cancer undergoing radical resection with or without adjuvant chemotherapy. Swiss Group for Clinical Cancer Research. Ann Oncol. 1999; 10(70):775–782.

55. Hwang S, Chang VT, Cogswell J, et al. Fatigue, depression, symptom distress, quality of life and survival in male cancer patients at a VA medical center. Proc Annu Meet Am Soc Clin Oncol. 1999; 18:A2294.

56. Sprangers MAG, Taal BG, Aaronson NK, et al. Quality of life in colorectal cancer. Stoma vs nonstoma patients. Dis Colon Rectum. 1995; 38:361–369.

57. DeCrosse JJ, Cennerazzo WJ. Quality of life management of patients with colorectal cancer. CA Cancer J Clin. 1997; 47:198–206.

58. Vordermark D, Sailer M, Flentje M, et al. Curative-intent radiation therapy in anal carcinoma: Quality of life and sphincter function. Radiother Oncol. 1999; 52:239–243.

59. Shibata D, Guillem JG, Lanouette BS, et al. Functional and quality of life outcomes in patients with rectal cancer after combined modality therapy, intraoperative radiation therapy, and sphincter preservation. Dis Colon Rectum. 2000; 43(6):752–758.

60. Sprunk E, Alteneder RR. The impact of an ostomy on sexuality. Clin J Oncol Nurs. 2000; 4(2):85–88.

61. Whyness DK, Neilson AR. Symptoms before and after surgery for colorectal cancer. Qual Life Res. 1997; 6:61–66.

62. Loseth DB. Changes in Spirituality of the Dying: A Longitudinal Study. Unpublished thesis. New Haven, CT: Yale University, 1991.

63. Ferrell BR, Grant MM. Quality of life and symptoms. In: King CR, Hinds PS, eds. Quality of Life: From Nursing and Patient Perspectives: Theory, Research and Practice. Boston, MA: Jones and Bartlett, 1998: 140–156.

64. Reed PG. Spirituality and well-being in terminally ill hospitalized adults. Res Nurs Health. 1987; 10:335–344.

65. Sodestrom KE, Martinson IM. Patient's spiritual coping strategies: A study of nurse and patient

perspectives. Oncol Nurs Forum. 1987; 14(2): 41–46.

66. Cella D. Quality of life as an outcome of cancer treatment. In: Groenwald SL, Frogge MH, Goodman M, et al., eds. Cancer Nursing: Principles and Practice, 4th ed. Boston, MA: Jones and Bartlett, 1997: 203–213.

CHAPTER 13 | Colon Cancer and Alcoholism

Russell Peter Berg

Almost 8 years ago, during the early hours of a Sunday in December of 1992, I was awakened by pain in my lower right abdomen. During the next hour, the pain slowly increased in severity, and I reluctantly decided that I had better go to the emergency room of Mary Washington Hospital in Fredericksburg, Virginia.

After a routine administrative check-in, subsequent physical examination, and x-rays, I was given some sort of sedative to ease my pain. Later, while lying on a gurney, a doctor stopped by, introduced himself, spoke some comforting words, informed me that I had an inflamed appendix, and that he would be performing an appendectomy around 1 P.M. Looking up at him in apprehension, and never having had any kind of operation before, my Yankee sense of humor kicked in and I inquired, "Have you ever done this sort of thing before?" As I recall, he suddenly looked somewhat askance and assured me that he had, and departed. That was my first encounter with one of the finest surgeons in the city, Dr. Richard N. Thompson, the man who saved my life, ultimately became a friend, and subsequently performed several other major surgeries on this old body of mine.

The next thing I can recall is waking up in a groggy state of mind. I was told that I was in the intensive care unit and that when the surgeon went in after the appendix, he discovered that there was a tumor coming out of the colon right next to it. After excising the appen-

dix, he had to make another long incision and open me up to examine the colon and all the other organs in the area, including the lymph nodes. Finding no more traces of the disease, he resected the entire right colon and closed me back up, using stainless steel staples. As stated, my mind was all muddled up at the time, and these things were related to me again when I came to in the surgical ward a day or so later.

On the first day in the surgical ward, a doctor of oncology, by the name of W. Angus Muir, visited me. He told me all about colon cancer and how important it was for me to begin treatment immediately after being released from the hospital. He also stated that he realized that I was still under the influence of opiates, that he had to catch a plane, but that his son, a medical student, would call later and talk to me at length. His son did so. As I recall, he was a very personable young man, but much of what he had to say was lost due to my still-befuddled state. However, the seriousness of the situation did register, and I realized that removal of my right colon did not mean that I was out of the woods.

My stay in the surgical ward was about 4 or 5 days, and despite the circumstances as to why I was there, it was a pleasant incarceration. After a couple of days, I discovered that a catheter, a Foley catheter to collect urine, was in place. Also, that my legs were wrapped in pressure leggings connected to a machine that made a lot of noise pumping air in and out. Additionally, there was a machine that dispensed morphine on demand through the IV tubes. I have a high threshold for pain, so I weaned myself off the morphine dispenser quickly. The nursing staff was excellent and very caring; one in particular, whose name is Rosie, was especially considerate, and I became very fond of her. At first I thought that she was a nurse's aide, but then one day she told me that she was going to remove the Foley catheter. I was embarrassed and alarmed, so I asked her whether she were "qualified" to do that. She laughed and responded, "Mr. Berg, if I can put one in, I can certainly take one out." Much to my amazement, she did so, quickly and painlessly. As soon as they removed the morphine dispenser from the IV tube, I was able to get up and go to the bathroom by myself. I also had my little "security blanket" folded up, which I held by one hand to my stomach so I could hold onto the mobile IV unit with the other. This way, I could take turns through the hallways for exercise.

I started my chemotherapy treatments at Dr. Muir's office the week following my release from the hospital. My attitude was positive and upbeat, and I was determined to complete the treatment successfully. I again met Dr. Muir, who explained the protocol and informed me that the treatment would take a whole year, and that I would be receiving chemotherapy infusions on a weekly basis for 52 weeks. I was encouraged by his words; he then took me to his chief oncology nurse, Lori, a "peach" of a lady whom I would later refer to as "Lori Darlin'." She was very compassionate, caring, and, like myself, had a great sense of humor. She inserted a shunt into a forearm vein, withdrew two tubes of blood, and then inserted another hypodermic containing the poisonous chemotherapy liquid into the shunt and slowly "pushed" in that awful fluid. I was given a prescription for Reglan "in case" of nausea.

Taking my leave, I thought to myself, "These treatments will not be so bad after all." Ha! Was I in for a rude awakening.

Shortly after starting these treatments—I cannot recall exactly when—Dr. Muir introduced me to another drug, called levamisole. He told me that it was used on animals and was only in the experimental stage for use in cancer patients; that it had not been officially approved by the Food and Drug Administration, but that they (oncologists) knew "it worked"; and that he wanted me to take it as an adjunct to my chemotherapy treatments. I took it three times a week, every other week. The mere thought that there could possibly be cancer cells lurking somewhere in my body made me jump at the chance to take it, or at any other thing that would be proposed. Later in my treatment, he informed me that levamisole had finally been approved for use in cases like mine. I also had a colonoscopy, which didn't reveal any other tumors, and an MRI body scan, which indicated that my liver and other organs appeared to be clear.

Initially, the chemotherapy manifested itself in nausea, headaches, chills, and a feeling of weakness in me that lasted a couple of days. After discussing this with Lori, we set my appointments so that I would be the last patient on Friday afternoons, just before the office closed at 2 P.M., so that I would be in shape to go to work on Monday mornings. Things got progressively worse, however, and after approximately 6 months into the program, my reactions became more severe, and it was Wednesday before the effects wore off. It was also taking its toll on my job performance. I was becoming extremely sick after the treatments, my morale dropped, and my appetite waned, as did my weight. The Reglan tablets were not helping the nausea, and my memory was going "bonkers." I was always cold and chilly, even when the heat was turned up. I itched all over and felt half dead, and knowing that the chemotherapy was killing good cells as well as bad ones didn't help my state of mind. My will to win was failing, and I was in complete despair. I concluded that I had just better take my chances and quit. I just couldn't take it any longer.

On checking in at my next visit to the clinic, I told the receptionist not to bother sending my records to Lori and asked to see the doctor so that I could inform him personally of my decision to stop treatment. Dr. Muir came right out, escorted me to his office, and we sat down. He asked me what my symptoms were. I described my reactions and told him that I was no longer living, merely existing. He quickly reviewed my records and then exclaimed, and I remember his words clearly, "I like those symptoms! I am going to reduce your dosage." We discussed the issues for a little while, and, fortunately for me, I still had a glimmer of hope. He convinced me to continue on. Thereafter, with the reduced dosages, my reactions became manageable, and I finished up the year, at which point "Lori Darlin' " pinned a "survivors pin" on me. After that I only went back for periodic check-ups, which, after a couple of years, were only on an annual basis.

Except for that one instance, when I was ready to chuck the program, my outlook and frame of mind had always been positive. I was determined that I would beat the cancer and knew that a positive frame of mind was very important to survival. Prior to my weekly visits, I would always stop at a bakery and buy some nonfattening "treats" for the office staff. My gregarious and cheerful attitude also manifested itself in the waiting room when I reported each week. When "Lori Darlin' " stuck her head out the door, I would boisterously make remarks such as, "I came back honey" and "Should I take all my clothes off out here now to save time?" One time, I exclaimed in front of everyone, "How come I have to strip naked when I get in there when you only take my blood?"

There were usually several patients in the waiting room, some of whom always looked very downcast, and this was my way of contributing a little bit of excitement and momentarily getting them out of their "dark thoughts." I always succeeded in getting a rise or laugh out of them, and sometimes I was a real clown. Lori told me more than once that they all, including Dr. Muir, looked forward to my visits, and the effect my arrival had on some of the patients.

Colon cancer did, however, have a devastating affect on my career in federal government in the national capitol region. I served in law enforcement and had worked all the way up from patrol officer to the rank of captain in a relatively short period of time, and was the commander of criminal investigations within the Department of Defense. Federal officers are required to carry weapons, are constantly in danger of becoming involved in armed physical confrontations and therefore must keep themselves highly physically fit. My operation left me with weak stomach muscles and hernias, thereby lowering my physical profile to a category that according to regulation "carriage of a weapon represented a danger to myself and others." Consequently, as I was no longer physically qualified to carry a weapon, I transferred, at the same pay grade, to a physical security specialist position within the department. But it wasn't the type of "law enforcement" that I loved, so I, somewhat reluctantly, decided to retire and move back to the state of Maine.

My lovely daughter-in-law, a registered nurse with many years of service in cancer research, recommended an oncologist close to my home. I went to see him and had my records transferred to his office. He was another grand guy, with a personality and a sense of humor to match my own. He gave me a thorough examination, and then had me come back for follow-ups every 6 months, then once each year, until one day he spoke the greatest words I have ever heard: "There has been no sign of cancer for

7 years, so I don't want to see you again unless you just want to come in and have a cup of coffee with me."

I would like to state here that, all of my life, I have respected and held the medical profession in the highest esteem. I am also a recovering alcoholic, and have been in the Alcoholics Anonymous program for over 21 years now. Many years ago, when I was drinking, in denial, and down in "my cups," I distinctly remember thinking, and hoping, that perhaps I might some day come down with a simple ailment, like appendicitis, and wind up in the hospital, where the doctors and nurses would recognize my drinking "problem" and help me. In some ways that fantasy materialized. My drinking "problem" was recognized, though that occurred before my "appendicitis." My medical ailment did not turn out to be simple. It was cancer! Today, I thank God for the support and treatments I've received for both my problems, as I would not be alive today and writing this chapter without them.

And that is why I entitled this chapter, "Colon Cancer and Alcoholism."

CHAPTER 14 | Advanced Disease: Symptom Management Strategies

Catherine M. Hogan, MN, RN, CS, AOCN

Deborah T. Berg, RN, BSN

Introduction

The etiology and management of symptoms associated with colorectal cancer may be conceptualized as resulting from the disease process, treatment, and/or a combination of these two broad categories. Several tenets guide the approach to the management of common symptoms. Perhaps the most basic is the most challenging. Patients and their lay caregivers must have access to a knowledgeable provider 24 hours a day, 7 days a week. Prevention and/or the minimization of side effects is a primary intervention. Further, caregivers must remain sensitive to the fact that discussions regarding gastrointestinal function are highly personal and may be a source of embarrassment and discomfort for the individual and the lay caregiver. The effective management of the symptoms associated with advanced colorectal cancer is derived from many sources, including a working knowledge of research-based inter-

ventions, creativity, and an appreciation of the concepts associated with caregiver burden and the demands of self-care.[1] In the current healthcare environment, nurses are pulled in many different directions. The goal of this chapter is to provide colleagues with a practical approach to the management of the common problems associated with this difficult disease.

Symptom Assessment

Effective symptom management is developed from an ongoing assessment of the experience and perception of the individual patient. The most important caveat related to assessment is that it remain a dynamic process. Rhodes and McDaniel[2] have eloquently refined the conceptualization of the process of symptom assessment. Their collaborative research serves as the foundation of this chapter.

A *symptom* is the individual's subjective ex-

241

perience of the physical and emotional disturbances related to the disease process and/or the treatment for the disease itself. While some symptoms, such as vomiting, may be objective in nature (i.e., observed), others, including nausea and pain, are not fully appreciated by any one other than the patient.

Symptom occurrence includes a variety of components, including frequency, duration, and severity. In the setting of colorectal cancer, this component of assessment merits particular attention. Symptoms such as anorexia, nausea, vomiting, diarrhea, and constipation may all be temporized as a result of treatment. Consequently, assessment of symptom occurrence also includes the following:

- *Onset of the symptom:* Is the symptom new, or has it occurred before? It is particularly important in the setting of advanced colorectal cancer to consider the onset of a symptom within the context of a temporal relationship to chemotherapy, radiation therapy, dietary intake, and analgesics.
- *Pattern of the symptom:* constant versus intermittent. In the context of colorectal cancer, the issue of pattern is particularly important in assessing symptoms such as nausea, vomiting, constipation, and diarrhea.
- *Location:* The individual's perception of the anatomic location of the symptom is an important component of pain assessment and bowel obstruction.
- *Aggravating and alleviating factors:* Ask simply, "What seems to make it worse and what seems to make it better?" These questions allow the nurse to evaluate self-care strategies, as well as the use of complementary therapies.
- *Severity:* This is perhaps the most elusive component of symptom assessment. Nurses who are familiar with clinical trials are educated regarding the National Cancer Institute's Common Toxicity Criteria.[3] While the

number of reported/measured/observed episodes of vomiting and diarrhea can be measured, subjective symptoms such as nausea, fatigue, and pain are far more difficult to equilibrate. The familiar "0–10 scale" (0 being "none" to 10 being "as bad as it can be") is a user-friendly measure. However, this tool does require that the patient have a perception of numeric function (i.e., the higher the number, the more severe the symptom). The effective, practical use of any scale, be it numerical (0–5, 0–10), descriptive (mild, moderate, severe, unbearable), or pictorial (happy to sad faces), is truly dependent on the consistent, culturally sensitive use of one scale between and among the patients and all care providers (physicians, inpatient providers, ambulatory care providers, home-care providers, hospice providers, lay caregivers). The nurse who assumes primary responsibility for the patient is in the best position to communicate the type of scale that is most efficacious for a particular patient.

- *Use of complementary therapies:* This includes the use of interventions such as chelation, herbs, macrobiotic diet detoxification, and natural substances. This component of assessment requires particular sensitivity, because many patients are reluctant to report the use of such therapies to traditional providers. The undisclosed use of these complementary therapies by individuals experiencing bowel dysfunction, particularly constipation or diarrhea, may result in iatrogenic complications. Consequently, it is incumbent on the nurse to foster an environment in which the patient is free to disclose the use of complementary therapies without fear of being maligned or misjudged.

Symptom distress has been described by Rhodes and Watson[4] as the amount of physical or mental upset or anguish that occurs as result of a symptom. More recently, Holland,[5] on behalf of the National Cancer Center Network (NCCN), also refined the concept of distress. The most important caveat related to the measurement of distress is that it does not consistently correlate with symptom severity. The practical measurement of distress is obtained by simply asking, "How much does the symptom (nausea, pain, vomiting, etc.) bother you (using the same numerical, descriptive, or pictorial scale used to elicit symptom severity)?" For example, one episode per day of a sudden onset of loose stool would well be considered a mild episode of diarrhea. Yet, for the professional sales representative who works and travels via car and suddenly has the immediate urge to defecate, without access to a bathroom, and who subsequently experiences fecal incontinence, the perception of distress is not limited to "mild."

Care of the Patient with Advanced Colorectal Cancer

The goal of the remainder of this chapter is to provide practical strategies for the management of the common problems associated with this difficult disease. A nursing-care format is utilized to illustrate the strategies (Table 14.1).

Table 14.1 Strategies for Managing Common Problems

Nursing Problem: Knowledge deficit regarding disease process and treatment plan
Expected Outcome: The patient will verbalize an understanding of the disease and the planned treatment.
Nursing Interventions:
1. Assess the patient's knowledge of colon or rectal cancer.
2. Assess the patient's understanding of the treatment options.
3. Ascertain the patient's and family's willingness to learn and comply with the treatment regimen.
4. Educate the patient regarding the following:
   - The treatment regimen's purpose and schedule
   - Common side effects of the prescribed treatment
   - Self-care measures to manage side effects
5. Review with the patient and family when to call for medical/nursing advice.

Symptoms Affecting the Upper Gastrointestinal Tract

Nursing Problem: Potential for nausea and vomiting from advanced disease and/or treatment
Expected Outcome: The patient will be without nausea and vomiting, or, if they do occur, they will be minimal.
Nursing Interventions:
1. Assess the likelihood of nausea and vomiting based on the following:
   - Emetogenic potential of the therapeutic regimen
   - Patient characteristics associated for high risk of nausea/vomiting: female gender, younger age, chronic alcohol intake, history of motion sickness[6]
2. Identify the underlying cause of the symptom, such as treatment-induced, constipation, opioid analgesia, hypercalcemia, or bowel obstruction, and initiate appropriate corrective measures.[7]
3. Administer antiemetics prior to therapy and regularly thereafter, with a regimen based on the emetogenic potential of the regimen.[6]
4. Assess the symptom and level of distress, encouraging the patient to record frequency of emesis.

(continues)

Table 14.1 *Continued*

5. Evaluate and adjust the antiemetic regimen according to patient tolerance.
6. Incorporate nonpharmacologic interventions, such as acupressure and guided imagery, as needed.[6,8]
7. Encourage dietary modifications[9]:
   • Eat small, bland meals.[6]
   • Foods should not be greasy, fatty, or rich or have unpleasant odors or tastes.
   • Cool or cold foods are often tolerated better, for example, crackers or dry toast.
   • Change the diet to clear liquids if vomiting is experienced.[10]
8. Suggest that the patient modify the environment to decrease stimuli (e.g., a well-ventilated area with low noise levels and without obnoxious sites and smells).[11]
9. Evaluate the potential impact of comorbid conditions, such as alterations in bowel habits due to progressing disease, dehydration, and electrolyte imbalance.

Nursing Problem: Potential mucositis or stomatitis related to side effects of chemotherapy treatment
   Expected Outcome: The patient will maintain intact, healthy mucosa and demonstrate good oral hygiene.
   Nursing Interventions:
   1. Perform a baseline oral mucosal examination.
   2. Identify the patient's normal oral hygiene practices and use of dental prostheses.[12]
   3. Consider cryotherapy for the prevention of 5-fluorouracil–induced mucositis; ask the patient to suck on ice chips for 5 minutes before the bolus injection and for at least 25 minutes afterward.
   4. Assess the patient's oral cavity for signs of redness, ulcerations, or other changes in appearance, which may initially occur 5 to 7 days after chemotherapy has started.[10]
   5. Teach the patient to perform the oral examination and to report any pain or burning in the mouth, difficulty swallowing, or white patches on the tongue, throat, or gums.[12]
   6. Instruct the patient to perform oral hygiene consisting of regular oral cleansing, which includes tooth brushing with a soft-bristled brush at least twice a day and rinsing with nonirritating, plain- or sterile-water mouth rinses three to four times during the day.[12,13]
   7. Alter the interventions if the mucositis is worsening.
   8. Consider the use of sucralfate, which may adhere to exposed mucosal tissue, providing a protective coating.
   9. Antifungal and antiviral agents can be added on an individual basis.
   10. Advise the patient to stop wearing dentures if oral ulcers are present.[12]
   11. Initiate topical or systemic pain medications, as ordered, to control discomfort and pain.
   12. Have the patient maintain nutritional intake, including soft or liquid foods high in protein.[10]
   13. The patient should avoid oral irritants such as tobacco, alcohol, citrus fruits and juices, spicy foods, and commercial mouthwashes.[10,13]
   14. Discuss the need for delay or dose modification with the physician.

Nursing Problem: Potential for taste changes, anorexia, and/or cachexia from advancing disease
   Expected Outcome: The patient will maintain a weight within 5% of the baseline state.
   Nursing Interventions:
   1. Assess the patient's baseline dietary intake and concomitant medications.
   2. Note any gastrointestinal symptoms or abnormalities at baseline.[14]
   3. Evaluate the patient's risk for developing taste changes, anorexia, or cachexia, such as the following[15]:
      • Older age
      • Alcoholism

Table 14.1 *Continued*

- History of smoking
- Anorexia
- Concomitant medications that cause diarrhea, nausea, vomiting, and taste alterations
- Malabsorption disorders
- Difficulty swallowing

4. Assess the etiology of symptoms, such as social (cultural influences), physical (mouth sores, ascites, early satiety), or general causes (pain, fatigue, hypercalcemia, treatment-induced side effects), and develop a plan to correct the underlying cause.[11]
5. Monitor the patient's weight and report any weight loss or gain.
6. Teach the patient to cleanse his or her mouth before and after meals to freshen the oral cavity, to reduce risk of irritation or infection, and to help stimulate the appetite.[16]
7. Suggest that the patient experiment with seasonings, salt, sorbitol, and sweetened candies to make food more appealing and palatable.[14]
8. Recommend mints, hard candy, or cough drops as a means of temporarily relieving taste changes.
9. Assess the patient for nausea prior to mealtime. If nausea is present, administer antiemetics before the food is served.
10. Encourage strategies to increase the caloric and nutritional value of oral intake[11,17]:
    - Eat small, frequent meals instead of three large meals.
    - Eat foods high in protein and calories, such as eggs, peanut butter, cheese, chicken, and fortified milkshakes.
    - Limit liquids during eating so as to increase the amount of food eaten.
    - Maximize intake when feeling the best, usually earlier in the day.
11. Encourage the patient to establish a pleasant, unhurried environment for mealtime.[11,18]
12. Advise the patient's family and friends against preparing and forcing the patient's favorite foods during periods of severe taste changes and/or nausea. These may be subsequently associated with the adverse symptoms.[14]
13. Encourage the patient to eat foods at room temperature or cold, because the smell of food cooking may exacerbate the symptoms.[17]
14. Offer liquid food supplements if the patient is not tolerating solid foods.[16]
15. Enteral and parenteral feedings in the terminal patient are controversial and are recommended carefully based on the patient's goals and current disease status.[19] The specific supplement offered requires a trial-and-error approach in terms of patient preferences.
16. Initiate pharmacologic interventions, such as corticosteroids, megestrol acetate, hydrazine sulfate, metoclopramide, and dronabinol, as ordered.[19]
17. Instruct the patient to avoid storing food in metal containers, and, if taste changes are severe, to consider using plastic utensils instead of metal ones.

Symptoms Affecting the Lower Gastrointestinal Tract

Nursing Problem: Potential for constipation caused by disease process, concomitant narcotic analgesia, or side effect of therapy
  Expected Outcome: The patient will move bowels at least once every 1 to 3 days.[18,20]
  Nursing Interventions:
  1. Assess the patient's baseline bowel habits and concomitant medications, especially narcotic analgesia.

(continues)

Table 14.1 *Continued*

2. Identify the underlying cause of constipation and initiate interventions based on cause.
3. Educate the patient about means to prevent constipation[21-23]:
   - Pharmacologic measures: stool softeners, laxatives
   - Fluid intake
   - Dietary alterations
   - Exercise
4. Advise the patient[21]
   - Not to strain with bowel movements
   - To respond immediately to the urge to defecate[10]
   - To create privacy and plenty of time for the bowel routine
5. Increase fiber intake, whole-grain foods, legumes, fresh foods, and raw vegetables, unless the patient is at risk for a narrow colonic lumen.[18,21,24]
6. Increase fluid intake; recommend 2 to 3 quarts of liquids, to include juices, water, and prune juice. A hot beverage first thing in the morning or at a time most likely to move the bowels may be helpful.[10,18,21,24]
7. Follow a prescribed bowel regimen to prevent or manage opioid-induced constipation as per the physician's or nurse's instructions.[7,21,24]
8. Report to the physician or nurse any changes in abdomen, stool, ease of defection, or lack of bowel movement for 3 days.
9. Assess the abdomen for bowel sounds, fecal impaction, and possible advancement to bowel obstruction.
10. Treat constipation with laxatives, bowel stimulants, enemas, or manual disimpaction, as required, based on the individual patient.[21,22]
11. Assess untoward effects of interventions such as abdominal cramping and diarrhea.[23]

Nursing Problem: Potential for diarrhea induced by treatment or progression of disease
Expected Outcome: The patient will be without diarrhea, or, if it does occur, it will be minimal.
Nursing Interventions:
1. Assess the patient's baseline bowel habits, concomitant medications, and the possibility of the chemotherapy regimen to induce diarrhea.
2. Teach the patient the dose and schedule of prescribed antidiarrheal medication, monitor to make sure the patient is taking the medications as required, and evaluate their effectiveness.[25]
3. Alter the antidiarrheal regimen, as appropriate.
4. Monitor electrolyte balance, especially potassium and sodium.
5. Advise the patient to document the elimination pattern: precipitating factors, onset of diarrhea, number of episodes, duration of diarrhea, and description of stools (color, consistency, etc.); report abnormalities to the physician or nurse.[25]
6. Assess bowel sounds and abdomen for any signs of abnormality.
7. Teach the patient about dietary and fluid recommendations.[26]
   - Foods and liquids to encourage:
     a. Bland, easily digested foods, such as the BRAT diet: *bananas, white rice, applesauce, toast*; gelatins, yogurt, sherbet; cooked foods at room temperature
     b. Small frequent meals
     c. Water, carbohydrate–electrolyte beverages, clear broth: Increase liquid intake to 2 to 3 quarts per day total.
     d. Such foods as boiled or baked potatoes, pasta, skinless baked chicken, and crackers: Increase these types of foods once diarrhea resolves.

Table 14.1 *Continued*

- Foods and liquids to avoid[26]:
  a. Foods that are raw or high in fiber or roughage
  b. Foods that are rich, seasoned, greasy, or very hot
  c. Milk products and milk, alcohol, caffeinated and very hot beverages
  8. Teach the patient about perianal skin care, sitz baths after each stooling, application of a skin barrier, and topical analgesics.[25]
  9. Assess perianal skin integrity.
  10. Discuss the need for delay or dose modification with the physician.

Symptoms Resulting from Progressive Disease

Nursing Problem: Potential for ascites from advancing disease
Expected Outcome: The patient will demonstrate prompt recognition of possible ascites.
Nursing Interventions:
1. Complete a baseline abdominal examination, noting girth.
2. Instruct the patient to report any changes in breathing; early satiety; abdominal bloating; new, unexplained weight gain; tight-fitting clothes; difficulty walking; and edema.[27–29]
3. Reevaluate the abdomen, noting girth, abdominal distention, bulging flanks, tympany at the upper and midabdominal areas, fluid wave, and shifting dullness.[27,29]
4. Monitor and maintain fluid and electrolyte balance; minimize sodium and fluid intake.[11,27]
5. Assess the patient for peripheral edema; utilize compression stockings and keep the patient's feet and legs elevated; avoid restrictive clothing.
6. Administer therapy to treat the underlying disease.
7. Assist with intermittent paracenteses and monitor for complications with each treatment, such as protein depletion, postural hypotension, electrolyte abnormalities, and infection.[29]
8. Along with the physician, assess the need for a intraperitoneal Tenchkoff catheter for drainage of fluid or peritoneovenous shunting to recirculate ascitic fluid into the intravascular space.[27–29]
9. Initiate pain management strategies, as appropriate.

Nursing Problem: Potential for bowel obstruction from advancing disease
Expected Outcome: The patient will have prompt recognition of alteration in bowel habits.
Nursing Interventions:
1. Assess the patient for signs and symptoms of bowel obstruction: nausea, sporadic vomiting, abdominal pain, worsening constipation, and lack of bowel sounds.[28,30]
2. Explain to the patient with suspected obstruction about the cause and the diagnostic work-up.
3. Initiate antiemetics, stool softeners, and a soft or liquid diet for early bowel obstruction.[7]
4. Intravenous fluids, antiemetics, electrolyte replacement, and nasogastric suctioning are recommended for severe obstruction and vomiting.[7,23]
5. Teach the patient about the rationale of nasogastric suctioning and parental fluids.
6. Assess the patient for complications of bowel obstruction, dehydration, peritonitis, bowel perforation, hypotension, hypovolemia, or septic shock.[23]
7. If appropriate, prepare the patient for surgery (i.e., colectomy, colostomy, gastrointestinal bypass, and gastric or intestinal tube placement).[31]
8. If the patient's cancer is inoperable, a gastrostomy tube or a percutaneous endoscopic gastrostomy tube may be placed for gastric decompression in addition to symptomatic measures to treat pain, nausea, and vomiting.[30]

(continues)

Table 14.1 *Continued*

Nursing Problem: Potential for ureteral obstruction due to advancing disease
Expected Outcome: The patient and a family member will demonstrate care of urinary stents or nephrostomy tubes.
Nursing Interventions:
1. Assess the patient for oliguria and elevated serum creatinine.[28]
2. If ureteral obstruction is suspected, educate the patient about the underlying cause and the diagnostic work-up.
3. Educate the patient about urinary stents or nephrostomy tubes, if inserted.[28,30]
   • Cleanse and dress the site according to hospital policy.
   • Tape tubes securely in place.
   • Assess the site for signs of infection, reduced urinary output, blockage, or bleeding. Report any changes to the physician or nurse.
   • Flush tubes, as ordered, according to hospital policy.
4. Monitor BUN, creatinine, and electrolytes. Notify the physician of abnormalities.[30]

Nursing Problem: Potential for pruritus due to advancing disease
Expected Outcome: The patient will not experience pruritus.
Nursing Interventions:
1. Monitor the patient's bilirubin levels and report abnormalities to the physician.
2. Differentiate between pruritus from an accumulation of bile salts and other etiologies of skin reactions.[28]
3. Administer therapy, as ordered, to treat the underlying malignancy.
4. Encourage the patient to increase fluid intake and to avoid alcohol and smoking.
5. Initiate symptomatic measures to control or prevent the patient's itching.
   • Apply topical anesthetic or corticosteroid preparations, as prescribed.[32]
   • Cholestyramine may relieve pruritus from hepatic abnormalities.[32]
6. Evaluate the effectiveness of the interventions.

Nursing Problem: Potential for pain from advancing disease or as a result of medical procedures
Expected Outcome: The patient will achieve adequate pain control.
Nursing Interventions:
1. Using a consistent assessment tool, assess the patient's pain: onset, location, severity, intensity, duration, and any associated symptoms.[9]
2. Evaluate conditions or interventions that alleviate the discomfort.
3. Initiate appropriate interventions based on assessment.[31]
   • Treat the underlying disease.
   • Diminish the emotional or reactive component of the patient's pain (e.g., relaxation, imagery).
   • Change the patient's perception or sensation of pain (e.g., analgesics, nerve blocks, neurosurgical procedures, acupressure, acupuncture).
4. Administer analgesics and routine and rescue medications on schedule, as prescribed. Morphine sulfate is the drug of choice for severe pain.[7]
5. Premedicate the patient with pain medication prior to a medical procedure.
6. Educate the patient about the common side effects of most pain regimens—constipation, dry mouth, drowsiness, nausea or vomiting, sedation, and respiratory depression—and self-care measures to treat them.[9]
7. Utilize nonpharmacologic methods to reduce pain: heat and cold, rest, music therapy, humor therapy, hypnosis, acupuncture, progressive muscle relaxation, guided imagery, and distraction.[7,9]
8. Evaluate the effectiveness of the interventions and alter the plan of care, as needed.

Table 14.1 *Continued*

Nursing Problem: Potential for thrombophlebitis and pulmonary embolism related to advancing disease process
  Expected Outcome: The patient will not develop deep vein thrombosis (DVT) or a pulmonary embolism.
  Nursing Interventions:
  1. Determine the patient's risk of developing DVT.[33] Risk increased with:
     • Diagnosis of colon or rectal cancer
     • Sedentary lifestyle
     • History of abnormalities in clotting or previous DVT
     • Injury or trauma to vasculature or extremity
     • Treatment used to treat malignancy (e.g., abdominal surgery, chemotherapy)
     • History of cigarette smoking
  2. Assess the patient for chest pain and/or shortness of breath.
  3. Assess the patient's calf for signs of thrombosis[33]:
     • Warmth
     • Pain
     • Redness
     • Unilateral swelling or edema
     • Positive Homans' sign (pain with flexion of the lower calf and dorsal flexing of the ankle)[33]
  4. Instruct the patient to wear antiembolism stockings when in bed and to perform leg exercises.
  5. Encourage regular exercise and ambulation to prevent stasis.
  6. Educate the patient about the radiographic work-up if DVT is suspected.
  7. Administer anticoagulant therapy, as prescribed, paying particular attention to dosing at consistent times, while monitoring coagulation parameters.
  8. Educate the patient about self-injection of anticoagulant therapy while at home.
  9. Assess the patient's compliance with prescribed interventions.

Nursing Problem: Potential for fear and anxiety related to progressing disease
  Expected Outcome: The patient will verbalize feelings about the probability and outcomes of disease progression.
  Nursing Interventions:
  1. Establish a trusting relationship with the patient.
  2. Assess the patient's levels of fear, anxiety, and psychosocial worries by asking general therapeutic questions, such as, "What are your concerns about your illness?"[34]
  3. Listen to and acknowledge the patient's and family's struggles and concerns about disease recurrence, further metastatic spread, how long he or she might live, and what will happen to their family in the future.[19,34]
  4. Determine the patient's and the family's perception of the disease to clarify misconceptions and develop realistic goals.[34]
  5. Assure the patient that he or she will receive palliative therapies, as appropriate.[19]
  6. Provide emotional support, consulting with a social worker and other healthcare providers, as needed.
  7. Encourage the patient to verbalize his or her feelings; emotion-focused coping mechanisms are more helpful than problem-focused coping mechanisms when little can be done to change the situation.[35]
  8. Assist the patient in managing emotional stress and maintaining equilibrium.[35]
  9. Refer the patient to professional counseling, as appropriate.

(continues)

Table 14.1   *Continued*

---

10. Provide and/or refer the patient for spiritual care and support.[19]
11. Encourage the patient to get his or her affairs "in order" legally.
12. Initiate a referral for a visiting nurse, home health aide, and hospice, as appropriate.

Miscellaneous Symptoms

Nursing Problem: Potential for alopecia induced by treatment
  Expected Outcome: The patient will verbalize feelings about hair loss and identify measures and resources to manage alteration in body image.
  Nursing Interventions:
  1. Educate the patient about the expected timing of hair loss, usually 10 to 21 days after the initiation of treatment.[10]
  2. Reinforce that hair loss is temporary, that it may involve thinning of body hair (eyebrows, eyelashes, facial hair, and pubic hair), and that hair will regrow at completion of the treatment plan.
  3. Encourage the patient to purchase head coverings—for example, wigs, caps, scarves, bandanas—prior to hair loss, to minimize the impact.[36]
  4. Head coverings should be worn year-round to protect the skin from sunburn in the summer and heat loss in the winter.[18]
  5. Encourage the patient to apply eyebrow pencil or false eyelashes, if helpful.[37]
  6. Educate the patient to avoid excessive or harsh hair treatments: chemical treatments (hair dye, bleach, permanent solutions), electric hair drying, curling irons, elastics, frequent shampoos, and excessive hair manipulation.[10,37]
  7. Encourage the patient to verbalize his or her feelings about hair loss, and provide emotional support.

Nursing Problem: Potential for fatigue from treatment or progressive disease
  Expected Outcome: The patient will maintain his or her activity level.
  Nursing Interventions:
  1. Assess the possible etiologies of fatigue, such as anemia, pain, emotional distress, insomnia, nutritional alterations, therapeutic regimen, and presence of advanced disease.[38]
  2. Develop a trusting relationship with the patient, so that he or she will discuss perceptions of fatigue openly.
  3. If there is a "treatable" etiology of the fatigue (e.g., anemia), prescribe treatment based on the underlying cause, and evaluate its effectiveness.[39]
  4. Teach the patient to rest, as needed, throughout the day, yet maintain normal bedtime patterns and rituals.[39]
  5. Encourage an individualized exercise program.[38]
  6. Instruct the patient to eat foods high in iron, such as liver, eggs, carrots, and raisins.[18]
  7. Advise the patient to do the following[40,41]:
     • Pace activities throughout day, avoiding overexertion.
     • Schedule the most important activities at times of maximal energy levels.
     • Delegate activities and responsibilities to family members and friends.
     • Create strategies to overcome "energy drainers": for example, eliminate stair climbing; get assistance, as needed, with personal hygiene and dressing; and allow friends and family members to prepare meals and do laundry.[39]
  8. Initiate a referral for a visiting nurse and home health aide, as appropriate.

Table 14.1 *Continued*

Nursing Problem: Potential alteration in sexual function related to disease process and/or treatment
  Expected Outcome: The patient will express feelings about the potential of sexual dysfunction due
  to disease or treatment. The patient will identify strategies and resources to minimize the adverse
  impact on his or her life. The patient and significant other will verbalize that they have achieved
  satisfactory sexual relations.
  Nursing Interventions:
  1. Establish a trusting relationship with the patient so as to maintain open lines of communication.
  2. Conduct a sexual history to establish a baseline status.
  3. Assess the patient's knowledge of the potential adverse effects of the colon or rectal cancer
      itself and/or its treatment on sexual function.[42]
  4. Review with the patient and significant other the potential alterations in sexual function that
      may occur because of the disease and the treatment.[43]
  5. Discuss behavioral strategies to minimize dysfunction.[44]
      • Create a sensual environment.
      • Explore alternative forms of sexual expression.
      • Use mechanical devices.
      • Use vaginal lubricants.
  6. Refer the patient and significant other for reproductive counseling, as appropriate.[42]

Conclusion

It is important that nurses strive to overcome barriers to symptom management. Basic research is needed to delineate the symptom, the distress it may cause, usual patterns, and the underlying pathophysiology. Until such research is available, patient assessment and therapeutic interventions must be complete and reevaluation must be frequent. This must be a dynamic process. The effective management of the symptoms associated with advanced colorectal cancer is derived from many sources, including a working knowledge of evidence-based interventions (where available), creativity, and an appreciation of the concepts associated with caregiver burden and patients' struggles with self-care. Additional tenets guide the approach to the management of symptoms associated with colorectal cancer. The nurse needs to take into consideration issues of cultural diversity and the wishes and goals of the patient.

While some of the interventions described in the prior nursing-care plans are not particularly dramatic (e.g., the use of mints, hard candy, or cough drops as a means of temporarily relieving taste changes), they do provide increased comfort. These interventions are limited largely to anecdotal and descriptive data, but when implemented on an individual basis, they do contribute to a reduction in distress. Most of all, they may decrease the stress of family caregivers who feel helpless as they attempt to do anything that will help their loved one eat.

In terms of cultural diversity, it is important to keep an open mind and to know the customs of the patient's culture. For example, a Korean patient cared for by one of the authors requested a traditional dish, Kim Chee. On the surface, this does not seem like an unusual request, except that the patient was experiencing moderate to severe mucositis. Kim Chee is a very spicy dish of fermented cabbage and hot red peppers. To the nurse, the spiciness of this food seemed a counterintuitive strategy in the setting of oral ulceration. To the patient, it was soothing, providing a decrease in her distress.

Clinical experience indicates that individual variations in symptomatology occur. Among the least helpful statements anecdotally reported by patients is to hear their healthcare provider utter phrases such as, "We don't usually see these types of problems with this regimen or protocol." For the individual or family member who remembers each and every conversation with providers and then proceeds to look for a hidden prognostic meaning, being labeled "different" from others with a similar disease is a source of great concern. It is also important to remember that the effective management of colorectal cancer–related symptoms is dependent on the management of concomitant conditions. For example, interventions for nausea and vomiting (arising from causes other than chemotherapy administration) should be developed within a framework that appreciates the cascade effect of taste changes, anorexia, nausea, and constipation.

As noted in the opening paragraph of this chapter, perhaps the most basic approach to the management of symptoms associated with colorectal cancer is the most challenging. Ferrell and colleagues[45] identified six themes that patients felt physicians and nurses should address to improve their care:

- Be accessible.
- Discover a cure.
- Provide support groups.
- Reinforce current education.
- Provide additional coping strategies.
- Increase patient participation in decision making.

Though this study was conducted with bone marrow transplant survivors, this list is applicable to any cancer patient. This study validated the need for nurses to be active with their patients throughout the patients' cancer experience and to be aware of the struggles that patients are facing every day.[45] Nurses are in a unique position to accomplish these six themes. We just need to remember that no matter how busy we are or how bad our day is, the patient surviving with cancer is facing a serious, probably life-threatening illness. By taking time to listen, being empathetic, and trying to provide the best physical and psychological care possible, we can make a great difference in the life of a patient.

References

1. Hogan CM. Cancer nursing: The art of symptom management. Oncol Nurs Forum. 1997; 24(8): 1335–1340.
2. Rhodes VA, McDaniel RW. The symptom experience and its impact on quality of life. In: Yarbo CH, Hansen MH, Goodman M, et al., eds. Cancer Symptom Management, 2nd ed. Sudbury, MA: Jones and Bartlett Publishers, 1999: 3–9.
3. National Cancer Institute Common Toxicity Criteria, Version 2.1999. Available at http://ctep .info.nih.gov/CTC3/ctc.htm Accessed March 1, 2001.
4. Rhodes VA, Watson PM. Symptom distress— the concept: Past and present. Semin Oncol Nurs. 1987; 3:242–247.
5. Holland JC. Standards for psychosocial cancer care under development. National Cancer Centers Network. Oncol News Int. 1999; 8(12). Available at www.cancernetwork.com Accessed March 1, 2001.
6. Wickham RS. Nausea and vomiting. In: Yasko JM, ed. Nursing Management of Symptoms Associated with Chemotherapy, 5th ed. West Conshohocken, PA: Meniscus Limited, 2001: 85–94
7. Crowley MJ. Symptom management and supportive care: Dying and death. In: Itano JK, Taoka KN, eds. Core Curriculum for Oncology Nursing, 3rd ed. Philadelphia, PA: W. B. Saunders Company, 1998: 96–114.
8. Wickham R. Nausea and vomiting. In: Groenwald SL, Frogge MH, Goodman M, et al., eds.

Cancer Symptom Management. Sudbury, MA: Jones and Bartlett Publishers, 1996: 218–251.

9. Swenson CJ. Pain management. In: Otto SE, ed. Oncology Nursing, 3rd ed. St. Louis, MO: Mosby, 1997: 746–785

10. Langhorne M. Chemotherapy. In: Otto SE, ed. Oncology Nursing, 3rd ed. St. Louis, MO: Mosby, 1997: 530–572

11. Berendt MC. Alterations in nutrition. In: Itano JK, Taoka KN, eds. Core Curriculum for Oncology Nursing, 3rd ed. Philadelphia, PA: W. B. Saunders Company, 1998: 223–258.

12. Miller SE. Oral and esophageal mucositis. In: Yasko JM, ed. Nursing Management of Symptoms Associated with Chemotherapy, 5th ed. West Conshohocken, PA: Meniscus Limited, 2001: 71–84.

13. Beck SL. Mucositis. In: Groenwald SL, Frogge MH, Goodman M, et al., eds. Cancer Symptom Management. Sudbury, MA: Jones and Bartlett Publishers, 1996: 308–323.

14. Wickham RS, Rehwaldt M, Kefer C, et al. Taste changes experienced by patients receiving chemotherapy. Oncol Nurs Forum. 1999; 26(4): 697–706.

15. Rust DM, Kogut VJ. Anorexia and cachexia. In: Yasko JM, ed. Nursing Management of Symptoms Associated with Chemotherapy, 5th ed. West Conshohocken, PA: Meniscus Limited, 2001: 41–62.

16. Tait NS. Anorexia–cachexia syndrome. In: Groenwald SL, Frogge MH, Goodman M, et al., eds. Cancer Symptom Management. Sudbury, MA: Jones and Bartlett Publishers, 1996: 171–196.

17. Rosenzweig MQ. Taste alterations. In: Yasko JM, ed. Nursing Management of Symptoms Associated with Chemotherapy, 5th ed. West Conshohocken, PA: Meniscus Limited, 2001: 63–70.

18. Burke MB, Wilkes CM, Ingwersen K. Cancer Chemotherapy: A Nursing Process Approach, 2nd ed. Sudbury, MA: Jones and Bartlett Publishers, 1996.

19. Brant JM. The art of palliative care: Living with hope, dying with dignity. Oncol Nurs Forum. 1998; 25(6):995–1004.

20. Murphy ME. Colorectal cancers. In: Otto SE, ed. Oncology Nursing, 3rd ed. St. Louis, MO: Mosby. 1997: 124–139.

21. Lin EM. Constipation. In: Yasko JM, ed. Nursing Management of Symptoms Associated with Chemotherapy, 5th ed. West Conshohocken, PA: Meniscus Limited, 2001: 95–108.

22. Curtis CP. Constipation. In: Groenwald SL, Frogge MH, Goodman M, et al., eds. Cancer Symptom Management. Sudbury, MA: Jones and Bartlett Publishers, 1996: 484–497.

23. Kuck AW, Ricciardi E. Alterations in elimination. In: Itano JK, Taoka KN, eds. Core Curriculum for Oncology Nursing, 3rd ed. Philadelphia, PA: W. B. Saunders Company, 1998; 259–278.

24. Camp-Sorrell D. Chemotherapy: Toxicity management. In: Yarbro CH, Frogge MH, Goodman M, et al, eds. Cancer Nursing Principles and Practice, 5th ed. Sudbury, MA: Jones and Bartlett Publishers, 2000: 444–486.

25. Berg DT. Diarrhea. In: Yasko JM, ed. Nursing Management of Symptoms Associated with Chemotherapy, 5th ed. West Conshohocken, PA: Meniscus Limited, 2001: 109–130.

26. Martz CH. Diarrhea. In: Groenwald SL, Frogge MH, Goodman M, et al., eds. Cancer Symptom Management. Sudbury, MA: Jones and Bartlett Publishers, 1996: 498–520.

27. Walczak JR, Heckman CS. Ascites. In: Groenwald SL, Frogge MH, Goodman M, et al., eds. Cancer Symptom Management. Sudbury, MA: Jones and Bartlett Publishers, 1996: 385–398.

28. Groenwald SL, Frogge MH, Goodman M, et al. Comprehensive Cancer Nursing Review. Sudbury, MA: Jones and Bartlett Publishers, 1998.

29. Works C, Maxwell MB. Malignant effusions and edemas. In: Yarbro CH, Frogge MH, Goodman M, et al., eds. Cancer Nursing Principles and Practice, 5th ed. Sudbury, MA: Jones and Bartlett Publishers, 2000: 813–830.

30. Ellis C, Saddler DAH. Colorectal cancer. In:

Yarbro CH, Frogge MH, Goodman M, et al., eds. Cancer Nursing Principles and Practice, 5th ed. Sudbury, MA: Jones and Bartlett Publishers, 2000: 1117–1137.

31. Polomano RC, McGuire DB, Sheidler VR. Management of cancer pain. In: Yarbro CH, Frogge MH, Goodman M, et al., eds. Cancer Nursing Principles and Practice, 5th ed. Sudbury, MA: Jones and Bartlett Publishers, 2000: 657–690.

32. Seiz AL, Yarbro CH. Pruritus. In: Groenwald SL, Frogge MH, Goodman M, et al., eds. Cancer Symptom Management. Sudbury, MA: Jones and Bartlett Publishers, 1996: 137–150.

33. Viale PH. Management of thromboembolism in patients with cancer. Oncol Nurs Forum. 1999; 26(10):1625–1632.

34. Klemm P, Miller MA, Fernsler J. Demands of illness in people treated for colorectal cancer. Oncol Nurs Forum. 2000; 27(4):633–639.

35. Zabalegui A. Coping strategies and psychological distress in patients with advanced cancer. Oncol Nurs Forum. 1999; 26(9):1511–1518.

36. Howser DM. Alopecia. In: Groenwald SL, Frogge MH, Goodman M, et al., eds. Cancer Symptom Management. Sudbury, MA: Jones and Bartlett Publishers, 1996: 261–268.

37. Chernecky CC. Alopecia. In: Yasko JM, ed. Nursing Management of Symptoms Associated with Chemotherapy, 5th ed. West Conshohocken, PA: Meniscus Limited, 2001: 181–190.

38. McDaniel RW, Rhodes VA. Fatigue. In: Yarbro CH, Frogge MH, Goodman M, et al., eds. Cancer Nursing Principles and Practice, 5th ed. Sudbury, MA: Jones and Bartlett Publishers, 2000: 737–753.

39. Madeya ML. Fatigue. In: Yasko JM, ed. Nursing Management of Symptoms Associated with Chemotherapy, 5th ed. West Conshohocken, PA: Meniscus Limited, 2001: 131–144.

40. Winningham ML. Fatigue. In: Groenwald SL, Frogge MH, Goodman M, et al., eds. Cancer Symptom Management. Sudbury, MA: Jones and Bartlett Publishers, 1996: 42–58.

41. Barnett ML. Fatigue. In: Otto SE, ed. Oncology Nursing, 3rd ed. St. Louis, MO: Mosby, 1997: 669–678.

42. Krebs LU. Sexual and reproductive dysfunction. In: Yarbro CH, Frogge MH, Goodman M, et al., eds. Cancer Nursing Principles and Practice, 5th ed. Sudbury, MA: Jones and Bartlett Publishers, 2000: 831–856.

43. Krebs LU. Sexuality and reproductive issues. In: Yasko JM, ed. Nursing Management of Symptoms Associated with Chemotherapy, 5th ed. West Conshohocken, PA: Meniscus Limited, 2001: 205–214.

44. Nishimoto PW. Sexuality. In: Itano JK, Taoka KN, eds. Core Curriculum for Oncology Nursing, 3rd ed. Philadelphia, PA: W. B. Saunders Company, 1998: 85–95.

45. Ferrell B, Grant M, Schmidt GM, et al. The meaning of quality of life for bone marrow transplant survivors. Part 2: Improving quality of life for bone marrow transplant survivors. Cancer Nurs. 1992; 15(4):247–253.

CHAPTER 15

Colorectal Cancer Resources for Patients, Families, and Professionals

Deborah T. Berg, RN, BSN

Introduction

This resource section is designed to help patients, families, and health professionals find information about colorectal cancer. The resources listed here represent a variety of options. It is not an exhaustive listing; rather, it is representative of the information available both in print and on the Internet. Some of the materials listed are free upon request, while others are for sale by publishing companies.

Early Detection and Screening Information

There is a growing body of evidence speaking to the importance of early detection and screening of colorectal cancer. It is important that the public become aware of this issue, both through public announcements and from their primary care providers.

Books

Title: *50 Ways to Prevent Colon Cancer*
Author: M. Sara Rosenthal
Source: Lowell House, 2000 (ISBN: 0737304596)
Cost: $13.95
Topics:
- Suggestions for people interested in cancer prevention and wellness in general
- Functions and malfunctions of the colon
- Examinations and prevention methods
- Selecting foods and fibers for optimal colon health

Title: *Colon Cancer and the Polyps Connection*
Authors: Stephen Fisher, David Fisher, and Robert D. Tufft
Source: Fischer Books (ISBN: 1555610803)
Cost: $16.95
Written by a colon cancer survivor and participant in the National Polyp Prevention Clinical Trial.
Topics:
  • How the colon works
  • Polyps and colon cancer
  • Symptoms
  • Early detection and screening
  • Diagnostic procedures and treatment
  • Finding the right doctor and hospital
  • Prevention through diet

Title: *Tell Me What to Eat to Help Prevent Colon Cancer*
Author: Elaine Magee, MPH, RD
Source: New Page Books, 2001 (ISBN: 156414514X)
Cost: $9.89
Written by a registered dietician.
Topics: Review of foods and how they may prevent colon cancer.

Other Materials

Title: *Colorectal Cancer Fact Sheet*
Source: American Digestive Health Foundation
www.gastro.org/adhf/co/canc2.html

Title: *Managed Care Organization Kit*
Source: American Digestive Health Foundation
www.Gastro.org/adhf/cc-letter.html
(301) 941-9786

Title: *Medicare Preventive Services Benefits*
Source: United States Government
www.medicare.gov/health/overview.asp

Title: *Screen for Life: National Colorectal Cancer Action Campaign*

Source: Centers for Disease Control and Prevention
www.cdc.gov/cancer/screenforlife/index.htm
(800) 311-3435

Title: *Women & Colorectal Cancer: What Are the Facts?*
Source: American Digestive Health Foundation
(800) 668-5237

Information Regarding Cancer, Colorectal Cancer, Diagnosis, and Treatment Options

Once the diagnosis of colorectal cancer has been made, patients and their families need to receive information as to how to proceed next. Treatment options, clinical trials, and side-effect management strategies are all crucial education elements and will vary depending on the stage of disease at the time of diagnosis. Treatment options are frequently presented to patients by their surgeon, primary care provider, or medical oncologist. The nurse is often in a position to help patients understand the information and to answer any questions. The following list of resources provides information on general cancer topics and on issues specific to colorectal cancer.

Pamphlets: General Cancer

Title: *After Diagnosis: Common Questions and Expectations*
Source: American Cancer Society (Publication #0406)
(800) ACS-2345
Cost: Free

Title: *Cancer Terms: A Guide for Your Patients with Cancer*
Source: Pharmacia, Inc.
Cost: Free

Title: *Chemotherapy and You*
Source: National Cancer Institute (NIH publication #94-1136)
(800) 4-CANCER
Cost: Free

Title: *Radiation Therapy and You*
Source: National Cancer Institute (NIH publication #95-2227)
(800) 4-CANCER
Cost: Free

Title: *Taking Part in Clinical Trials: What Patients Need to Know*
Source: National Institutes of Health
(800) 4-CANCER
Cost: Free

Title: *Tumor Markers: A Guide for Your Patients with Cancer*
Source: Pharmacia, Corp.
Cost: Free

Title: *What You Need to Know about Cancer*
Source: National Cancer Institute
Cost: Free

Books: Cancer in General

Title: *50 Essential Things to Do When the Doctor Says It's Cancer*
Source: Plume, 1993; revised 1999 (ISBN: 0452269547)
Cost: $11.95
Written by a cancer survivor.
Topics:
 • Holistic approach to living with cancer
 • Determining your treatment program
 • Healing your lifestyle
 • Healing with your mind
 • Total wellness

Title: *2001 Oncology Nursing Drug Handbook*
Authors: Gail Wilkes, Karen Ingwersen, and Margaret Barton-Burke
Source: Jones and Bartlett Publishers, 2000 (ISBN: 076371478x)
Cost: $52.95
Topics: Covers drugs used in chemotherapy and side-effect management.

Title: *Cancer Clinical Trials Experimental Treatments and How They Can Help You*
Author: Robert Finn
Source: O'Reilly & Associates, Inc., 1999 (ISBN: 1-56592-566-1)
Cost: $14.95
Topics:
 • Reasons to participate in clinical trials
 • Clinical trial regulations and guidelines
 • The informed consent document
 • Understanding what is involved

Title: *Cancer Facts and Figures—2000*
Source: American Cancer Society
Cost: Free
Topics:
 • Facts and general information
 • Early detection
 • Psychosocial and support services
 • Treatment options

Title: *Cancer Management. A Multidisciplinary Approach: Medical, Surgical, and Radiation Oncology*
Author: Richard Pazdur, MD, ed.
Source: Publisher Research and Representation, 2000 (ISBN: 1891483056)
Cost: $49.95
Topics:
 • Medical textbook covering the screening, diagnosis, staging, and treatment of cancer, including colorectal cancer
 • Patient management section

Title: *Cancer Nursing Principles and Practice, 5th ed.*

Authors: Connie H. Yarbro, Margaret H. Frogge, Michelle Goodman, and Susan L. Groenwald, eds.

Source: Jones and Bartlett Publishers, 2000 (ISBN: 0763711640)

Cost: $138.95

Topics: Nursing textbook covering the screening, diagnosis, staging, treatment, and patient management of cancer patients.

Title: *Cancer Treatments Your Insurance Should Cover*

Source: Association of Community Cancer Centers, cosponsored by the Oncology Nursing Society and the National Coalition for Cancer Survivorship

Cost: Free

Topics:
- Payment denials
- Steps to obtain coverage
- Steps to reverse denials

Title: *The Activist Cancer Patient: How to Take Charge of Your Treatment*

Authors: Beverly Zakarian and Ezra M. Greenspan, MD

Source: John Wiley & Sons, 1996 (ISBN: 047112026X)

Cost: $15.95

Written by a cancer survivor and an oncology physician.

Topics:
- Case studies, personal stories, and the author's own experiences to illustrate how to take an active role in treatment
- Guidance on finding state-of-art and experimental therapies

Title: *The Cancer Dictionary*

Authors: Roberta Altman and Michael J. Sarg, MD

Source: Checkmark Books, 1999 (ISBN: 0816039542)

Cost: $19.95

Topics: A dictionary with listings on cancer symptoms, procedures, drugs, side effects, risk factors, diagnostic tests, and prevention.

Title: *The Chemotherapy & Radiation Therapy Survival Guide*

Authors: Judith McKay, RN, OCN, and Nancee Hirano, RN, MS, AOCN

Source: New Harbinger Publications, Inc., 1998 (ISBN: 1-57224-070-9)

Cost: $14.95

Written by two oncology nurses.

Topics:
- Chemotherapy and radiation therapy, including a listing of the drugs commonly associated with treatment
- Review of blood tests
- Coping with side effects and practical survival techniques
- Dealing with changes in sexuality and fertility
- Relaxation and stress-reduction techniques

Pamphlets: Colorectal Cancer

Title: *What You Need to Know about Cancer of the Colon and Rectum*

Source: National Cancer Institute (NIH publication #98-1552)

(800) 4-CANCER

Cost: Free

Books: Colorectal Cancer

Title: *Colon and Rectal Cancer*

Author: Peter S. Edelstein, ed.

Source: John Wiley & Sons, 2000 (ISBN: 0471351458)

Cost: $95.00

Topics: Clinician's guide to recent improvements in diagnosis, treatment, and follow-up.

Title: *Colon and Rectal Cancer: A Complete Guide for Patients and Families*
Author: Lorraine Johnston
Source: O'Reilly and Associates, Inc., 1999 (ISBN: 1-56592-633-1)
Cost: $24.95 (U.S.); $36.95 (Canada)
Topics:
- Colorectal cancer and its prognosis
- Symptoms, testing, diagnosis, and staging
- Treatments and clinical trials
- How to find a doctor and treatment facility
- What to expect from different treatment options
- Coping with side effects
- Dealing with stress, support, insurance, employment, and financial issues
- Life after treatment, including late effects and disease recurrence

Title: *Colorectal Cancer: A Thorough and Compassionate Resource for Patients and Their Families*
Author: Bernard Levin, MD
Source: Random House, 1999 (ISBN: 0679778136)
Cost: $14.95
Topics:
- Colorectal cancer development
- Screening and early detection
- Staging
- Treatment options: surgery, chemotherapy, and radiation therapy
- Prevention of disease with diet
- American Cancer Society Recommendations for Nutrition and Cancer Prevention

Title: *Myths and Facts about Colorectal Cancer*
Authors: Richard Padzur, MD, and Melanie Royce, MD
Source: Unknown, 1998 (ISBN: 0964182394)
Cost: $9.95

Written by two medical oncologists.
Topics:
- Colorectal cancer and its causes
- Detection and diagnosis
- Colorectal cancer treatment
- Follow-up care of patients
- Coping with the diagnosis
- Resources and glossary

Title: *Sexuality and Fertility after Cancer*
Author: Leslie Schover, PhD
Source: John Wiley & Sons, 1997 (ISBN: 0-471-18194-3)
Cost: $15.95
Written by a clinical psychologist and sex therapist.
Topics:
- Resource for colon cancer survivors facing sexual issues before, during, and after treatment
- Possible sexual and psychosexual changes during diagnosis and treatment
- Physical and emotional feelings regarding the cancer diagnosis
- Communication
- Specific physiologic sexual problems and how to resolve them
- Fertility and pregnancy

Title: *The Complete Cancer Survival Guide*
Authors: Peter Teeley and Philip Bashe
Source: Main Street Books, 2000 (ISBN: 0385486057)
Cost: $19.95
Written by a colon cancer survivor (with assistance).
Topics:
- Review of the 25 most common types of cancers
- Staging, diagnosis, treatment options, and quality-of-life issues
- Second opinions
- Where to get care
- What to expect during treatment

- Controlling symptoms, side effects, and complications
- Emotional health
- Support systems
- How to handle insurance, finances, and employment issues

Title: *The Ostomy Book: Living Comfortably with Colostomies, Ileostomies, and Urostomies*
Authors: Barbara Dorr Mullen and Kerry Ann McGinn
Source: Bull Publishing, Co., Palo Alto, CA, 1992 (ISBN: 0-923521127)
Cost: $16.95
Written by an ostomate and registered nurse.
Topics:
- Medical, practical, and psychological information for people living with ostomies
- Descriptions of different surgical procedures and ostomy supplies
- Illustrations, resources, and glossary

Title: *The Wellness Community Guide to Fighting for Recovery from Cancer*
Author: Harold H. Benjamin, PhD
Source: Putnam, 1995
Cost: $7.50
Topics: Information on overcoming the cancer experience.

Title: *What to Do if You Get Colon Cancer: A Specialist Helps You Take Charge and Make Informed Choices*
Authors: Paul Miskovitz, MD, and Marian Betancourt
Source: John Wiley & Sons, 1997 (ISBN: 0-471-15984-0)
Cost: $15.95
Topics:
- Overview of colorectal cancer
- Risk factors and symptoms
- Diagnosis and staging

- Selecting a physician and treatment center
- Finding emotional support
- Treatment options: surgery, chemotherapy, and radiation therapy
- Recovery and follow-up care

Personal Accounts

Title: *Don't Die of Embarrassment: Life after Colostomy and Other Adventures*
Author: Barbara Barrie
Source: Fireside, 1999 (ISBN: 0684846241)
Cost: $12.00
Topics: First-hand account of the author's experience with colon cancer.

Title: *Recovering Life*
Authors: Charisse and Darryl Strawberry
Source: Plough Publishing, 1999 (ISBN: 0874869889)
Cost: $25.00
Topics: Conversation with Darryle Strawberry and his wife about his experience with colon cancer.

Titles: *Second Act: Life after Colostomy and Other Adventures*
Author: Barbara Barrie
Source: Scribner, 1997 (ISBN: 0684835878)
Cost: $23.00
Topics: Candid discussion about the author's battle with colon cancer and a colostomy.

Diet and Nutrition

Pamphlets

Title: *Eating Hints for Cancer Patients*
Author/Source: National Cancer Institute
Cost: Free

Books

Title: *The Cancer Survival Cookbook*
Author: Donna L. Weilhofen, RD
Source: John Wiley and Sons, 1997 (ISBN: 0471346683)
Cost: $16.95
Written by a nutritionist.
Topics:
- Practical eating hints
- Cancer-fighting fruits and vegetables
- Neutropenic precautions diet
- Recipes

Psychosocial Support Resources

Pamphlets

Title: *Caring for the Patient with Cancer at Home: A Guide for Patients and Families*
Source: American Cancer Society (Publication #4645)
(800) ACS-2345
Cost: Free

Title: *Facing Forward: A Guide for Cancer Survivors*
Source: National Cancer Institute (NIH publication # 94-2424)
(800) 4-CANCER
Cost: Free

Title: *It Helps to Have Friends When Mom or Dad Has Cancer*
Author: Carol Lindberg
Source: American Cancer Society (Publication #4654)
(800) ACS-2345
Cost: Free

Title: *Listen with Your Heart—Talking with the Cancer Patient*
Author/Source: American Cancer Society (Publication #4557)
(800) ACS-2345
Cost: Free

Title: *Sexuality and Cancer: For the Woman Who Has Cancer and Her Partner* and *Sexuality and Cancer: For the Man Who Has Cancer and His Partner*
Source: American Cancer Society
(800) ACS-2345
Cost: Free

Title: *Taking Time: Support for People with Cancer and the People Who Care about Them*
Source: National Cancer Institute (NIH Publication #98-2059)
(800) 4-CANCER
Cost: Free

Title: *What about Me? A Booklet for Teenage Children of Cancer Patients*
Author: Linda Leopold Strass
Source: Cancer Family Care, Inc.
(513) 731-3346

Title: *When Someone in Your Family Has Cancer*
Source: National Cancer Institute (NIH Publication #96-2685)
(800) 4-CANCER
Cost: Free

Books

Title: *The Paper Chain*
Author: Claire Blake
Source: Health Pr. (ISBN: 0923173287)
Cost: $8.95
Topics: Story to help young children understand their parent's cancer diagnosis and treatment.

Title: *When Life Becomes Precious: A Guide for Loved Ones and Friends of Cancer Patients*
Author: Elise Needell Babcock
Source: Bantam Books, 1997 (ISBN: 0553378694)
Cost: $14.95

Topics:
- How to interact with cancer patients
- Resources for patients, their partners, and family members
- Understanding your feelings when a family member is diagnosed with cancer
- Giving without giving out
- How to ask the physician to speak in lay terms

Audiovisual Materials

Title: *Cancer Survival Toolbox*
Source: National Coalition for Cancer Survivorship, cosponsored by the Oncology Nursing Society
Call (301) 206-9789 or (301) 650-9127 to order
Cost: Free
Content: Six audiotapes discussing communication, information finding, decision making, problem solving, negotiating, and your rights.

Title: *Kids Tell Kids What It's Like When Their Brother or Sister Has Cancer*
Source: Cancervive
(800) 4-TO-CURE
Cost: Free
Content: Videotape of children talking about how it feels to have a sibling with cancer.

Title: *Kids Tell Kids What It's Like When Their Mother or Father Has Cancer*
Source: Cancervive
(800) 4-TO-CURE
Cost: Free
Content: Videotape of children talking about how it feels to have a parent have cancer.

Title: *Screening for Colorectal Cancer: An Easy Step to Save Your Life* (video)
Source: American Digestive Health Foundation
Call (800) 668-5237 to order

Content:
- Profiles people who have been screened for colorectal cancer
- Value of screening
- Who and when to be screened

Title: *Spouse to Spouse. What It's Like When Your Partner Has Cancer*
Source: Cancervive
(800) 4-TO-CURE
Cost: Free
Content: Profiles couples talking about what it is like when your spouse has cancer.

Resources for Colorectal Cancer Information

There are many organizations that can provide information on cancer in general and colorectal cancer in particular. The types of organizations listed here provide a variety of services, from professional-only publications to public awareness services. Each listing includes a short statement about the organization's interests and services.

American Association for Cancer Research
Public Ledger Building, Suite 816
150 South Independence Mall West
Philadelphia, PA 19106-3483
(800) 477-7127; (215) 440-9300
Web site address: www.aacr.org
Supports public awareness of opportunities in cancer research.

American Cancer Society
National Headquarters
1599 Clifton Road, NE
Atlanta, GA 30309
(800) ACS-2345
Web site address: www.cancer.org
Local chapters listed in telephone book

Provides patient educational materials, support programs, prevention and cancer awareness information, and treatment center referrals. Cancer Profiler, a new tool to help determine the best treatment option.

American College of Gastroenterology
4900B South 31st Street
Arlington, VA 22206
(703) 820-7400
Web site address: www.acg.gi.org
Provides information and referrals regarding colorectal cancer and other digestive conditions.

American College of Radiology
1891 Preston White Drive
Reston, VA 20191
(800) ACR-LINE (800-227-5463)
Web site address: www.acr.org
E-mail address: info@acr.org
Provides information about current developments in diagnostic and therapeutic radiation.

American College of Surgeons
633 North Saint Clair Street
Chicago, IL 60611-3211
(312) 202-5000
Web site address: www.facs.org
E-mail address: postmaster@facs.org
Public information about issues related to surgery, finding a surgeon, second opinions, cost issues, and surgeon credentials. Links to the National Cancer Data Base and other cancer organizations.

American Digestive Health Foundation
7910 Woodmont Avenue, Suite 700
Bethesda, MD 20814-3015
(301) 654-2635
Web site address: www.gastro.org
E-mail address: dlee@gastro.org
Provides education information about colo-

rectal cancer and other disorders of the gastrointestinal tract.

American Institute for Cancer Research
1759 R Street, NW
Washington, DC 20009
(800) 843-8114
Web site address: www.aicr.org
Supports cancer research; provides educational materials on nutrition and cancer.

American Society of Clinical Oncology
225 Reinekers Lane, Suite 650
Alexandria, VA 22314
(703) 299-0150
Web site address: www.asco.org
E-mail address: asco@asco.org
National organization for oncologists and researchers worldwide; supports cancer research in prevention, treatment, and supportive care; provides educational programs and materials; cancer information available to the public through the Internet; published the "Recommendations for Colorectal Cancer Surveillance Guidelines by the American Society of Clinical Oncology."

American Society of Colon and Rectal Surgeons
85 W. Algonquin Road, Suite 550
Arlington Heights, IL 60005
(847) 290-9184
Web site address: www.fascrs.org
Patient information available regarding colon and rectal surgery and other gastrointestinal conditions.

American Society for Gastrointestinal Endoscopy
13 Elm Street
Manchester, MA 01944-1314
(978) 526-8330
Web site address: www.asge.org
Patient information about the use of endoscopy

to diagnose and treat gastrointestinal diseases.

American Society of Therapeutic Radiation and Oncology
12500 Fair Lakes Circle, #375
Fairfax, VA 22033-3882
(800) 962-7876; (703) 502-1550
Web site address: www.astro.org
Provides information about cancer and radiation oncology.

Cancervive
6500 Wilshire Boulevard, Suite 500
Los Angeles, CA 90048
(213) 655-3758
Many services available to cancer survivors.

Collaborative Group of the Americas on Inherited Colorectal Cancer (ACG-ICC)
85 W. Algonquin Road, Suite 550
Arlington Heights, IL 60005
(847) 290-9184
Web site address: www.fascrs.org/ascrs-cancer-reg.html
Provides a listing of hereditary colon cancer registries and information on clinical and chemoprevention clinical trials.

Hereditary Cancer Institute
Creighton University
2500 California Plaza
Omaha, NE 68178
(402) 280-2942
Provides educational materials and evaluations for families with possible hereditary cancers.

Hereditary Colorectal Cancer Polyposis Registry
Johns Hopkins Hospital
550 North Broadway, Suite 108
Baltimore, MD 21205
(410) 955-3875

A registry for people with hereditary colorectal cancer polyposis.

International Agency for Research on Cancer (IARC)
150 cours Albert Thomas
F-69372 Lyon Cedex 08
France
+33 04 72 73 84 85
Web site address: www.iarc.fr
Part of the World Health Organization; coordinates and conducts cancer research involving cancer control methods and the causes of cancer; links to other cancer sites.

International Union Against Cancer (UICC)
3 Rue du Conseil General
1205 Geneva, Switzerland
+41 22 809 1811
Web site address: www.uicc.org
Involved in all aspects of the worldwide fight against cancer by advancing knowledge, research, prevention, early detection, and treatment.

National Cancer Institute Cancer Information Service (CIS)
(800) 4-CANCER
Web site address: rex.nci.nih.gov
Provides information on cancer, treatment, clinical trials.

National Comprehensive Cancer Network
50 Huntingdon Pike, Suite 200
Rockledge, PA 19046
For patient information: (888) 909-NCCN, or e-mail: patientinformation@nccn.org
(215) 728-4788
Web site address: www.nccn.org
An alliance of leading cancer centers, providing patient information, treatment guidelines, and referral service.

Oncology Nursing Society
501 Holiday Drive
Pittsburgh, PA 15220-2749
(412) 921-7373
Web site address: www.ons.org
National organization promoting excellence in
oncology nursing and quality cancer care;
provides information related to nursing practice, technology, education, and research;
supports nursing research; presents educational programs and materials.

*The Society of Gastroenterology Nurses and
Associates*
401 North Michigan Avenue
Chicago, IL 60611-4267
(800) 245-7462; (312) 321-5165 in Illinois
Web site address: www.sgna.org
Provides information to promote awareness
about colorectal cancer.

*WCET–World Council of Enterostomal
Therapists*
P.O. Box 48099, 60 Dundas Street East
Mississauga, Ontario, Canada, L5A 468
(905) 848-9400
International organization of enterostomal
therapists.

Wound Ostomy and Continence Nurses Society
2755 Bristol Street, Suite 110
Costa Mesa, CA 92626
(714) 476-0268
National organization of enterostomal therapy
nurses; local referrals available.

Patient and Caregiver Support

Organizations listed here not only provide information, but may also provide specific types
of services, such as transportation assistance;
insurance, employment, and financial services;
hospice referrals; medication assistance pro-

grams; and support and counseling programs.
Again, this is not an all-inclusive listing, so it
is important to check with local organizations
regarding additional programs and resources.

AirLineLine
National Office
50 Fullerton Court, Suite 200
Sacramento, CA 95825
(877) AIRLIFE; (916) 641-7800
Web site address: www.airlifeline.org
E-mail address: staff@airlifeline.org
Volunteer pilots fly cancer patients, free of
charge, to specialists, hospitals, and clinics
for their treatment.

Cancer Care, Inc.
1180 Avenue of the Americas
New York, NY 10036
(800) 813-HOPE; (212) 302-2400
Web site address: www.cancercare.org
Patient information, counseling, and support
groups available; referrals available.

Cancer Family Care
7162 Reading Road, Suite 1201
Cincinnati, OH 45237
(513) 731-3346
Web site address: www.cancerfamilycare.org
E-mail address: info@cancerfamilycare.org
Provides information on various medical tech-
nologies.

Cancer Hope Network
2 North Road, Suite A
Chester, NJ 07930
(877) HOPENET; (907) 879-4039 (within New
Jersey)
Web site address: www.cancerhopenetwork.org
Trained cancer survivor volunteers provide
one-to-one support to cancer patients and
their families.

Colon Cancer Alliance
175 Ninth Avenue
New York, NY 10011
(212) 627-7451
Web site address: www.ccalliance.org
Educational information on a variety of colorectal cancer topics; support groups; news articles; links to other cancer organizations.

Colorectal Cancer Association of Canada
180 Bloor Street West, Suite 904
Toronto, Ontario M5S 2V6
(888) 318-9442
Web site address: www.ccac-accc.ca
Dedicated to supporting people with colorectal cancer, their families, and caregivers; increase quality of life and cancer awareness.

Corporate Angel Network
Westchester County Airport, 1 Loop Road
White Plains, NY 10604
(914) 328-1313
Web site address: www.corpangelnetwork.org
E-mail address: info@corpangelnetwork.org
Provides free plane transportation for cancer patients undergoing treatment at cancer treatment centers.

Gilda's Club
195 West Houston Street
New York, NY 10014
(212) 647-9700
Web site address: www.gildasclub.org
Locations across the United States and in Toronto and Montreal; listed in telephone book.
Provides social and emotional support to patients, families, and friends.

Kids Konnected
27071 Cabot Road, Suite 102
Laguna Hills, CA 92653
(800) 899-2866; (949) 582-5443
Web site address: www.kidskonnected.org

Provides support, education, and counseling to children who have a parent with cancer.

National Association of Hospital Hospitality Houses, Inc.
P.O. Box 18087
Asheville, NC 28814
(800) 542-9730; (828) 253-1188
Web site address: www.nahhh.org
E-mail address: helphomes@nahhh.org
Provides information on lodging.

National Coalition for Cancer Survivorship
1010 Wayne Avenue, Suite 505
Silver Spring, MD 20910
(877) 622-7037; (301) 650-9127
Web site address: www.cansearch.org
E-mail address: info@cansearch.org
Advocacy organization for insurance, employment, and legal rights for cancer survivors.

National Family Caregivers Association
10400 Connecticut Avenue, Suite 500
Kensington, MD 20895
(800) 896-3650; (301) 942-6430
Web site address: www.nfcacares.org
E-mail address: info@nfcacares.org
Provides education, respite care, counseling, and advocacy for caregivers.

National Insurance Consumer Helpline
1001 Pennsylvania Avenue, NW
Washington, DC 20004
or
110 William Street
New York, NY 10038
(800) 942-4242
Web site address: www.iii.org
Provides assistance in finding insurance coverage; information on various issues and consumer complaint services.

National Patient Advocate Foundation
National Managed Care Resource Network

753 Thimble Shoals, Suite B
Newport News, VA 23606
(800) 532-5274
Web site address: www.patientadvocate.org
E-mail: patient@pinn.net
Provides legal counseling and referral services for patients denied insurance, employment discrimination, and/or need of support in public assistance negotiations.

Needy Meds
c/o Libby Overly
Mobile, AL 36693
Web site address: www.needymeds.com
E-mail address: LibOverly@pobox.com
Provides information on pharmaceutical company medication assistance programs.

The Chemotherapy Foundation
183 Madison Avenue, Suite 403
New York, NY 10016
(212) 213-9292
Provides information on clinical research.

The Wellness Community
National Office
35 East 7th Street, Suite 412
Cincinnati, OH 45202
(888) 793-WELL; (513) 421-7111
Web site address: www.wellness-community.org
E-mail address: help@wellness-community.org
Locations also in Arizona, California, Delaware, Florida, Georgia, Indiana, Kentucky, Maryland, Massachusetts, Nevada, Ohio, Pennsylvania, Tennessee, and Washington, DC.
Provides educational materials, psychosocial support, stress management, and social activities to patients and families. A comprehensive, well-written source of information on the many aspects of colorectal cancer is "Frankly Speaking," available from the Wellness Community.

United Ostomy Association
19772 MacArthur Blvd., Suite 200
Irvine, CA 92612
(800) 826-0826; (714) 660-8624
Web site address: www.uoa.org
Provides information, support, and advocacy for people with ostomies.

End-of-Life Support

Choice in Dying
1035 30th Street, NW
Washington, DC 20007
(800) 989-WILL
Web site address: www.choices.org
Advocates for the protection of patients' end-of-life rights; information and support regarding preparation of living wills and healthcare durable powers of attorney.

Hospice Education Institute/Hospicelink
190 Westbrook Road
Essex, CT 06426
(800) 33101620; (860) 767-1620
E-mail address: hospiceall@aol.com
Provides information and referrals regarding hospice and palliative care.

National Hospice Organization
1700 Diagonal Road, Suite 300
Arlington, VA 22314
(800) 338-8619
HELPLINE: (800) 658-8898
Web site address: www.nho.org
E-mail address: drsnho@cais.com
Provides information and referrals to local hospitals, advocacy groups, and professional organizations.

Internet Resources

As we become more computer literate, we turn to the Internet as a source of information on a variety of topics affecting our lives. In addition to accessing the Internet from home, many public libraries, hospitals, and physician's offices have computers for public use.

Information can be found by going to specific sites, using an electronic address, and as part of a general search for information, using search engines such as Yahoo, Alta Vista, Infoseek, and Excite. Using a specific term, such as *colon cancer*, will yield a different set of Internet sites, compared with using a broad term like *cancer*. There is a tremendous amount of information available on the Internet, but some of it may not be reliable. It is important to consider the source of information obtained from the Internet before using it in the decision-making process. Chat rooms or discussion groups are also becoming popular. Some of the web sites listed below include such forums. Each of the sites listed has been reviewed for content, readability, and timely information. Many organizations listed previously also have web sites, so they are not listed again in this section. The web site address is included with the organization's listing.

Site name: American Cancer Society Ostomy
    Rehabilitation Program
Web site address: www.cancer.org
Links to information about the ostomy rehabilitation program and other services from the ACS.

Site name: American Institute for Cancer
    Research
Web site address: www.aicr.org
Information in the area of diet, nutrition, and cancer prevention.

Site name: Association of Cancer Online
    Resources
Web site address: www.acor.org
Colon Cancer Discussion List
Web site address: www.acor.org/colon.html

Cancer information system offering information, support, and access to Internet mailing lists and web-based resources. The colon cancer discussion list is an exchange of information for people dealing with colorectal cancer.

Site name: Association of Community Cancer
    Centers
Web site address: www.ASSOC-Cancer-Centers.org
Information regarding cancer centers, basic insurance information, treatments, and standards.

Site name: Black Health Net
Web site address: www.blackhealthnet.com/articles/9711/colorectal.asp
Health information for African Americans.

Site name: CancerNet Information
Web site address: www.ncc.go.jb/cnet
Information from PDQ, CANCERLIT communication, access to information for NCI's Office of Cancer Communication.

Site name: CancerSource.com
Web site address: www.cancersource.com
In-depth information on cancer in general and specific cancers, including colorectal cancer, symptom management information, news items, message boards, and live-chats on a variety of topics.

Site name: Cancer Survivors Network
Web site address: www.cancersurvivorsnetwork.org
Means to communicate about survivorship issues.

Site name: Center for Cancer Nutrition
Web site address: www.cancernutrition.com
Certified nutritional specialist provides information about cancer and nutrition.

Site name: Center Watch
Web site address: www.centerwatch.com
Clinical trials listing service (national and international), listing of recently approved drugs, research center profiles, health-related web sites, industry profiles.

Site name: Clinical Cancer Genetics Resource Directory
Web site address: cancernet.nci.nih.gov/genesrch.shtml
Provides information about genetics research.

Site name: Colorectal Cancer Network
Web site address: www.colorectal-cancer.net
Provides information about treatment options and disease management to people with cancer, their families, friends, and caregivers.

Site name: Colon and Rectum Cancer Resource Center
Web site address: www3.cancer.org/cancerinfo/load_cont.asp
General information on colorectal cancer, risks, diagnosis, and treatment.

Site name: Family Caregivers Association
Web site address: nfcacares.org
Provides information for people caring for their loved ones.

Site name: Harvard Center for Cancer Prevention
Web site address: www.yourcancerrisk.harvard.edu
Risk assessment for the public.

Site name: Hereditary Colon Cancer Association
Web site address: www.hereditarycc.org
Provides support and information for patients with an inherited colon cancer disorder and their families.

Site name: Medicine Online's Colon Cancer Library
Web site address: www.meds.com/colon/colon.html
In-depth information on colorectal cancer.

Site name: MSNBC: What's Your Risk for Colon Cancer?
Web site address: www.msnbc.com/modules/quizzes/0910_coloncancer.asp
Questionnaire about regular screening.

Site name: National Cancer Institute CancerNet Information Service
Web site address: www.icic.nci.nih.gov/icichome
Access to *Cancerlit* articles; information on screening, prevention, treatment, clinical trials, and supportive care; sections for patients, professionals, and basic researchers.

Site name: National Cancer Institute Office of Cancer Survivorship
Web site address: dccps.nci.nih.gov/ocs
Defines and coordinates research to improve the quality of life and health of cancer survivors and their families.

Site name: National Center for Complementary and Alternative Medicine
Web site address: nccam.nih.gov
Information on complementary and alternative practices.

Site name: National Colon Cancer Research Alliance
Web site address: www.nccra.org
Information on colon cancer and research efforts.

Site name: National Institutes of Health
Web site address: www.nih.gov
Access to National Cancer Institute Data Base,

clinical trials database, CancerNet, patient information, and cancer information service.

Site name: National Institutes of Health Cancer Information Service/PDQ
Web site address: cancernet.nci.nih.gov or rex.nci.nih.gov
(800) 4-CANCER
Nationwide telephone service with personnel trained to provide up-to-date information about cancer; web site is also a source of information; wide variety of free publications in English and Spanish.

Site name: OncoLink
Web site address: oncolink.upenn.edu/disease/ colorectal
General information about cancer; specific questions and answers about colorectal cancer, treatment options, news items, links to colorectal cancer sites, recommendations for screening, risk factors, prevention, and genetics; information on support groups.

Site name: ONS on-line
Web site address: www.ons.org
Access to discussion forums, journal abstracts, book reviews, information on prevention and detection; resource for ONS members.

Site name: PDQ-NCI's Comprehensive Cancer Database
Web site address: www.cancernet.nci.gov/pdq
Information regarding screening, prevention, treatment, clinical trials, and supportive care, sites for public and professionals.

Site name: PhRMA America's Pharmaceutical Companies
Web site address: www.phrma.org

Provides information about prescription medications, including a directory of prescription drug patient-assistance programs and medicines in development.

Site name: Quackwatch, Inc.
Web site address: www.quackwatch.com/ 00AboutQuackwatch/altseek.html
A nonprofit organization that provides information about health-related fraud, myths, and fallacies.

Site name: Score against Colon Cancer
Web site address: www.scorecec.com
(877) SCORE-123
A national public awareness campaign to promote colorectal cancer screening and early detection.

Site name: U.S. Social Security Administration
Web site address: www.ssa.gov/odhome/ odhome.htm or, for written material, www .ssa.gov/pubs/englist.html
Information for disabled individuals.

Site name: WWW Cancernet
Web site address: www.arc.com/cancernet/ cancenet
Alternative access to NCI database, Oncolink, and University of Pennsylvania Cancer Center Resource.

Conclusion

Patients, families, and health professionals all seek to keep abreast of the latest available information. There are a variety of mechanisms for which to do this, many of which are listed in this resource section.

INDEX

Page numbers followed by f and t represent figures and tables respectively. Photographic images are represented by *P-1* through *P-8*.

www.ingramcontent.com/pod-product-compliance
Lightning Source LLC
Chambersburg PA
CBHW061340210326
41598CB00035B/5840